third edition

Psychiatric and Mental Health Nursing

A Commitment to Care and Concern

Joanne E. Perko, R.N., B.S.N., M.N.Ed., Ed.D.
Associate Professor
Cleveland State University
Cleveland, Ohio

Helen Z. Kreigh, R.N., B.S.N.Ed., M.A., Ed.D.
Former Professor
Cuyahoga Community College
Cleveland, Ohio

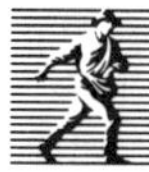

APPLETON & LANGE
Norwalk, Connecticut/San Mateo, California

0-8385-8005-X

Notice: The author(s) and publisher of this volume have taken care that the information and recommendations contained herein are accurate and compatible with the standards generally accepted at the time of publication.

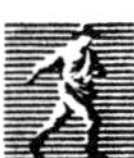

88 89 90 91 92 / 10 9 8 7 6 5 4 3 2 1

Prentice-Hall of Australia, Pty. Ltd., Sydney
Prentice-Hall Canada, Inc.
Prentice-Hall Hispanoamericana, S.A., Mexico
Prentice-Hall of India Private Limited, New Delhi
Prentice-Hall International (UK) Limited, London
Prentice-Hall of Japan, Inc., Tokyo
Prentice-Hall of Southeast Asia (Pte.) Ltd., Singapore
Whitehall Books Ltd., Wellington, New Zealand
Editora Prentice-Hall do Brasil Ltda., Rio de Janeiro

Library of Congress Cataloging-in-Publication Data
Perko, Joanne E.
Psychiatric and mental health nursing.

Kreigh's name appears first on the earlier edition.
Includes bibliographies and index.
1. Psychiatric nursing. I. Kreigh, Helen Z.
II. Title. [DNLM: 1. Psychiatric Nursing. WY 160 P451p]
RC440.P425 1988 610.73'68 87-22957
ISBN 0-8385-8005-X

Production Editors: Michael Duford, Bellamy Printz
Designer: Kathleen Peters Ceconi

PRINTED IN THE UNITED STATES OF AMERICA

third edition

Psychiatric and Mental Health Nursing

A Commitment to Care and Concern

To Richard and Mike for their continued support and encouragement

CONTENTS

PREFACE

Our third edition, like its predecessors, was undertaken out of our desire to present what we believe to be helpful guidelines for the development and improvement of practice skills in psychiatric–mental health nursing. We also believe that our text speaks for our practice and identifies us to our colleagues as educators and practitioners who are both committed to caring for students and patients and concerned with their development as people. Therefore, this revision continues to be grounded in a humanistic philosophy, with emphasis on the nurse as a professional who through her empathic approach uses her knowledge and skill to plan for and implement patient care.* We continue to maintain that learning and knowledge without skillful application results in disservice to patients and reflects a lack of commitment to care and concern for patients as people. Thus, we reaffirm that there remains a genuine need to emphasize the practical aspects that demonstrate how learning is transferred and how knowledge is applied to the real situations encountered by the nurse in her everyday practice.

Clarity, readability, and brevity continue to be salient features of the text. No text can encompass all that is known or needs to be known about a subject. Faculty, as facilitators of learning, must guide and stimulate the learner's quest for the most recent and vital knowledge available in the field. A textbook provides basic guidance, while research provides enrichment and future direction for application.

Essentially, the format adopted in the second edition has been carried forward in this third edition. Changes that the reader will encounter are related to the clarification, expansion, and addition in content. We have included an introduction in which we identify our

*To ensure consistency in the text, the term *man* refers to humankind in general, while the pronoun *she* refers to the nurse and *he* to the patient, client, and resident. Please note also that the words patient, client, and *resident* are used interchangeably throughout the text. No gender bias against the nursing profession or its patients is intended by the use of these terms.

personal philosophy and the conceptual framework on which this text is based. In Part I, we have elaborated on the contemporary role of the nurse, emphasized ethical considerations in practice, and included the most recent Standards for Professional Practice. In Part II, we have added the strategy of conflict resolution and have completely rewritten the chapter on stress and crisis in living. In Part III, we have reorganized some of the tables emphasizing nursing concepts and principles, while Part IV remains as originally presented. In Part V, we have addressed the concept of contracting with patients and clarified the use of a nursing diagnosis as a basis for planning care. In Part VI, we have added a new chapter that speaks to nursing intervention for those clients who experience alterations in and interruptions of their daily pattern of living and have detailed specific interventions for those clients for whom seclusion, restraint, or both have been identified as a therapeutic necessity. The case presentation and the progressive care plan contained in Part VII have been modified to demonstrate the nursing process.

As the major divisions indicate, we have moved through what appears to us a logical sequencing of the content the learner is likely to encounter within an educational, experiential learning program. In addition, much of the case material presented has been garnered from our own experience while working directly with both clients and students in acute care settings. Although a large segment of these examples, as well as some of the identified nursing interventions, relate specifically to the institutionalized client, the reader should note that the principles exemplified can be applied in community settings, outpatient departments, emergency rooms—in any facility or treatment program in which the nurse chooses to practice. Furthermore, the text is intended to provide a basic orientation to psychiatric nursing from which specialization can develop.

Students and practitioners alike frequently comment that the ideal presented within the classroom is not possible to implement in the workplace and, furthermore, that educators are out of touch with the stressors encountered in daily clinical practice. The reader might be interested to know that the authors, concurrent with the initiation of this revision, returned to staff nursing for a 3-month period of time. During this experience, the staff nurses' reality became our reality. The stressors they experienced, we experienced—overwork, staff shortages, disputes with medical colleagues, ethical dilemmas, as well as numerous psychiatric and medical emergencies. This experience allowed us to implement the nursing process within the context of a psychiatric setting and provided data to substantiate many of the nursing care principles and interventive strategies we have detailed within this text. Moreover, the interpretation of our joint observations of our colleagues functioning within the practice setting revealed that professional practice can and does exist.

We wish specifically to acknowledge the dedicated and skillful secretarial services of Mary Claire Novy and Joan Mindzora in the preparation of manuscript for our third edition.

We would also like to take this opportunity to express our appreciation for the support, encouragement, and helpful comments received from our colleagues and, in particular, those who were involved in the review of our manuscript prior to publication.

INTRODUCTION

Professional practice is influenced by a personal belief system, that is, a philosophy of nursing. It is further directed by the conceptual framework used to operationalize a philosophy in practice. And, lastly, practice is modified by the experiences encountered in the actual delivery of care.

We acknowledge that each individual reader may not share equally in our philosophy or framework, but we felt the need to affirm our position, since we are strongly committed to the idea that practice is a direct outcome of one's beliefs, theoretical considerations, and applied principles.

Nursing is a profession involving the care of people. We believe nursing to be a goal-directed process in which the primary objective is to develop a relationship between the care provider (nurse) and the care receiver (patient) for the purpose of maintaining a level of health, preventing illness, and restoring an individual to an optimal level of functioning. Nursing, using a scientific, theoretical framework, focuses on the uniqueness and individuality of the person. It takes into account the biological, psychosocial, and environmental contexts of the patient. Nursing makes use of the interaction between the patient and those with whom he comes in contact. It concerns itself with the significant aspects of the patient's total life experiences. Nursing requires the assessment of individual needs on a personal, interpersonal, and intrapersonal level. Nursing modifies the environment to meet the needs of the individual. It produces within the patient a change in attitudes, expectations, and possible outcomes. Nursing employs evaluation and judges its effectiveness on the application of the principles derived from the theoretical framework.

We believe that the practice of psychiatric–mental health nursing requires that the nurse commit herself, without reservation, to the basic concepts implicit within the nursing process: namely, that the patient is a person who has a right to the best possible care and a right to be included in the planning of that care. When we say that the patient is a person, we mean that he is a human being entitled to *all* the basic needs, whether these needs be physical, psychosocial, or spiritual—fulfillment of which enables the individual to function in his entirety. Examples of such needs include, but are not limited to, physical comfort and safety, physiological equilibrium, love, understanding, communication, respect, and fulfillment. Nursing care is designed to utilize these needs in assisting the individual to move toward actualization of his inherent potential. This belief is the cornerstone on which the psychiatric nurse must build her practice. We think that the fundamental satisfaction and gratification the nurse achieves are based on implementation and realization of this philosophy.

To say that a patient has a right to be included in the planning of his care is merely extending the idea that the patient is a person, that he has a right to exert control over his environment and the conditions affecting that environment in an effort to achieve self-actualization. He is entitled to participate and strive toward the fulfillment of his physical and emotional well-being. We maintain that a patient is cared for in terms of his totality and not in terms of his parts. If we believe that patients are human, then we cannot talk around, above, or beneath them, nor can we talk to, for, or about them, but rather, we must talk with them.

Another concept which we believe is important in developing criteria for care is that behavior has meaning. Here again, we look at the totality of the individual, that is, his spoken words plus the nonverbal ways in which he portrays himself. The two key words of this concept are behavior and **meaning**. A broad definition of behavior is that which a person says and does. It includes everything! When we use the word meaning, we are looking at the implications of the behavior. Meaning may be broadly defined as the way in which an individual attempts to convey the expression of his innermost feeling. We, as nurses, must never lose sight of the fact that what a patient says and does is in response to perceived external and internal stimuli. While the speech and actions of the patient may appear to be without purpose and meaning, they do hold purpose and meaning for the patient. Intervention requires that the nurse be vitally concerned with finding meaning in what is being communicated.

We reemphasize the concept that the nurse has an obligation to render the best possible care. Students and staff have been taught the rudiments of what makes up good patient care; however, it is the term **obligation** which they sometimes may not perceive. We defined obligation as a form of responsibility that demands the nurse's personal investment. It implies the courage of one's convictions, the willingness to give of oneself, the ability to communicate through action, and the desire to invest effort into care. The idea of obligation entails the knowledge of what quality care is and how it is provided.

Psychiatric–mental health nursing is based on a theoretical framework that incorporates and reflects the theoretical constructs, concepts, and principles developed within nursing and the allied disciplines of medicine, psychology, sociology, cultural anthropology, and the physical sciences. To date, the body of knowledge specific to the practice of the profession has been limited. This limitation has produced within the profession a tendency to draw rather heavily upon the knowledge base of the above-mentioned disciplines. However, the literature reflects that movement toward identifying and defining nursing theory is in progress.

Even though there is a paucity of clearly identified and workable theoretical formulations, for us there is in existence a viable theoretical framework upon which the current practice of psychiatric–mental health nursing is based. We have identified at least four basic components of psychiatric nursing theory. These include a holistic concept of man; the identification of an interactive relationship occurring between man and his universe; adaptation as a means of self-fulfillment; and the interactive–interventive process existing between nurse and client(s).

HOLISTIC CONCEPT OF MAN

The *holistic concept of man* designates man as a unified whole—a complete entity in and of himself, separate and unique from all other men. As such, man is viewed as an integrated being and not merely as a composite of fragmented, interlocking parts. The holistic concept recognizes that man in his totality is a complex being whose makeup involves physical, mental, emotional, social, and cultural interdependent aspects and components that are irrevocably linked and related one to the other.

This holistic concept is not limited to the client alone, but also includes the nurse as she implements her professional roles. By this we mean that although a particular situation may demand the enactment of a specific role, such as counselor or teacher, successful intervention requires that the total self be actively involved. Therefore, aspects of all other roles are always present. The nurse cannot compartmentalize self in the delivery of care, for it is the totality of self that is the therapeutic tool.

MAN AND HIS UNIVERSE

The *concept of man in relationship to his universe* implies that man is in a constant state of interaction with his environment—internal and external, proximal and distal. Environment is understood to represent the totality of living experience. This totality is inclusive, consisting of interaction between man and his self-system as well as man and other men, as in a family, group, community, culture, or society. Moreover, this concept implies continuous interchange between the internal and external aspects of environment. Within this interchange man attempts to maintain personal identity, integrity, worth, and equilibrium. To facilitate a harmonious interchange, man makes use of adaptive mechanisms.

ADAPTATION

The *concept of adaptation* connotes man's ability to vary his responses acccording to his perceived needs and the internal or external demands of his environment. Adaptation is a protective, dynamic mechanism aimed toward preservation and survival.

In addition, adaptation is a process of change that can facilitate the person's fulfillment as a self-actualized being. As such, adaptation is a response mechanism that occurs as the individual encounters stressors and attempts to minimize, neutralize, or eliminate the debilitating effects of stress. Adaptation can be either positive or negative. **Positive adaptation** is defined as effective coping and occurs when the integrity and equilibrium of the individual is preserved. Adaptation is viewed as negative when the coping responses fail to contribute to or maintain homeostasis. Negative adaptation is often referred to as **maladaption**.

Various terms have been used to describe and differentiate between aspects of adaptation. Some terms appear to be mutually exclusive, while others appear to connote some degree of overlap. These terms include **intrinsic, automatic, intuitive, learned,** and **planned**. These descriptors may be used singly or in any combined form, and their use is an attempt to categorize response behavior as man interacts with his environment.

Intrinsic adaptation is an inherent coping response that pertains to a person's internal self and is reflective of the person's individuality and uniqueness as a human being. An intrinsic adaptive response of one person can never be identical to that or any other person. An example of an intrinsic adaptation may be an idiosyncratic reaction to medication. Another example may be seen in a person's physiological reaction to anxiety. Two students are confronted with the same testing situation; one student complains of "butterflies" in her stomach, while the second breaks out in a "cold sweat." This type of adaptation may result from a person's constitutional composition, be associated with specific genetic factors peculiar to him, emerge as a manifestation of internal physiological functioning, or occur as an outgrowth of the person's developing self-system.

Automatic adaptation is a natural phenomenon that occurs without thought or conscious effort. It is an instantaneous, involuntary response reaction that is predicated on immediacy of need and is operationalized regardless of consequences. This type of adaptation involves the calling forth of an organized set or system of coping devices that are or have become an integral part of man. The antigen–antibody reaction, the use of mental mechanisms, or the reaction of a person walking down the street who experiences a chilling wind, shivers, and draws his coat more closely about him are examples of automatic adaptation.

Intuitive adaptation is a response that comes into operation without the benefit of conscious thought or reasoning. In essence, it results from what a person feels or senses. For instance, a nurse has completed an assessment and routine check of a patient having a Blakemore tube in place; vital signs are consistent with previous monitoring; there is no observable evidence of physical distress; intravenous therapy is in accordance with schedule and orders; the patient is responding verbally and giving no indication of subjective discomfort; the nurse leaves the room, gets halfway down the hall, experiences a prickly feeling that something is not right, goes back to check, and finds the patient hemorrhaging. Thus, intuitive adaptation is a response to a hunch or gut-level feeling. It may, in fact, be a response to another dimension that we have not as yet been able to identify, much less articulate.

Learned adaptation is born out of man's ability to think, to feel, to perceive, to acquire knowledge and skill, to act, to react, and to interact. As knowledge increases and cognitive functioning expands, the data base affecting ability to adapt changes. An example to demonstrate learned adaptation occurs when a child registers fear of the dark and dark places and refuses to enter a closet, observes his mother repeatedly going in and returning unharmed, and subsequently follows her inside.

In **planned adaptation**, a goal has been identified and the individual employs cognitive strategies to attain the goal. It involves choice and the directing of volitional behavior. A situation portraying planned adaptation is one in which a person recognizes within himself a need for further education. As a result, he actively engages in behavior designed to fulfill and gratify this perception: he explores avenues for acquiring the education, makes appointments for interviews, collects facts about programs, determines financial requirements, reaches a decision and makes a selection, marshalls supporting resources, and makes application to the program and institution of his choice.

Adaptation in and of itself may not always be in man's best interest. In order for adaptation to be position, it must provide man with a sense of well-being, a feeling of satisfaction and comfort, and an optimistic and hopeful future outlook. Furthermore, successful adaptation leads man toward an optimal level of functioning whereby he can make use of his total potential and capabilities in his efforts to achieve self-actualization. Successful adaptation is not and can never be the same for each individual, since it is predicated on the awareness of the contextual framework surrounding each individual. Thus, the implication for nursing is that there is no standard or set of interventions that can be applied to all persons in similar situations. Nurses must be cognizant of the fact that each situation and each person demands recognition of uniqueness in adaptation. Yes, there are generalities. Yes, there are commonalities. Yes, there are similarities. But nursing practice must consciously and actively explore the differences with each person and each situation. For example, why does aspirin, an antipyretic agent, when administered to two patients with an elevated temperature, produce a reduction of temperature in the first while the second person breaks out in hives? The answer: an idiosyncratic response—a difference. In another instance, where similarity seems most apparent and adaptation a foregone conclusion, we find two people are experiencing a toothache. The one chooses to seek dental care for relief, while the other chooses to doctor self and accepts limited relief rather than submit to the perceived greater pain of sitting in a dentist's chair. Again, the answer is a difference between individuals and their pattern of adaptation.

THE INTERACTIVE–INTERVENTIVE PROCESS

The concept of the **interactive–interventive process** describes in dynamic terms the alliance that exists between the nurse and her client. In this process each participant is actively involved in pursuing therapeutic endeavors that are directed toward assisting the client to maximize his human potential while adapting to life's exigencies. The interactive–interventive process is synonymous with the nurse–patient relationship. This process is used with individuals and with groups and serves as the base for all nursing practice, since effective intervention is predicated on effective interaction. The interactive–interventive process implies a basic therapeutic goal; that is, the outcome is directed toward assisting man in his process of adaptation.

The belief statements presented together with the major concepts identified, makeup what we envision as the foundation for the practice of psychiatric–mental health nursing. It is from this perspective that the content of this text flows.

third edition

Psychiatric and Mental Health Nursing

A Commitment to Care and Concern

I

THE PROFESSION

A Commitment to Care and Concern

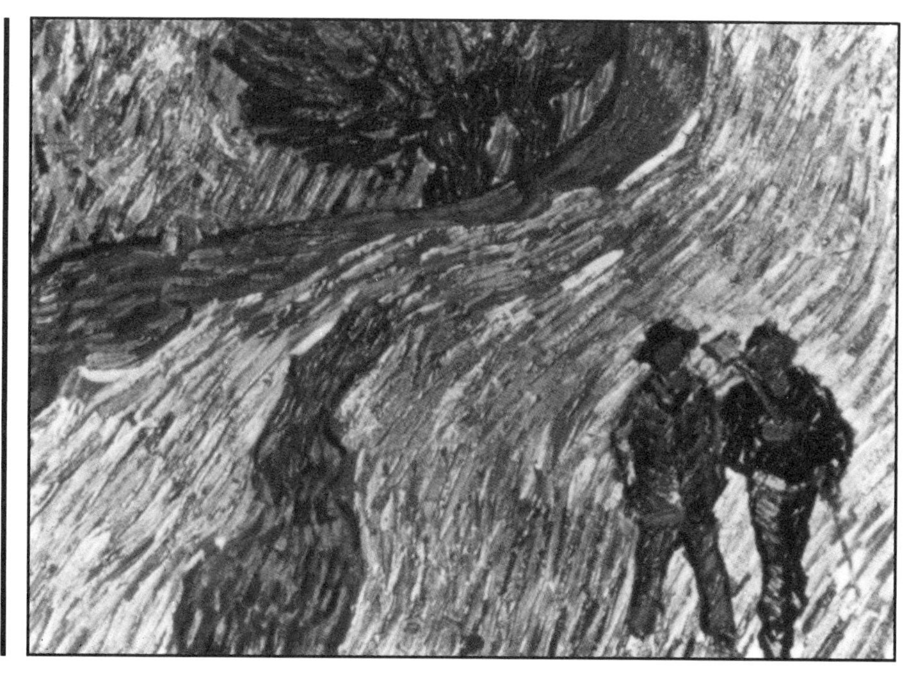

1

PSYCHIATRIC–MENTAL HEALTH NURSING PRACTICE

What Was It? What Is It? What Might It Become?

LEARNING OBJECTIVES

On completion of this chapter the reader should be able to:

1. List a minimum of five individuals who have made a significant contribution to the field of psychiatry, psychiatric nursing, and mental health.
2. State one major contribution for each of the identified individuals in the first objective.
3. Define the term **psychiatric–mental health nursing**.
4. Identify the basic philosophy and framework of psychiatric–mental health nursing practice.
5. Identify and describe a minimum of two current issues facing psychiatric nurses in practice.
6. Identify and describe a minimum of two challenges confronting psychiatric nurses in the future.

A GLIMPSE AT THE PAST

Universally, the care and treatment of the mentally ill have been influenced by man's belief about himself, his world, and his fellow man. In preliterate societies, those afflicted were often segregated, cast out, and abandoned. Fear and dread were the prevailing emotions exhibited by those confronted with the unknown, the misunderstood and the unexplained. Anthropologists tell us that primitive peoples held the belief that those stricken with illness of any kind were possessed by malevolent demons. Demonic possession was viewed as a form of punishment for sins committed—illness a "just outcome"; the afflicted were objects to be avoided. Treatment meted out was based on the need of the group to drive out the demons from their midst. Other forms of treatment designed to rid the afflicted of possession were starvation, beatings, burnings, trephines, and amputations. Each form of treatment was undertaken with the firm conviction that the corporeal body would no longer be a suitable habitat for the demon.

As centuries advanced, the treatment scene changed, as did to some extent the beliefs. The afflicted were no longer treated in caves or open fields but rather were brought to the temples and temple courtyards. Treatment was no longer the exclusive province of the designated leader but now came under the control of the magician-physician and his helpers. The concept of demonic possession as the underlying cause of illness still held sway, but the beliefs were now divided. Some held that the demons were evil, and therefore the afflicted must be shunned; others espoused the concept that the demons could also be benevolent, and therefore the afflicted should be revered as holy objects. The early treatments, although essentially unchanged, were now accompanied by chants, mystic rites, burnt offerings, and special incantations.

Gradually, as the pendulum of time moved forward, man began the quest for scientific knowledge and truth; a period of experimental investigation ensued. **Pythagoras** (580–510 B.C.) developed the concept that the brain is the seat of intellectual activity. He also is credited as the first to regard mental disorders as an illness of the mind. A hundred years later (460–370 B.C.), **Hippocrates** entered the scene systematizing and describing the mental disorders of hysteria, depression, and mania. **Plato** (427–347 B.C.), the searcher of the good, the true, and the beautiful, identified the psychosomatic relationship between the mind and the body. He advocated prophylactic measures to strengthen these two separate yet integral components of man. Another 200 years passed before a staunch advocate appeared to prescribe humane treatment for the mentally ill. **Asclepiades**, the father of psychiatry, whose emblem, the caduceus, is still used today by the medical profession, condemned the use of mechanical restraints and encouraged the use of simple hygienic measures. He recommended that attention be paid to the diet and that soothing baths and massages be employed to keep the pores open. To these basic treatments he added the use of emetics and the practice of bloodletting. As the doctrine of these initial proponents of enlightened health care spread, treatment sites shifted slightly, moving away from the temples and into the centers of learning. Some accepted, but many rejected the new ideas and held fast to their superstitious beliefs.

Vestiges of these innovative modes of treatment, begun so long ago, find their modern counterparts among the various treatments and modalities currently in use. For example, music therapy finds its antecedent in the harmonious music of the flute, lyre, and choral singing of the past. Likewise, the use of gently flowing water from springs and fountains coupled with peaceful aesthetic surroundings can be considered a forerunner of hydrotherapy and the concept of a therapeutic environment. To soothe the spirit and stimulate the mind, the ancients endorsed the pursuit of reading, particularly poetry—the bibliotherapy of today. Occupational, recreational, and physical therapy also find their beginnings in the past when the afflicted were encouraged to participate in simple tasks, gymnastics, and massage, while hypnosis finds its genesis in temple sleep. It seems incredible that with such a glorious beginning mankind was forced to wait almost 2000 years for these simple, yet effective, treatments to be rediscovered and refined.

As Christianity began to spread, ministering to the sick and needy became a sacred duty. The early deaconesses of the Church took the first tentative steps towards organizing nursing care. Although these early attempts at organized care, however minimal, were both needed and beneficial, caring, in and of itself, was only a secondary objective of the care providers. Nursing as a primary goal did not really emerge until well into the 19th century.

While Christianity brought with it increased emphasis on caring for man's physical and mental well-being, it also gave rise to an attitude of condemnation for scientific discovery, which persisted throughout the Middle Ages until the period of the Renaissance and Reformation. It was during this intervening period, between the early and late Middle Ages, that organized nursing activity flourished. Two major influences, religious and military, guided this development. The military contributed order, routine, and regimentation, while the religious created centers for care under a doctrine of humanitarianism. Three similar yet distinct types of nursing orders evolved: the military orders, whose inception grew out of the need to care for soldiers felled in battle; the religious orders, which resulted from the work begun by the deaconesses of the early church; and lastly, the secular orders, whose primary commitment was to the sick rather than to the

Church, although they were organized under Church sanction. Remnants of these nursing orders are still found today.

As Western civilization evolved and became technically more proficient, man's attitude toward mental health and mental illness took several giant steps backwards. A moralistic view of illness prevailed, with health being equated with "good," while illness was equated with "bad." Shame, guilt, and fear were predominant feelings. Interestingly, as medical practice began to adopt and utilize the scientific discoveries of the 17th and 18th centuries, nursing activity as a "public good" declined and degenerated. By and large, the mentally ill during this period were often subjected to torture, ridicule, or incarceration in attic rooms or dungeons, or simply driven away from any community in which they tried to seek refuge. Almshouses, jails, asylums abounded and were filled with poor, pitiful creatures whose only "crime" was being different.

Probably the most benign way to describe the care of the mentally ill would be to state that it was **custodial**. Yet the term hardly applies from our more modern outlook. The laws governing the care of those designated as mentally ill provided that they be sheltered and given food and clothing but little else. The actual conditions under which they were forced to exist and the type of treatment to which they were subjected can only be termed barbaric. The law concerned itself far more with the disposition of the individual's property than with the treatment of the person. A typical example of such a philosophy in operation was found in 1756 at St. Mary's of Bethlehem (Bedlam) in London where, for the price of a penny, a visitor could spend a "very amusing" afternoon and come away with many tales to tell about the "loonies." Inside Bedlam the visitor was provided with a glimpse of the horrific, yet socially acceptable, treatment of mental disease. The grisly living conditions, slovenly attendants, and the bizarre treatments that prevailed were products of the times in which the social conscience of man paid scant attention to the needs of his fellow man.

However, glimmers of hope penetrated this murky gloom with the outstanding contributions made by such enlightened men and women as William Tuke, Philippe Pinel, Benjamin Rush, and Dorothea Lynde Dix. In 1792, **William Tuke**, a Quaker and tea merchant, built a private asylum, the York Retreat, so that those afflicted by mental illness could be treated along more humane lines. **Philippe Pinel**, a French doctor, convinced that the destructive behavior of the mentally ill was due, in large part, to their filthy living conditions and cruel treatment, made history in 1793 by acting on his beliefs. He unchained 12 men and a year later 12 women. **Benjamin Rush** (1745–1831), the father of American psychiatry, urged the building of special hospitals for the care of the mentally ill and published in 1812 the first American textbook on psychiatry. This text remained in use for over 70 years.

Between the years 1841 and 1887, **Dorothea Lynde Dix** was responsible for spearheading a movement to stimulate public interest in building state mental hospitals and in educating the public on the needs of the mentally ill.

As indicated earlier, the function of nursing probably has been a part of man's existence since the beginning of time. Its emergence as a professional pursuit did not occur until the mid to late 19th century. At this time, in both Europe and America, it was recognized that specifically educated persons were needed to care for the sick and infirm. Thus, between 1860 and 1900, the development of formal education for nursing began. In the United States, the first school to prepare nurses to care for the mentally ill opened at McLean Hospital in Waverly, Massachusetts, in 1880. By 1890, this school had graduated 90 psychiatric nurses.

During the period between 1850 and 1930, psychiatry was primarily descriptive and psychiatric nursing care, custodial. Psychiatrists were essentially interested in classifying observable behaviors, while nursing concerned itself with solidifying the principles delineated by Florence Nightingale. This nursing focus led to improved conditions within institutions. The psychiatric nurse of this era possessed few psychological skills and confined the practice of the profession to the care and supervision of the physical well-being of patients. Among the professional functions considered to lie within the province of the nurse were administration of drugs; the application of wet packs, cold or hot tubs, and Scotch douches; the supervision of diet; and the organizing of simple activities for patients. Yet the profession did not remain stagnant but rather moved forward with the times. Leaders in the profession began to emerge. Among these were two nurses who made outstanding contributions to the field of psychiatric nursing—Linda Richards and Harriet Bailey. **Linda Richards**, who is often credited with being the first American psychiatric nurse, devoted a significant part of her career to establishing standards of care within institutions. In 1920, **Harriet Bailey**, a leading educator and administrator of her time, published *Nursing Mental Diseases*, one of the first textbooks in psychiatric nursing. This text received great praise as a needed addition to the neophyte practice field of psychiatric nursing and remained a standard text for the next 20 years.

Gradually, the emphasis in psychiatry moved from a descriptive approach to that of a dynamic approach. The term **dynamic** as applied to psychiatry indicated a change in concern. Attention was now focused on the unconscious mental forces motivating behavior and on the interpersonal aspects of living. In the forefront of this change were such men as Eugene Bleuler, Sigmund Freud, Adolf Meyer, Harry Stack Sullivan, Clifford Beers, and Maxwell Jones. Each made a significant contribution to the practice of present-day psychiatry.

In 1912, **Eugene Bleuler** (1857–1939), a Swiss psychiatrist, introduced the diagnostic term **schizophrenia**. He described the schizophrenic process as a splitting off of emotions from thinking and saw this disease as primarily psychogenic in origin. He believed that psychiatry should focus its attention on the interpretation of abnormal behavior and not on the mere description of symptoms.

Sigmund Freud (1856–1939), a Viennese neurologist, is credited with initiating a historic intellectual revolution in man's view of man. His major premise, derived from extensive work with psychoneurotic patients, proposed the concept that man's unconscious forces were highly significant in the cause of mental and emotional illness. Freud's exploration of the emotional basis of neurotic conditions led to the definition of, and differentiation between, the levels of consciousness and the function of the psyche. The result of his work led to the establishment of the psychoanalytic approach to psychiatric care.

Adolf Meyer (1866–1950), a Swiss pathologist and contemporary of Freud, became the first head of the Department of Psychiatry at Johns Hopkins University, holding this position from 1910 to 1940. He viewed most mental disorders as failures in adaptation and taught that this inability was produced by interpersonal trauma. Furthermore, he advocated the patient–therapist relationship as an integral component of the therapeutic process in assisting the patient to gain insight into interpersonal problems and achieve resolution of emotional conflicts. He developed a theoretical system known as "Common Sense Psychiatry."

Harry Stack Sullivan (1892–1949) was an American psychoanalyst who, although trained by Freud, deviated somewhat from the basic Freudian psychoanalytic approach. In effect, he altered the approaches developed by both Freud and Meyer and added to their theoretical framework his concept regarding the importance cultural influences have on man's development. He saw the need to establish a closer patient–therapist bond as an essential part of the therapeutic process. Thus, he evolved what is today referred to as the **interpersonal** approach to psychiatry.

Clifford Beers (1876–1943), a layman who himself had been hospitalized for psychiatric illness, wrote of his experiences and the inhumane conditions that existed in both private and state mental institutions. His book, *A Mind That Found Itself*, did much to arouse public interest in psychiatry at a time when the public's social conscience was demanding new welfare legislation and enacting child labor laws. In 1909, Beers helped to establish and became the first Executive Secretary of the National Committee for Mental Hygiene, which later became known as the National Association for Mental Health.

In 1953, **Maxwell Jones** impacted the treatment scene inside psychiatric facilities when his book, *The Therapeutic Community*, was published. His focus was on the social environment of the patient as a significant part of the therapeutic experience. This dynamic change in approach to treatment provided the means whereby the patient became an active participant in the total treatment process. The concept of the therapeutic community spread rapidly and today is the preferred mechanism around which treatment programs are developed. The contributions made by these individuals and many others such as Alfred Adler, Hippolyte Bernheim, Abraham Brill, Anna Freud, Karen Horney, Ernest Jones, Carl Jung, Emil Kraeplin, Kurt Lewin, and Max Werthheimer have made the practice of dynamic psychiatry what it is today.

As the cycles of reform affected the growth, development, and expansion within the field of psychiatric medicine, so too did these societal reforms influence the growth, development, and expansion of psychiatric–mental health nursing. The 1930s and 1940s found that the nature of psychiatric nursing was gradually undergoing change. The professional focus shifted from primarily custodial care, from efforts to merely safeguard and maintain the status quo, to an awakened awareness of the nurse's role in developing the interpersonal environment designed to promote recovery. To meet the need for advanced preparation, collegiate nursing programs were developed, basic psychiatric principles were included within the general nursing curriculum, and a separate course in psychiatric nursing became part of the total nursing program. These advancements in education in conjunction with the rapid development of somatic therapies such as insulin (1933) and electroshock (1938) influenced the growth and expansion of psychiatric nursing as a significant component of the profession.

Following the Second World War, with its increased postwar demand for better and more efficient psychiatric services, the need for psychiatric nurses with advanced preparation became more acute. In 1946, Congress enacted the National Mental Health Act, which authorized the creation of the National Institute for Mental Health along with a program and funding to provide for the training of psychiatric personnel. Psychiatric nursing was one of the mental health service groups specified under this act to receive economic support. This paved the way for federal monies to be allocated toward collegiate institutions in order for them to promote baccalaureate and graduate education in the field of psychiatric nursing. Despite the rapid growth of such programs, today's need far exceeds the supply.

During the 1940s and the 1950s, the concept of **milieu**, that is, the creation of the therapeutic interpersonal environment, together with the involvement of psychiatric nurses and the development of therapeutic relationships with patients on a one-to-one basis formed the foundation for present-day psychiatric nursing practice. In 1952, a leading exponent in the field of psychiatric nursing, **Hildegard Peplau**, published her book, *Interpersonal Relations in Nursing*, which identified and described the essential skills, functions, and roles of the psychiatric nurse. In this work Peplau detailed the four major phases of the therapeutic nurse–patient relationship and provided the first systematic, theoretical framework for the practice of psychiatric nursing.

The next decade saw further changes take place. For example, the use of the nursing process became the basis for the development of a more refined and better understood definition of the complex functioning of the psychiatric nurse. In addition, a clearer distinction was made between the general practitioners who were staff nurses within a psychiatric setting and the psychiatric nurses who, because of their advanced preparation, brought to the patient care situation special skills and expert clinical capability. Subsequently, the expansion of the nurse's role grew to include involving psychiatric nurses as leaders in group psychotherapy. This period of growth and refinement of clinical skills was instrumental in assisting the psychiatric nurse to move beyond the confines of institutional walls and out into the community. Thus, during this decade, psychiatric nurses demonstrated an expanded and more meaningful scope of practice and were able to assume an equal, contributing role on the interdisciplinary team wherever and whenever their particular expertise was needed.

The 1960s saw the beginning of intense work by nurse leaders to define levels of practice and delineate standards for that practice. Under the auspices of the American Nurses' Association (ANA), a conference group was created in 1961. By 1963, a special task force was established to help address the emergent need of the profession for identity and autonomy of action. The task force is credited with the development of the first tentative statement of philosophy and the identification of the basic assumptions underlying practice. Their efforts resulted in a nationwide polling of nurses in the field. The solicited reactions and suggestions for modification resulted in the ANA's adoption in 1973 of a statement on psychiatric nursing practice and the publication of the first Standards for Psychiatric and Mental Health Nursing Practice.

Further refinement of the Standards of Practice and the emergence of nursing as an autonomous discipline characterized the late 1970s and early 1980s. Within this context, nurses have become articulate about independent, dependent, and interdependent functioning, and have succeeded, through the use of the nursing process, in demonstrating the effectiveness of interventions in the rendering of nursing care. Moreover, a concurrent emphasis on the development of nursing theory as a basis for professional practice, together with a heightened awareness of a professional identity, has assisted nursing to assume a coparticipative position with other disciplines and the patient in the delivery of health care on a primary, secondary, and tertiary preventative basis.

CONTEMPORARY PRACTICE

Psychiatric–mental health nursing is identified as a specialized field within the practice of nursing. The uniqueness attributed to this specialized field is the priority given to and the emphasis placed on the skillful use of the interpersonal process in the attainment of therapeutic goals. The focus of psychiatric–mental health nursing is both corrective and preventative. It is corrective in that it provides individuals, families, or groups who are experiencing various degrees of emotional or psychosocial disequilibrium an opportunity to engage in a therapeutic interactional process. It is preventative in that it endeavors through the educative aspect of the interpersonal process and role model exemplification to preserve equilibrium, promote optimal mental health, encourage early identification and intervention, and provide opportunities for rehabilitation. Therefore, **psychiatric–mental health nursing** may be defined as a specialized field of practice within nursing that utilizes the interpersonal process to provide the individual, family, group, or community with corrective and preventative life experiences that enhance human potential and delimit maladaptive functioning.

From a historical perspective, psychiatric nursing, as a specialized field of practice, is literally in the "early childhood" stage of development. It has come into being and is in a state of transition. Maturation has been and continues to be a painful process characterized by upheaval, chaos, and conflict. In spite of or perhaps because of this process, psychiatric nursing remains viable and healthy. Progression over a relatively short period of time has demonstrated movement and growth.

Psychiatric nurses began at Point A, providing custodial care and focusing their attention and concern on the physical well-being of patients. From this position they advanced to Point B, where priority was given to the development of psychological skills. Between Points B and C, nurses concentrated on refining their interpersonal skills and therapeutic techniques of communication. During this span of time they also expanded the scope of therapeutic relationships to include the practice of group therapy.

Contemporary professional practice has arrived at Point D, where the previously recognized concept of the therapeutic alliance has been extended to incorporate the idea of coparticipation. Coparticipation stresses equality between the client and the therapist. Within this context, recognition is given to the client as a purchaser and consumer of services. As such, the client has a right to verbalize what is expected from the professional and from the treatment plan. This concept further implies that both therapist and client alike share responsibility and accountability for their actions within the interactive–interventive process.

Thus, contemporary psychiatric nursing practice finds the practitioner engaged in a diverse number of settings using a wide range of skills and treatment modalities. The psychiatric nurse can be found in the traditional in-patient psychiatric treatment facilities providing direct patient care by creating a therapeutic living situation for patients, by engaging in therapeutic relationships with individuals, families, and groups, and in utilizing the dynamics of small group process to facilitate adaptation, communication, socialization, and reeducation.

In the general hospital, psychiatric nurses have developed a liaison role. Within this role, they have moved off the designated psychiatric unit and out into the mainstream of general nursing care units. They can be found in the cardiac unit supporting and guiding staff in caring for patients manifesting a cardiac psychosis. They are on the surgical unit acting as consultants when postsurgical depression inhibits patient recovery.

Other settings that challenge the scope of the psychiatric nurses' capabilities include halfway houses, day hospitals, night hospitals, ambulatory care centers, emergency rooms, mental health clinics, and private practice. All in all, contemporary practice is a far cry from the custodial care that characterized the beginning of the 20th century.

To ensure uniformity in practice and to provide continued quality care, the American Nurses' Association published in 1982 the third revision of Standards of Psychiatric–Mental Health Nursing Practice. These standards provide a framework for operation. They establish a baseline that identifies the nurse's scope of practice and sets forth guidelines to encourage and to facilitate an equitable, holistic, and humane approach to client care. This revised document has increased specificity that provides structure, process, and outcome criteria against which practice can be measured.

The Standards of Psychiatric–Mental Health Nursing have been divided into two major sections; the first addresses professional practice, while the second addresses professional performance. Thus, Standards I through VI give direction to the manner in which the nursing process is to be applied, while Standards VII through IX set the parameters of accountability for the professional. These Standards apply to both the generalist and the specialist. In essence, the Standards of Practice serve as an outline detailing and directing the nurse's scope of responsibility for her practice. Each of the Standards, plus the rationale on which each standard is based, is reprinted here to serve as a ready reference and to give direction to learning.

PROFESSIONAL PRACTICE STANDARDS*

Standard I. Theory: THE NURSE APPLIES APPROPRIATE THEORY THAT IS SCIENTIFICALLY SOUND AS A BASIS FOR DECISIONS REGARDING NURSING PRACTICE.
Rationale. Psychiatric and mental health nursing is characterized by the application of relevant theories to explain phenomena of concern to nurses, and to provide a basis for intervention and subsequent evaluation of that intervention. A primary source of knowledge for practice rests on the scholarly conceptualizations of psychiatric and mental health nursing practice and on research findings generated from intradisciplinary and cross-disciplinary studies of human behavior. The nurse's use of selected theories provides comprehensive, balanced perceptions of clients' characteristics, diagnoses, or presenting conditions.

Standard II. Data Collection: THE NURSE CONTINUOUSLY COLLECTS DATA THAT ARE COMPREHENSIVE, ACCURATE, AND SYSTEMATIC.
Rationale. Effective interviewing, behavioral observation, and physical and mental health assessment enable the nurse to reach sound conclusions and plan appropriate interventions with the client.

Standard III. Diagnosis: THE NURSE UTILIZES NURSING DIAGNOSES AND/OR STANDARD CLASSIFICATION OF MENTAL DISORDERS TO EXPRESS CONCLUSIONS SUPPORTED BY RECORDED ASSESSMENT DATA AND CURRENT SCIENTIFIC PREMISES.
Rationale. Nursing's logical basis for providing care rests on the recognition and identification of those actual or potential health problems that are within the scope of nursing practice.

Standard IV. Planning: THE NURSE DEVELOPS A NURSING CARE PLAN WITH SPECIFIC GOALS AND INTERVENTIONS DELINEATING NURSING ACTIONS UNIQUE TO EACH CLIENT'S NEEDS.
Rationale. The nursing care plan is used to guide therapeutic intervention and effectively achieve the desired outcomes.

Standard V. Intervention: THE NURSE INTERVENES AS GUIDED BY THE NURSING CARE PLAN TO IMPLEMENT NURSING ACTIONS THAT PROMOTE, MAINTAIN, OR RESTORE PHYSICAL AND MENTAL HEALTH, PREVENT ILLNESS, AND EFFECT REHABILITATION.

---

*Reprinted by permission from the American Nurses' Association, Division on Psychiatric and Mental Health Nursing Practice: Standards of Psychiatric and Mental Health Nursing Practice. Kansas City, Mo.: ANA, 1982.

Rationale. Mental health is one aspect of general health and well-being. Nursing actions reflect an appreciation for the hierarchy of human needs and include interventions for all aspects of physical and mental health and illness.

Standard V-A. Intervention: Psychotherapeutic Interventions: THE NURSE USES PSYCHOTHERAPEUTIC INTERVENTIONS TO ASSIST CLIENTS IN REGAINING OR IMPROVING THEIR PREVIOUS COPING ABILITIES AND TO PREVENT FURTHER DISABILITY.
Rationale. Individuals with and without mental health problems often respond to health problems in a dysfunctional manner. During counseling, interviewing, crisis or emergency intervention, or daily interaction, nurses diagnose dysfunctional behaviors, engage clients in noting such behaviors, and assist the client in modifying or eliminating those behaviors.

Standard V-B. Intervention: Health Teaching: THE NURSE ASSISTS CLIENTS, FAMILIES, AND GROUPS TO ACHIEVE SATISFYING AND PRODUCTIVE PATTERNS OF LIVING THROUGH HEALTH TEACHING.
Rationale. Health teaching is an essential part of the nurse's role with those who have mental health problems. Every interaction can be utilized as a teaching-learning situation. Formal and informal teaching methods can be used in working with individuals, families, groups, and the community. Emphasis is on understanding principles of mental health as well as on developing ways of coping with mental health problems. Client adherence to treatment regimens increases when health teaching is an integral part of the client's care.

Standard V-C. Intervention: Activities of Daily Living: THE NURSE USES THE ACTIVITIES OF DAILY LIVING IN A GOAL-DIRECTED WAY TO FOSTER ADEQUATE SELF-CARE AND PHYSICAL AND MENTAL WELL-BEING OF CLIENTS.
Rationale. A major portion of one's daily life is spent in some form of activity related to health and well-being. An individual's developmental and intellectual levels, emotional state, and physical limitations may be reflected in these activities. Nurses are the primary professional health care providers who interact with clients on a day-to-day basis around the tasks of daily living. Therefore, the nurse has a unique opportunity to assess and intervene in these processes in order to encourage constructive changes in the client's behavior so that each child, adolescent, and adult can realize his potential for growth and health or maintain that level previously achieved.

Standard V-D. Intervention: Somatic Therapies: THE NURSE USES KNOWLEDGE OF SOMATIC THERAPIES AND APPLIES RELATED CLINICAL SKILLS IN WORKING WITH CLIENTS.
Rationale. Various treatment modalities may be needed by clients during the course of illness. Pertinent clinical observations and judgments are made concerning the effect of drugs and other somatic treatments used in the therapeutic program.

Standard V-E. Intervention: Therapeutic Environment: THE NURSE PROVIDES, STRUCTURES, AND MAINTAINS A THERAPEUTIC ENVIRONMENT IN COLLABORATION WITH THE CLIENT AND OTHER HEALTH CARE PROVIDERS.
Rationale. The nurse works with clients in a variety of environmental settings such as inpatient, residential, day care, and home. The environment contributes in positive and negative ways to the state of health or illness of the client. When it serves the interest of the client as an inherent part of the overall nursing care plan, the setting is structured and/or altered.

Standard V-F. Intervention: Psychotherapy: THE NURSE UTILIZES ADVANCED CLINICAL EXPERTISE IN INDIVIDUAL, GROUP, AND FAMILY PSYCHOTHERAPY, CHILD PSYCHOTHERAPY, AND OTHER TREATMENT MODALITIES TO FUNCTION AS A PSYCHOTHERAPIST, AND RECOGNIZES PROFESSIONAL ACCOUNTABILITY FOR NURSING PRACTICE.
Rationale. Acceptance of the role of psychotherapist entails primary responsibility for the treatment of clients and entrance into a contractual agreement. This contract includes a commitment to see a client through the problem presented or to assist the client in finding other appropriate assistance. It also includes an explicit definition of the relationship, the respective role of each person in the relationship, and what can be realistically expected of each person.

Standard VI. Evaluation: THE NURSE EVALUATES CLIENT RESPONSES TO NURSING ACTIONS IN ORDER TO REVISE THE DATA BASE, NURSING DIAGNOSES, AND NURSING CARE PLAN.
Rationale. Nursing care is a dynamic process that implies alterations in data, diagnoses, or plans previously made.

PROFESSIONAL PERFORMANCE STANDARDS

Standard VII. Peer Review: THE NURSE PARTICIPATES IN PEER REVIEW AND OTHER MEANS OF EVALUATION TO ASSURE QUALITY OF NURSING CARE PROVIDED FOR CLIENTS.
Rationale. Evaluation of the quality of nursing care through examination of the clinical practice of nurses is one way to fulfill the profession's obligation to ensure that consumers are provided excellence in care. Peer review and other quality assurance procedures are utilized in this endeavor.

Standard VIII. Continuing Education: THE NURSE ASSUMES RESPONSIBILITY FOR CONTINUING EDUCATION AND PROFESSIONAL DEVELOPMENT AND CONTRIBUTES TO THE PROFESSIONAL GROWTH OF OTHERS.
Rationale. The scientific, cultural, social, and political changes characterizing our contemporary society require the nurse to be committed to the ongoing pursuit of knowledge that will enhance professional growth.

Standard IX. Interdisciplinary Collaboration: THE NURSE COLLABORATES WITH OTHER HEALTH CARE PROVIDERS IN ASSESSING, PLANNING, IM-

PLEMENTING, AND EVALUATING PROGRAMS AND OTHER MENTAL HEALTH ACTIVITIES.
Rationale. Psychiatric nursing practice requires planning and sharing with others to deliver maximum mental health services to the client and the community. Through the collaborative process, different abilities of health care providers are utilized to communicate, plan, solve problems, and evaluate services delivered.

Standard X. Utilization of Community Health Systems: THE NURSE PARTICIPATES WITH OTHER MEMBERS OF THE COMMUNITY IN ASSESSING, PLANNING, IMPLEMENTING, AND EVALUATING MENTAL HEALTH SERVICES AND COMMUNITY SYSTEMS THAT INCLUDE THE PROMOTION OF THE BROAD CONTINUUM OF PRIMARY, SECONDARY, AND TERTIARY PREVENTION OF MENTAL ILLNESS.
Rationale. The high incidence of mental illness in our contemporary society requires increased effort to devise more effective treatment and prevention programs. Nurses must participate in programs that strengthen the existing health potential of all members of society. Such concepts as primary prevention and continuity of care are essential in planning to meet the mental health needs of the community. The nurse uses organizational, advisory, advocacy, and consultative skills to facilitate the development and implementation of mental health services.

Standard XI. Research: THE NURSE CONTRIBUTES TO NURSING AND THE MENTAL HEALTH FIELD THROUGH INNOVATIONS IN THEORY AND PRACTICE AND PARTICIPATION IN RESEARCH.
Rationale. Each professional has responsibility for the continuing development and refinement of knowledge in the mental health field through research and experimentation with new and creative approaches to practice.

Progress, change, and growth are not achieved without cost. This cost is made manifest in the apparent lag or dichotomy that prevails between the knowledge and skill base psychiatric nurses possess and the translation and application of this data base and expertise to actual practice. That is to say, there exists in today's practice of the profession an observable discrepancy between the ideal that nurses verbalize and the real that they practice.

Many factors impact the current concept of what psychiatric nursing is, how it should be delivered, what part it plays, and where it fits within the total scheme of the mental health care system. These factors account, in part, for this discrepancy. Some of these factors include: the lack of visibility and low profile projected by practitioners; the paucity of prepared, qualified psychiatric nurses to meet society's increasing demand for services, producing, as a result, a higher nurse–patient ratio; the lack of a cohesive bond between and among professional nurses; increased reliance on the use of group process to meet client needs; decentralization of services, which has the potential for fragmenting patient care; and the diminishing amount and scarcity of financial resources committed to the support and subsidization of health services and of professional education, which has, in effect, prioritized expediency and lauded quantity over quality to the detriment of client need.

Furthermore, the development of psychiatric nursing over the past 40 years has been so rapid and in such a constant state of flux that the resultant changes have been difficult to assimilate. Consequently, nurses have displayed resistance to change along with a need to maintain the status quo. Both the desire to maintain equilibrium and the desire to progress have produced stress as evidenced by feelings of dissatisfaction, helplessness, powerlessness, apathy, and burnout.

Our present posture demonstrates an awareness of the issues and the challenges they represent. Current practice does reflect the fact that inroads have been made in dealing with some of the major problems. For example, with respect to visibility, there is the growing trend of psychiatric nurses to move out of traditional settings and become more active, assertive, and involved in community health issues, agencies and organizations. And, too, the number of psychiatric nurse practitioners in private practice is increasing despite the system's reluctance to compensate them for their services under third-party payment programs. Moreover, the concepts of collegiality and cooperative effort between and among mental health disciplines are evidence of the growing recognition of the psychiatric nurse's unique contribution to client care. In addition, two assessment mechanisms, peer group review and nursing audits, have given some indication that psychiatric nurses are actively engaged in fulfilling their direct and indirect care functions. The practice of psychiatric nursing is moving from Point D, the present, to Point E, the future—today! Hope and vitality as clinical entities lie within the scope of the future, where the care and commitment of the present will spur the profession to close the gap, thereby making tomorrow's "real" more closely resemble today's "ideal."

RECOMMITMENT TO CARE AND CONCERN—A FUTURE DIRECTION

In reviewing the past and present status of the field of psychiatric nursing, it seems hard to believe that so much has been accomplished in such a short span of time. At the same time, so much remains to be accomplished—needs must be met and goals fulfilled. It can be stated unequivocally that the past and the present have provided a firm foundation for continued expansion and growth. Realistically, no one can predict what the future will be, since to make such projections entails voyaging into new and unchartered waters. However, what has gone on before can furnish some indications about what should be, needs to be, and hopefully will be accomplished in the future.

Planning for the future involves close examination of resource networks to provide the necessary economic and human support systems to promote and increase ongoing research and education activities. Further, as the profession struggles with finding solutions to the problems of the present, there is a definite need to prioritize concerns so that systematized, organized, innovative, and creative activity can be undertaken to assure progress. Along with prioritizing comes the need to evaluate and resynthesize that which already exists in order to give direction to future endeavors. The impetus for forward movement must come from within and be under the control of the profession and the professionals. If the profession permits the exercise of external control by others, it places itself in a position of jeopardy, that is, in a situation which may potentially result in its dissolution.

Although future needs confronting psychiatric nurses are many and varied, several seem most pressing. First, there is a need to establish solidarity within the practice field—a unanimity that not only acknowledges the expertise of its members but makes use of this expertise in a collective and organized manner. Second, there is the need for professionals to stand up and be counted. This entails clearly articulating our position, defining our domain for ourselves and others, and demonstrating that we do possess the ability to consistently implement and refine our practice skills.

Third, there is the need for practitioners in the field to publish and share their experiences, skills, opinions, beliefs, and ideas with their colleagues. And fourth, there is the need for psychiatric nurses to become more politically active within their communities, to assume a political posture regarding the problems, concerns, and issues involving funding, scope of service, legal ramifications, and rights of those we are committed to serve. Carried a step further, there is a fifth need; that is, psychiatric nurses must continue to participate in the decision-making process governing the formulation of national mental health policy, both from the standpoint of the consumer and from the standpoint of the profession.

The future must be spearheaded by rededication and recommitment. This revitalization is essential to combat apathy if a humanistic, holistic system of care and caring is to be responsive to and responsible for individuals and groups struggling to cope with a broad spectrum of human problems. The profession and its members must be willing to give to others and to accept within themselves the credit, respect, and understanding that are reflective of the philosophy so readily stated.

SUMMARY

The practice of psychiatric–mental health nursing can trace its antecedents back to the dawn of time. However, the past 50 years have seen the emergence of psychiatric–mental health nursing as a specialized field of nursing practice that utilizes the interpersonal process to provide the individual, family, group, or community with both corrective and preventative life experiences that enhance human potential and delimit maladaptive functioning. The psychiatric nurse is grounded in theory, uses current research findings in the delivery of care, is guided by standards of professional practice, and continues to define and clarify her place in the field of psychiatric–mental health care.

SUGGESTED READINGS

Andrulis, D.P., & Mazade, N.A. American Mental Health Policy: Changing Directions in the 80's. *Hospital and Community Psychiatry*, Vol. 34, No. 7 (July, 1983), 601–606.

Benfer, B.A. Defining the Role and Function of the Psychiatric Nurse as a Member of the Team. *Perspectives in Psychiatric Care*, Vol. 18, No. 4 (July/August, 1980), 166–177.

Chamberlain, J.G. The Role of the Federal Government in Development of Psychiatric Nursing. *Journal of Psychosocial Nursing and Mental Health Service*, Vol. 21, No. 4 (April, 1983), 11–18.

Church, O.M., & Buchwalter, K.C. Harriet Bailey—A Psychiatric Nurse Pioneer. *Perspectives in Psychiatric Care*, Vol. 18, No. 2 (March/April, 1980), 62–66.

Covert, A.B. Community Mental Health Nursing: The Role of the Consultant in the Nursing Home. *Journal of Psychiatric Nursing and Mental Health Services*, Vol. 17, No. 7 (July, 1979), 15–16, 19.

Creighton, H. Negligence in Releasing Psychiatric Patient. *Nursing Management*, Vol. 14, No. 11 (November, 1983), 53–54.

Cushing, M. A Judgment on Standards. *American Journal of Nursing*, Vol. 81, No. 4 (April 1981), 797–798.

Cutler, D.L. Clinical Care Update: The Chronically Mentally Ill. *Community Mental Health Journal*, Vol 21, No. 1 (Spring, 1985), 3–12.

Delgade, M. Hispanic Natural Support Systems: Implications for Mental Health Services. *Journal of Psychosocial Nursing and Mental Health Services*, Vol. 21, No. 4 (April, 1983), 19–24.

Division on Psychiatric and Mental Health Nursing Practice. *Standards of Psychiatric and Mental Health Nursing Practice*. Kansas City, Mo.: American Nurses' Association, 1982.

Edwards, L.H. Health Planning Opportunities for Nurses. *Nursing Outlook*, Vol. 31, No. 6 (November/December, 1983), 322–325.

Ellison, E. Social Networks and the Mental Health Caregiving System: Implications for Psychiatric Nursing Practice. *Journal of Psychosocial Nursing and Mental Health Services*, Vol. 21, No. 2 (February, 1983), 18–24.

Fife, B. The Challenge of the Medical Setting for the Clinical Specialist in Psychiatric Nursing. *Journal of Psychosocial Nursing and Mental Health Services*, Vol. 21, No. 1 (January, 1983), 8–13.

Gammonley, J. New Direction for Mental Health Education. *Journal of Psychiatric Nursing and Mental Health Services*, Vol. 16, No. 12 (December, 1978), 40–44.

Hart, C. A. Psychiatric Mental Health Nursing Consultation: A Two-Model System in a General Hospital. *Issues in Mental Health Nursing*, Vol. 4, No. 2 (April–June, 1982), 127–148.

Janetakos, J. & Schissel, C. Partners: Nurse Practitioner and Social Worker. *American Journal of Nursing*, Vol. 79, No. 8 (August, 1979), 1434–1435.

Kane, C. The Outpatient Comes Home. *Journal of Psychosocial Nursing and Mental Health Services*, Vol. 22, No. 11 (November, 1984), 19–25.

Karasu, T.B. Recent Developments in Individual Psychotherapy. *Hospital and Community Psychiatry*, Vol. 35, No. 1 (January, 1984), 29–38.

Kuntz, S., Stehle, J., & Marshall, R. The Psychiatric Clinical Specialist: The Progression of a Specialty. *Perspectives in Psychiatric Care*, Vol. 18, No. 2 (March/April, 1980), 90–92.

Lamb, H.R., & Peterson, C.L. The New Community Consultation. *Hospital and Community Psychiatry*, Vol. 34, No. 1 (January, 1983), 59–64.

Lancaster, J. Community Treatment for Mental Health's Forgotten Population. *Journal of Psychiatric Nursing*, Vol. 17, No. 7 (July, 1979), 20–26.

Lego, S.M. The One-to-One Nurse-Patient Relationship. *Perspectives in Psychiatric Care*, Vol. 18, No. 2 (March/April, 1980), 67–89.

Leone, D., & Zahourek, R. Aloneness in a Therapeutic Community. *Perspectives in Psychiatric Care*, Vol. 12, No. 2 (April/June, 1974), 59–63.

Mark, B. From "Lunatic" to "Client": 300 Years of Psychiatric Patienthood. *Journal of Psychiatric Nursing and Mental Health Services*, Vol. 18, No. 3 (March, 1980), 32–35.

Mericle, B.B. The Male as Psychiatric Nurse. *Journal of Psychosocial Nursing and Mental Health Services*, Vol. 21, No. 11 (November, 1983), 28–34.

Meyerson, A.T., & Herman, G.S. What's New in Aftercare? A Review of Recent Literature. *Hospital and Community Psychiatry*, Vol. 34, No. 4 (April, 1983), 333–342.

Morrissey, J.P., & Goldman, H.H. Cycles of Reform in the Care of the Chronically Mentally Ill. *Hospital and Community Psychiatry*, Vol. 35, No. 8, (August, 1984), 785–793.

Munjas, B.A. Chronicity in Mental Illness: Does "Nursing Care" Maintain It? *Issues in Mental Health Nursing*, Vol. 2, No. 3 (March, 1980), 1–13.

Nelson, J.K.N., and Davis, D.S. Educating the Psychiatric Liaison Nurse. *Journal of Nursing Education*, Vol. 18, No. 8 (October, 1979), 14–20.

Pearlmutter, D.R. Recent Trends and Issues in Psychiatric–Mental Health Nursing. *Hospital and Community Psychiatry*, Vol. 36, No. 1 (January, 1985), 56–62.

Peplau, H.E. The Psychiatric Nurse—Accountable? To Whom? For What? *Perspectives in Psychiatric Care*, Vol. 18, No. 3 (1980), 128–134.

Pesarcik, G., et al. Psychiatric Nurses in the Emergency Room. *American Journal of Nursing*, Vol. 79, No. 7 (July, 1979), 1264–1266.

Powers, K.A. Nursing Home Ombudsman: A Challenge Accepted. *Nursing & Health Care*, Vol. 5, No. 1 (January, 1984), 32–33.

Romano, C.A. Computer Technology and Nursing: A Futuristic View. *Computers in Nursing*, Vol. 3, No. 2 (March–April, 1985), 85–87.

Rubenfeld, M.G., et al. The Nurse Training Act: Yesterday, Today, and. . . . *American Journal of Nursing*, Vol. 81, No. 6 (June, 1981), 1202–1204.

Rupp, A., Steinwachs, D.M., & Salkever, D.S. The Effect of Hospital Payment Methods on the Pattern and Cost of Mental Health Care. *Hospital and Community Psychiatry*, Vol. 35, No. 5 (May, 1984), 456–459.

Schoolcraft, V. *Nursing in the Community*. New York: Wiley, 1984.

Shaffer, F. Nursing Power in the DRG World. *Nursing Management*, Vol. 15, No. 6 (June, 1984), 28–30.

Sills, G.M. Research in the Field of Psychiatric Nursing, 1952–1977. *Nursing Research*, Vol. 26 (November, 1977), 1201–1207.

Spitz, H.I. Contemporary Trends in Group Psychotherapy: A Literature Survey. *Hospital and Community Psychiatry*, Vol. 35, No. 2 (February, 1984), 132–141.

Thurer, S.L. Deinstitutionalization and Women: Where the Buck Stops. *Hospital and Community Psychiatry*, Vol. 34, No. 12 (December, 1983), 162–163.

Theodo, G.C., & Scarry, K.D. Networking Community Services: Politics of Hospice Development. *Nursing and Health Care*, Vol. 4, No. 10 (December, 1983), 568–572.

Tringali, R. The Role of a Psychiatric Nurse Consultant on a Burn Unit. *Issues in Mental Health Nursing*, Vol. 4, No. 1 (January–March, 1982), 17–24.

2

MENTAL HEALTH–MENTAL ILLNESS

A Perspective in Caring

LEARNING OBJECTIVES

On completion of this chapter the reader should be able to:

1. Define and differentiate between **mental health** and **mental illness.**
2. Recognize the implications mental illness has for an individual and for society.
3. Recognize the implications that an awareness of mental health and mental illness has for the practice of nursing.
4. Identify and discuss the major indications for psychiatric hospitalization.
5. Distinguish between voluntary and involuntary hospitalization.
6. Differentiate between conditional and absolute discharge.
7. Identify a minimum of five patient rights.
8. Discuss the implications of statutory laws on nursing practice.
9. Discuss the importance of ethical considerations in practice.

MENTAL HEALTH-MENTAL ILLNESS: A DICHOTOMY

In the psychiatric–mental health field, much of the literature points toward the existence of a continuum between **mental health** and **mental illness**. This view of health and illness implies linear movement from one extreme of the continuum to the other. At any given time in an individual's life, his functioning is reflected by a specific point along the continuum. Where the point lies depends on the individual's ability to satisfy his needs. The position changes as the individual responds and reacts to the impact of his current reality, thereby affecting his functioning. Correspondingly, the statement is made that no one has absolute health or is "completely normal." However, seldom does one hear or see a disavowal of the claim of absolute illness. The individual is either mentally ill or not; that is, the person is identified as having a specific set of symptoms and is therefore labeled as having a specific clinical condition. This distinction between health and illness does not seem to satisfy all prevailing conditions, however. For example, there exist many individuals who are identified as having chronic conditions. If one looks at where they might fit along a linear plane between health and illness, where exactly are they placed? Are they placed more toward the healthy side of the continuum, or are they placed toward the unhealthy side? A linear concept for a distinction between health and illness presupposes a definite point of demarcation. The existence of such a point is questionable; therefore, for us, this way of explaining an individual's ability to cope is not completely satisfactory.

An alternative way of expressing an individual's relationship to himself, to others, and to his environment is to state that both health and illness exist on separate and distinct continua. Thus, on the health continuum there are specific criteria used in the assessment of variations in mental functioning and in identifying the degree of maturity. On the illness continuum there are specific behaviors that manifest the existence of a pathological process and are indicative of its severity.

In keeping with this viewpoint, when a healthy individual encounters crisis and is temporarily unable to satisfactorily resolve the crisis, he remains a healthy person but moves toward the lower end of the health continuum. If, on the other hand, a healthy individual is subjected to sustained stress or crisis over a prolonged period of time, he moves from the health continuum to the illness continuum. In the first instance, where the healthy individual moves from one extreme of the health continuum to the other, he remains able to initiate coping devices or learn alternative means of adaptation, usually without therapeutic intervention. This is not so in the second instance, where the individual moves from the health continuum to the illness continuum. This individual will need therapeutic intervention. *The goal of therapeutic intervention is to return the individual to optimal functioning along the health continuum.*

Mental health is an evolving process in which the individual's internal demands and needs are brought into harmonious relationship with the reality of the environment in which he lives. Its achievement is obtained through successful adaptation. Successful adaptation in daily living requires that an individual establish a point of equilibrium between wants, needs, abilities, ambitions, values, and feelings and the real or perceived expectations of the society and surrounding environmental influences in which the individual operates. Consequently, the individual is able to function independently without distorting reality while gaining mastery over self and environment. Thus, a **mentally healthy person** is one who possesses the ability to make adjustments that enable him to remain unhampered by emotional conflict and free from pathological symptomatology: confirm and follow a philosophy of living; find satisfaction and fulfillment in exercising and expanding his potential; and establish and maintain meaningful relationships with others.

Mental illness is a personal as well as a social problem. It is disruption, disorganization, dysfunction or disintegration. As a personal problem, **mental illness** is maladjustment in living. It produces a disharmony in a person's thoughts, feelings, and actions. In mental illness, the individual loses his ability to respond according to the expectation he has for himself and the demands that society has for him. In essence, mental illness is a failure on the part of the individual to adapt and vary responses within the context of current reality. In mental illness, the individual's reaction to self, others, and the environment are usually inadequate, inappropriate, and unacceptable, reflecting the extent of emotional, psychological, and physical dysfunction.

The presence of mental illness and the extent of its influence produce an economical and political threat to society. Economically, mental illness decreases society's productivity by (1) reducing either the numbers or the efficiency of the labor force, thus affecting the gross national product, and (2) placing budgetary constraints on the general economy because of the need to allocate a substantial amount of available funds toward treatment facilities and programs. Politically, the ramifications of social deviance, nonconformity, and the unpredictable nature of mental illness undermine the power structure of society through their psychological impact on all the members of society. Society is not concerned so much with the presence of disability as it is concerned with the presence of deviance, which in turn generates increased tension, disruption, and fear. Thus, mental illness is a complex problem which in its broadest sense implies an all-encompassing umbrellalike concept used to designate psychological, emotional, and social disequilibrium.

The two illustrations in Figures 2–1 and 2–2 are symbolic representations of mental health and mental illness. They depict the outcome of what happens to an individual who is exposed to either sustained positive nurturing or sustained negative experiences.

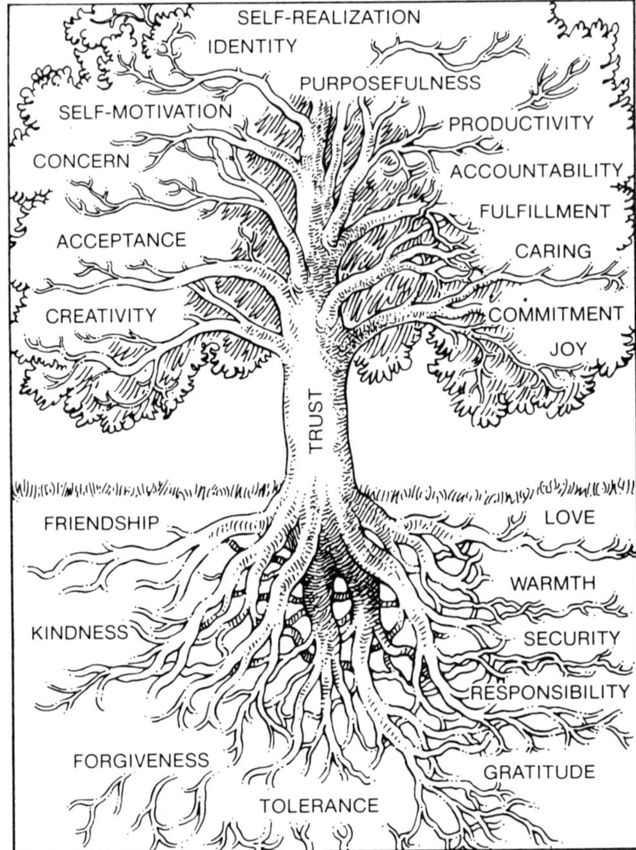

Figure 2–1. Tree of Mental Health

CHARACTERISTIC DIFFERENCES BETWEEN MENTAL HEALTH AND MENTAL ILLNESS

To provide the reader with a clear, concise overview of the major, significant, descriptive elements distinguishing a mentally healthy person from a mentally ill person, we have made the following comparisons in Table 2–1. These comparisons are based on the relationships that the self maintains toward the self, toward others, and with the environment. The reader should note that an element of unreality exists when an attempt is made to distinguish artificially between absolutes. Life is full of gray areas. This Table, then, is an effort to identify the extremes that personify the absolutes. Every so-called

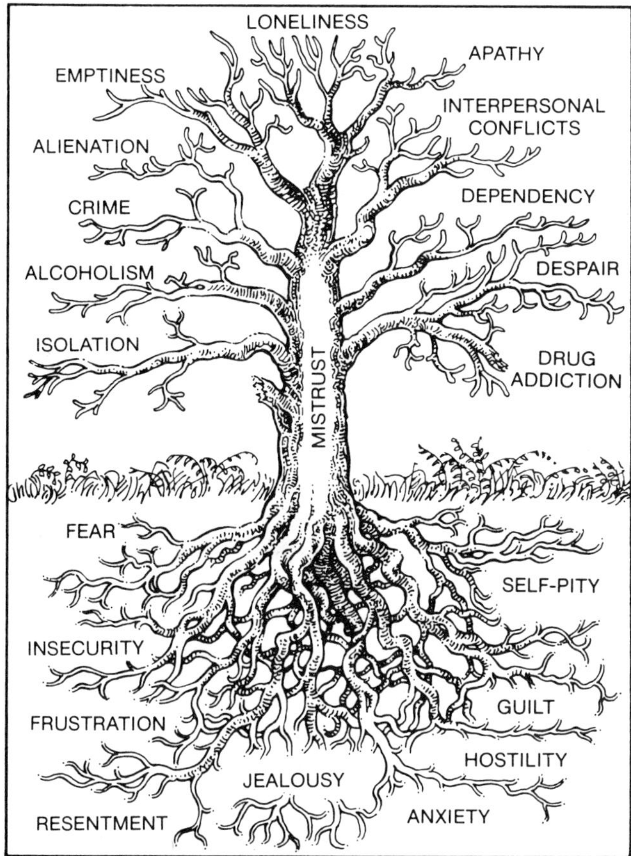

Figure 2–2. Tree of Mental Illness

healthy person has at one time or other displayed one or more of the characteristics ascribed to mental illness. Conversely, every individual who is identified as being mentally ill possesses some of the characteristics of mental health.

To summarize, the mentally healthy person is an individual who has self-awareness, who likes, respects, and accepts himself for what he is, and who acknowledges his limitations and seeks improvement. The reader should be aware that failure to possess one or more of the elements listed under mental health does not connote mental illness. Immaturity or lack of specific elements merely points out areas of inadequacy and decreased potential for optimal functioning.

TABLE 2-1. COMPARISON BETWEEN MENTAL HEALTH AND MENTAL ILLNESS

Mental Health	Mental Illness
Relationship with Self	
Possesses self-knowledge and a sense of identity.	Self-identity is is distorted and not based in reality.
Accepts self, both strengths and weaknesses.	Unable to accept strengths or weaknesses.
Accepts criticism.	Rejects or denies criticism.
Meets or postpones gratification of basic needs.	Depends on others to meet basic needs.
Sets appropriate short- and long-term goals and moves toward actualization.	Inappropriate goal setting with ineffective organization and planning.
Establishes a value system.	Value system fluctuates indiscriminately.
Uses past experience to illuminate the present and to plan for the future.	Focuses on the past; has a limited awareness of before-and-after effects.
Assumes responsibility for self-learning.	Demonstrates limited incentive to learn and is negativistic.
Values productivity; achieves satisfaction and enjoyment from work.	Uses work to avoid involvement and responsibility in the growth process; work is nonproductive.
Integrates thoughts, feelings, and actions.	Displays disharmony among thoughts, feelings, and actions.
Resolves conflict.	Unable to make choices; exercises poor judgment; avoids conflicts.
Relationship with Others	
Establishes and maintains positive relationships.	Unable to establish or maintain relationships; uncomfortable with others.
Assumes responsibility for terminating those relationships that may be harmful or detrimental.	Unable to evaluate or terminate threatening relationships.
Validates feelings.	Denies or projects.
Works collaboratively.	Is defensive or destructive; isolates self.
Accepts compromises when appropriate.	Refuses to compromise; maintains rigidity and resistance.
Communicates directly.	Secretive, suspicious, and distrustful.
Uses body gestures to enhance or facilitate communication.	Uses body gestures instead of verbal language.
Varies content of communication appropriate to the situation.	Seldom talks about self or focuses entirely on self and content of communication is limited in scope.
Respects others.	Disdains others.
Relationship with Environment	
Organizes environment.	Operates in a disorganized fashion.
Exerts control over or modifies immediate environment.	Exerts minimum or excessive control; creates a new environment.
Adapts to change.	Unable to retain objectivity.
Engages in planned, thoughtful, responsible activity.	Behaves impulsively and irresponsibly.
Resolves power struggles through cooperation and collaboration.	Unable to deal with the concept of power and authority, resulting in dysfunction and disintegration.

IMPLICATIONS FOR NURSING PRACTICE

The total spectrum of mental health and mental illness—the identifiable criteria for health and specific symptoms of illness—their significant differences and the vast variations in degrees, the endless possibilities of interpretations of behavior, and the deceptive nuances that pervade the communication of thoughts and feelings serve as a background for the practice of nursing. An awareness of the subtleties involved in human behavior influences the practitioner in the kind of care, the quality of care, and the commitment to caring provided. The nurse's role involves a dual responsibility not only for the treatment of illness but, equally important, for the prevention of illness.

INDICATIONS FOR HOSPITALIZATION

The primary goal of hospitalization is to provide an individual with an opportunity to preserve and enhance personal and social functioning. Indications for hospitalization include needs for safety, diagnosis, treatment, asylum, burden sharing, insight, and partnership. If any one or combination of these factors is present within the life situation of the individual, then hospitalization generally becomes the most appropriate vehicle for assisting the person to deal with presenting problems.

Safety

Safety, as an indication for hospitalization, refers to the personal well-being of the individual, or to the well-being of others. In the first instance, we are talking about violations of the individual's biological integrity. One example of a situation in which safety plays a significant role would be the case of a patient who has emotionally regressed to the point where basic biological needs, such as eating or sleeping, are no longer perceived or met. Another example might be the individual for whom life has become meaningless and who therefore views suicide as the one and only alternative. A third example is the individual whose preoccupation with hand-washing rituals have left his hands raw and bleeding. In the second instance, regarding the safety of others, a classic example might be the homicidal individual whose acting out might tend to place the lives of others in jeopardy. A further example might involve the person who feels severely threatened by "the voices" to the point where he believes that his neighbors are in tune with "cosmic beings" and are directing their rays at him. He feels compelled to protect himself by attacking them before they can "get him." In each of the five cases cited, the individual manifests an inability to care for self or to care about the welfare of others in a reasonable, logical, and beneficial manner. In addition, there is a marked diminution in the necessary cognitive or perceptive ability to exercise discriminatory judgment, thereby placing the individual's physical and mental well-being in jeopardy.

Diagnosis

People can often behave in strange and bizarre fashions, either on impulse or as the result of quite careful planning. Behaving in such a manner is not necessarily an indication of mental illness, yet when a person, his relatives, or other members of society become aware that discrepancies exist between the individual's ability to think, feel, and act in a manner consistent with the usual expectations and norms of his society, then that individual is in need of diagnostic assessment. The need for diagnosis becomes manifest when, for example, an individual displays unreasonable fear that his thoughts can be the cause of another's death; or when feelings of helplessness or hopelessness reach the point where the only thing the person can do all day and all night is to sit in a chair and rock; or when a person, despite evidence to the contrary, firmly believes that he is "Superman" and can tackle any situation singlehandedly. In many cases, an accurate appraisal of the individual's condition and awareness of his unique personal characteristics to determine his true mental status can only be accomplished within the confines of a hospital setting. Adequate psychological evaluation requires time to test and time to observe interpersonal functioning.

Treatment

The need for treatment presents itself when the person's capacity to adapt becomes markedly diminished and the only viable alternative left open is a retreat or movement away from reality. In other words, coping with reality has become so complex, so threatening, so unbearable that fantasy becomes "livable" reality in which the pain is less acute and the living conditions less stressful. Theoretically, primary prevention should be initiated long before an individual reaches this crisis point. However, in point of fact, acute onset of debilitating symptomatology often occurs before the need is recognized by the person or by others within the immediate environment and treatment is sought. Once hospitalized, the initiation of an optimal treatment plan depends on an accurate appraisal of the individual's condition and awareness of his unique personal characteristics.

Asylum

The need for asylum, that is, for a protective, nurturing environment, eventuates when the individual requires time out to regroup his resources away from the demands of his current life situation. Asylum may meet many needs. For instance, it might provide the individual with an opportunity to learn about himself and how he responds to people and, in turn, how they respond to him. He may come to realize that there are alternative solutions to dealing with specific problems, and he may learn new ways of coping with adverse situations, if they should arise. Asylum may also meet a need for peace, a reduction in the pressures encountered in daily life. It may provide an opportunity for dependency needs to be met in a constructive, supportive manner that otherwise might not occur. Asylum may also provide an opportunity, perhaps for the first time, for the individual to recognize assets and strengths, instead of focusing only on deficits and areas of weakness. Thus, meeting the overall need for asylum through hospitalization allows the individual to retreat from life's stressors when they become overpowering. Asylum provides the person with breathing space.

Burden Sharing

Burden sharing, as an indication for hospitalization, occurs when family members and friends need relief from the stresses produced by the presence of a person who manifests an inability to cope with the usual routine aspects of life and living. At first, this idea may sound revolting and heartless. It may even cause the reader to view the hospital as a sort of dumping ground for society's rejects—a place to hide away those who are unwanted, unloved, or unproductive. However, in reality, the complete reverse is true. Families and friends who have been supportive in the past, who wish to continue to keep their loved one with them in the future, and who are willing to participate and share in caring view hospitalization as a viable alternative to isolation, rejection, and renunciation. In meeting this need for continued involvement, maintenance, support, and caring, the hospital and the significant others enter into a relationship designed to relieve stress. Stress reduction preserves the supportive functioning of the individual's family constellation and reduces the chance of producing negative attitudes toward the individual, resulting in ultimate rejection by that constellation. In essence, just as asylum allows the patient time out for regrouping and reorganizing resources, burden sharing allows significant others to pull themselves together, reduce stress and conflict, and remobilize their positive strengths and assets.

Insight

Insight is an awakening awareness that assistance is required. It arises as the individual begins to acknowledge that something is wrong, that his functioning is not appropriate, that his feelings are out of proportion to the event, that his thoughts are illogical, disjointed, and confused. When an individual reaches this point and comes to the realization that a problem does indeed exist, whether or not he possesses knowledge regarding the full extent of the situation, then that individual, either with or without encouragement, makes a move toward seeking appropriate assistance. A patient may find his way to the hospital through direct admission from an emergency room, as an outcome of visits to a mental health clinic, because of a need for continuation of treatment begun in the therapist's office, or as a "walk-in" stating that he has a problem and is in need of help. Whatever the mode of referral, the individual has sufficient awareness to recognize disparity in functioning and takes appropriate steps to meet an identified need.

Partnership

Partnership is the assumption of responsibility for care on the part of both the patient and the hospital. Partnership involves the realization on the part of the individual that the hospital represents a source of clinical help. It presupposes that the person seeking assistance recognizes and is willing to assume coresponsibility in the pursuit of therapy. Partnership requires commitment, involvement, cooperative effort, trust, and compliance along with a sincere desire to decrease, modify, change, or eliminate problems that prevent effective, optimal functioning as an independent and self-actualized individual.

Effects of Social Changes

If any one or more of these seven indications for hospitalization are present within the life situations of the individual, then hospitalization is perhaps the most appropriate method of assisting the person to deal with presenting problems. In the foreseeable future, the hospital will most likely continue to play a significant role as a viable treatment facility within the context of our societal structure. However, it must be noted that over the past decade we have observed change leading to a shift in emphasis and a resultant alteration in purpose. That is, we are beginning to see movement away from using the psychiatric hospital as an extended, long-term, chronic treatment facility and toward a greater emphasis on its use as an acute care setting. This change in function reflects society's attitudinal change toward the care and treatment of the mentally ill. There is an attitudinal stance that now accepts, encourages, and even mandates with increasing frequency the return of the individual to the broad spectrum of community living and involvement. This attitudinal shift results not so much from enlightenment and understanding of the problems faced by the mentally ill or even from an acute awareness of the need for societal concern from a humane or altruistic basis, but rather, unfortunately, from society's concern and preoccupation with the personal and legal rights of individuals.

Furthermore, we see another major social issue impinging on this attitudinal change, that of a growing sense of dashed hopes and distrust of established, traditional systems within our societal structure. Other elements affecting this attitudinal change include: the increasing concern about autonomy; the almost phobic reaction of fear to governmental intrusion and control; the questioning and subsequent churning of values, which has led to the adoption of rules to replace responsibility; the dwindling of resources, which has aroused questions concerning the appropriate, effective utilization and disbursement of funds to produce the greatest good; the uncovering and highlighting of racism and its subtle practices; as well as a generalized feeling of uneasiness regarding the relationship that is supposed to exist between the care provider and the care receiver.

We have identified the preceding factors as having produced an effect on the changing purpose of psychiatric hospitalization. We believe these factors, forces, and attitudinal shifts have also had an impact on the whole field of psychiatric–mental health care and the future of its delivery both in kind and scope as well as for whom, when, under what circumstances, and by whom the health care can be delivered.

CARING—RIGHTS AND RESPONSIBILITIES

Institutional policies and procedures governing the admission and discharge of clients are based on statutory laws. By and large, these statutes are concerned with three major issues: types of admissions; protection of the client's civil rights; and factors determining the length of time and circumstances under which an individual may be detained. Most states recognize two categories of psychiatric hospitalization—**voluntary** and **involuntary**.

Admission

Voluntary admission status stipulates that an individual or his parents or guardian make direct application to the institution for service. Under this type of admission, the client retains his right to request and obtain release. The request for release must be presented in writing. Generally, what follows is that a "period of grace" is invoked. A grace period is a timeout period in which both the client and the institution have an opportunity to consider and examine the request. It varies from state to state. In some instances, the client, having acted impulsively, may subsequently rescind the request. On the part of the hospital, the grace period enables the institution to obtain a data base to document the client's mental health status and act accordingly. The action taken may result in the client's immediate release or may result in a recommendation that the client's admission status be changed from voluntary to involuntary.

Involuntary admission implies that the individual is institutionalized against his wishes. Such action also requires that formal written application be made on behalf of the patient. Here again, each state dictates what constitutes sufficient criteria and cause for commitment to a psychiatric facility. This type of admission can be instituted or authorized by a private citizen, the court, an administrative tribunal, or the requisite number of physicians. Each initiator has determined that the person's mental status meets the statutory criteria and the person is therefore in need of care. Involuntary commitment is usually subdivided into three categories—emergency, temporary or observational, and extended or indeterminate.

Emergency hospitalization is a temporary, time-limited provision for short-term treatment and care. This type of admission is brought about at the instigation of any private citizen, police officer, health officer, court, or physician. It is generally applied where an individual is clearly and consistently manifesting behavior that could be considered injurious to self or others.

Temporary commitment is short-term hospitalization for a specified period of time, generally 60 to 90 days. This type of admission provides an opportunity for observation and data collection so that a definitive diagnosis can be made and needed treatment prescribed. Usually, hospitalization of this type can be initiated at the request of any private citizen, family member, law officer, or physician. Specifics related to admission criteria, length of time, and initiator of application are regulated by the laws of each state. There are normally three potential outcomes of temporary hospitalization. First, the patient may be discharged; second, the individual's admission status may change from involuntary commitment to that of voluntary hospitalization; or, third, the physician in charge of treatment may file an application for extended or indeterminate commitment.

Indeterminate commitment is, as its name implies, hospitalization over an extended period of time ranging from 60 to 180 days. This type of commitment results from either court action or medical certification. Generally, throughout this process, the individual retains his right to contest such action, and he may in most states request that he be represented by legal counsel. Usually, before such action is undertaken, a medical review of the patient's case is carried out. At this time, medical evidence is presented to support application for extended hospitalization. In a number of states, the individual retains his right to request a review of his current status to determine the need for continued hospitalization. In those states where this right is not clearly spelled out, there are provisions mandated for periodic review, usually on a yearly basis.

Discharge

Discharge, like admission, is governed by statutory laws. Within our current system, two types of discharge predominate—conditional and absolute. A **conditional discharge** is one that imposes certain prerequisites or stipulations with which the patient is expected to comply. If compliance is beyond the ability of the individual, the client may be reinstitutionalized without having to undergo another legal admission procedure. Trial visits are an example of conditional discharge. In this situation, the patient is released from the hospital under the condition that if the trial visit goes well he need not return and will be discharged. Successful trial visits are usually related to the individual's ability to continue taking medication as prescribed, to adjust to activities of daily living, or to keep scheduled out-patient appointments. Another example of conditional discharge is that described as **against medical advice (A.M.A.)**. In this situation, a voluntarily hospitalized patient requests release. In the professional opinion of his treatment physician, interruption of therapy would not be advantageous. The physician will honor the request but indicate disagreement with the client's decision. A waiting period between reception of and action on the patient's request is usual. This allows time for the patient to reconsider and for the physician to provide documentation, if in his judgment continued hospitalization is necessary.

Absolute discharge implies a complete and final severing of the partnership that existed between client and hospital. If reinstitutionalization is required, the client must reapply and undergo all admission procedures. Generally, absolute discharge may occur in one of three ways: as the outcome of an administrative decision made by hospital officials; as an outcome of legal proceedings that result in a court order demanding release; or as an outcome of a petition made to the courts to have the patient released on a writ of habeas corpus.

Patient Rights

It has only been within the past 15 years that society as a whole has evidenced concern and that the legal profession has become more actively involved in safeguarding the basic civil rights of psychiatric patients. From the standpoint of the nursing profession, recognition of rights has always been acknowledged; however, sensitivity and persistence in application have been somewhat lacking. This professional inconsistency is not surprising, as it has merely been a reflection of prevalent societal attitudes. Certainly, mental health legislation along with statements from professional organizations, such as the American Nurses' Association and the National League for Nursing, have urged nurses to become directly involved in assuring that the human and legal rights of patients are respected and preserved. Legislation and statements of professional conduct are in and of themselves not sufficient motivators. What is needed is an attitudinal change within the practitioner, which no legal body or court can impose. Thus, for the beginning practitioner, it becomes imperative to cultivate a philosophical approach to care and caring that reflects a humanistic outlook valuing the rights of self and others.

It is currently a common practice for hospitals to publish and issue to incoming clients a document listing the rights of patients. Furthermore, many institutions display these rights on bulletin boards throughout the hospital. Although there is no universal "Bill of Rights" and variations exist from institution to institution and from state to state, most professionals are in agreement that the following list encompasses the fundamental framework of human and civil rights to which the patient is entitled.

- The right to treatment
- The right to treatment in the least restrictive setting
- The right of informed consent
- The right to legal representation
- The right to periodic review of status
- The right to be free of unnecessary mechanical restraints
- The right to privacy and confidentiality
- The right to communicate with people outside the hospital
- The right to send and receive mail without censorship
- The right of access to a telephone
- The right to see visitors
- The right to wear personal clothing
- The right to keep and use personal possessions
- The right to religious freedom
- The right to enter into contractual agreements
- The right to manage and dispose of property
- The right to marry and divorce
- The right to execute wills
- The right to vote
- The right to make purchases
- The right to engage in legal proceedings
- The right to retain and maintain licenses
- The right to refuse treatment
- The right not to perform institutional labor

To simply have developed a statement of rights and to supply a copy of those rights to patient and to professional alike does not guarantee the enactment of these rights. We believe that a salient question each professional nurse must ask herself after reviewing these rights is: Do I believe in them? If the answer is yes, then to what extent? If the answer comes back no, then why not? Let us look at the right to vote as an example. In our society, we supposedly value this right, but does this value translate into action within the institutional or community setting? Do we arrange or assist the client to arrange for transportation to polling places? Do we assist the client in securing an absentee ballot? Do we even know if the client is a registered voter? If we have a client who manifests severe psychotic symptoms, does anyone point out to him that election time is near? In other words, is this right to vote applied in all cases or is it only available to those, who in our professional opinion, are capable of rational thinking and discriminative judgment?

Looking beyond the questions generated from this example, we may pose additional questions with respect to rights and their application. For example, are rights upheld and applied equally without discrimination? How are the rights of clients implemented and monitored? Does each care provider have a personal and professional responsibility for implementation? Is it nursing's responsibility alone to safeguard rights, or do we share responsibility with other health care disciplines? If we share responsibility, to what degree? Is it equal, 60-40, 90-10? Does fear of litigation or personal risk best influence professional judgment as to which rights will be supported most consistently and which will receive less attention?

The identified list of rights came into being out of societal concern for patients who might be in a dependent or vulnerable position. The fear, and rightly so, was and is that clients may be taken advantage of by unthinking, unfeeling, or unscrupulous care providers. These rights were developed with good intent, but their conception may have occurred without foresightedness in identifying limitations, exceptions, or potential adverse outcomes and without regard for expert professional judgments as to the appropriateness of application with a given person or situation. Furthermore, it appears that no attempt was made either to distinguish priority of rights or to establish the relationship of one right to another, or even to decide whether each right is mutually exclusive of all other rights. Moreover, apparently no attempt was made to identify a right as inherent by virtue of personhood versus a right that is conferred on a person by society by virtue of being a member of that society.

Let us look at the right to be free of unnecessary mechanical restraint. Questions that might arise in any discussion concerning the application of mechanical restraints might very well include: Who defines "unnecessary"—client, professional, society? If mechanical restraints are viewed as a form of therapeutic intervention, does their application impinge on the patient's right to refuse treatment? If so, when, under what conditions? If not, why not? How does the professional, in light of the client's refusal to accept restraint, safeguard, preserve, and implement the right to informed consent? There appears to be some dichotomy. This dichotomy gives rise to unresolved ethical dilemmas.

To have merely compiled a list of patient rights is meaningless if the process eventuates in only philosophical discussion rather than the use of such identified rights as a guide for the delivery of humane care. For example, the patient has a right to wear personal clothing. On admission, however, a certain patient did not come with any clothes other than pajamas, and has had no visitors or made any outside contact. Three days later, this patient is still attired in hospital clothing. Who is responsible for seeing that the right to wear personal clothing is exercised by the patient? Does this right only apply if the patient has clothing immediately available, or does the patient have the option to refuse what has been identified as his right? This brings us to another very salient question. What is the limit of responsibility for a health care professional when a client says, "No, I don't want to exercise that right"? The identification of rights is all well and good, but if the rights are not respected, if the rights are not safeguarded and upheld, if the rights are not incorporated as part of the plan of care, and if the rights and manner in which they are implemented are not periodically reviewed and evaluated, then the identification of rights lacks meaning and substance.

Therefore, we advocate that each professional nurse must closely examine the list of identified rights in light of her personal beliefs and value system, as well as examining them in light of her practice. Such an examination will permit the nurse to determine for herself the extent to which congruence exists between what is said to be valued and what is actually carried out and most importantly, if congruence is found to exist, to determine its basis. Does congruity exist out of fear—fear of legal entanglements and censure—or does it exist as an outcome of a humanistic philosophy of caring that demands an acceptance of responsibility and personal accountability?

In conclusion, it should be noted that practitioners in the mental health field are being held more and more accountable for the exercising of their clinical judgments, resultant behaviors, and treatment outcomes. Consequently, the nurse must possess a knowledge of the laws relating to the care of the mentally ill and an awareness of what constitutes patient rights, and must make sound clinical judgments with respect to the implications that laws and rights have on practice. If there is doubt about the community's concern for liability, one only has to pick up the daily newspaper to read an account of a lawsuit involving questions arising from denial and violation of rights, inadequate or incompetent treatment, negligence, or even flagrant misuse and abuse of the psychiatric patient. Ignorance of the law is no longer an acceptable curtain behind which the professional can hide.

ETHICAL CONSIDERATIONS

Another aspect of nursing practice is the ethical and moral considerations inherent in each nursing action. Broadly, the question of ethical–moral behavior in practice deals with the nurse's perceived rightness and wrongness, that is, the goodness or badness of an act, set of acts, judgment, or decision. Basically, ethics dictate which human actions are justifiable. Ethics portray the conscience of the professional and the profession. Ethics reflect beliefs and belief systems and are the guiding principles governing our daily lives.

Each nursing action has an ethical component that must be addressed by the practitioner. In the nurse–patient relationship, for example, thoughtful deliberation must be given to such basic issues as informed consent, privacy, confidentiality, the right of self-determination, and power. With respect to restraints, for instance, the nurse needs to resolve such questions as first, whether or not their application is an infringement of a person's right to freedom of movement and self-control; second, whether or not the safety of the individual takes precedence over the safety of the majority; third, whether or not the use of restraint is intrinsically dehumanizing, whatever the cause or end; and fourth, whether or not the application of restraints stems from therapeutic or punitive motivation.

In fact, any therapeutic endeavor undertaken by the nurse, such as administering psychotropic drugs, engaging in behavior modification, answering questions and giving information, or recording observations, precipitates the need for reflection involving at least two major issues, control and goals of treatment. Control is an issue because most people view it in a negative light, that is, as an imposition of the will of one over the will of another. In this context, control also negates a basic value and right—freedom of choice. With respect to goals, we generally understand these to mean the client's goals for his treatment; however, on initial contact, the client's goals and the nurse's goals may be at variance, resulting in conflict. Ideally, resolution of this conflict brings both the nurse and the client into mutual agreement.

Ethical considerations present a challenge to the nurse. Implementation of the ethical component demands an awareness and understanding of human needs and rights, respect for human justice and caring, knowledge of values and beliefs, and a commitment based on active involvement.

Guidelines exist that give direction to ethical decisions. For example, the profession has adopted a Code of Ethics, which describes the expected behavior of the nurse; the Constitution contains a Bill of Rights that speaks to beliefs about the person; and a Standard of

Practice has been developed to direct the delivery of nursing care. These documents do not provide solutions to the complex, multidimensional issues or questions faced by the practitioner, but they do form the foundation from which problems can be addressed.

Ethical dilemmas exist, and the fact that they are described as dilemmas is indicative of the state of uncertainty regarding their resolution. We are not always in the position to know what is the most right thing to do, but the fact that we question what is right is of paramount importance. Ethical practice demands that the choices made by each and all of us as practitioners can be justified in a rational, thoughtful manner and be based on viable principles rather than be founded or reside in an appeal to emotion. It is our belief that nurses must openly discuss with one another the ethical issues and implications of their daily practice. Each of us must be willing to risk disclosure of our beliefs, values, and opinions in our search for the "rightness" of our professional actions.

SUMMARY

This chapter presents the significant aspects of human functioning that can be used to differentiate mental health from mental illness. In addition, this chapter discusses the indications that may necessitate hospitalization and focuses the reader's attention on some of the legal and ethical aspects involved in the delivery of care.

SUGGESTED READINGS

Adams, G.L., et al. Primary Mental Health Care: An Innovative Model. *Journal of Psychiatric Nursing and Mental Health Services*, Vol. 18, No. 1 (January, 1980), 26–30.

Alexis, A. Body Serches and the Right to Privacy. *Journal of Psychosocial Nursing and Mental Health Services*, Vol. 24, No. 11 (November, 1986), 21–25.

Aroskar, M.A. Ethics of the Nurse-Patient Relationship. *Nurse Educator*, Vol. 5, No. 2 (March/April, 1980), 18–20.

Aroskar, M.A. Are Nurses' Mind Sets Compatible with Ethical Practice? *Topics in Clinical Nursing*, Vol. 4, No. 4 (April, 1982), 22–23.

Atkinson, G.M. Medical-Moral Dilemma: Crisis Care vs. Health Maintenance. *Ethics and Medics*, Vol. 4, No. 2 (February, 1979), 1.

Atkinson, G. Medical-Moral Dilemma: Involuntary Hospitalization. *Ethics and Medics*, Vol. 3, No. 3 (May/June, 1978), 1–4.

Bandman, E.L., & Bandman, B. *Bioethics and Human Rights*. Boston: Little, Brown, 1978.

Bandman, E.L. & Bandman, B. Do Nurses Have Rights? *American Journal of Nursing*, Vol. 78, No. 1 (January, 1978), 84–86.

Benoliel, J.Q. Ethics in Nursing Practice and Education. *Nursing Outlook*, Vol. 31, No. 4 (July/August, 1983), 210–215.

Beranzweig, E.P. 7 Questions About Nursing Negligence. *Nursing Life*, Vol. 4, No. 4 (July/August, 1984), 23.

Bevilacqua, J. Voodoo—Myth or Mental Illness. *Journal of Psychiatric Nursing and Mental Health Services*, Vol. 18, No. 2 (February, 1980), 17–23.

Brooks, N.E. Behind the Heavy Metal Door. *American Journal of Nursing*, Vol. 79, No. 9 (September, 1979), 1546–1550.

Brucolierer, T.M. That Fine Line. *Nursing 78*, Vol. 8, No. 10 (October, 1978), 136.

Carper, B.A. The Ethics of Caring. *Advances in Nursing Science*, Vol. 1, No. 3 (April, 1979), 11–20.

Curtin, L., & Flaherty, M.J. *Nursing Ethics*. Bowie, Md: Robert J. Brady Co., 1982.

Cushing, M. Informed Consent—An M.D.'s Responsibility? *American Journal of Nursing*, Vol. 84, No. 4 (April, 1984), 437–440.

Davis, A.J. Informed Consent: How Much Information Is Enough. *Nursing Outlook*, Vol. 33, No. 1 (January/February, 1985), 40–42.

Dolan, M.B. By The Rules. *American Journal of Nursing*, Vol. 83, No. 5 (May, 1983), 815, 819.

Egbert, E. Concept of Wellness. *Journal of Psychiatric Nursing and Mental Health Services*, Vol. 18, No. 1 (January, 1980), 9–12.

Fenner, K.M. *Ethics and Law in Nursing: Professional Perspectives*. New York: D. Van Nostrand Co., 1980.

Finkel, N.J. *Therapy and Ethics*. New York: Grune & Stratton, 1980.

Fromer, M.J. *Ethical Issues in Health Care*. St. Louis: C. V. Mosby Co., 1981.

Fry, S.T. Dilemma in Community Health Ethics. *Nursing Outlook*, Vol. 31, No. 3 (May/June, 1983), 176–179.

Goleman, D. Who's Mentally Ill? *Psychology Today*, Vol. 11, No. 8 (January, 1978), 34–41.

Gregory, B., & Gouge, R.L. Disfigured by a Violent Patient: A Case . . . and Comment. *R.N.*, Vol. 42, No. 3 (March, 1979), 61–62, 65, 72.

Halleck, S.L. *The Politics of Therapy*. New York: Harper & Row, 1971.

Hamilton, P.A. *Health Care Consumerism*. St. Louis: C. V. Mosby, 1982.

Hannah, G.T., Christian, W.P., & Clark, H.B. (eds.) *Preservation of Client Rights*. New York: Free Press, 1981.

Hemelt, M.D., & Mackert, M.E. *Dynamics of Law in Nuring and Health Care*. Reston, Va.: Reston Publishing Co., 1978.

Jourard, S.M. *Healthy Personality: An Approach from the Viewpoint of Humanistic Psychology*. New York: Macmillan, 1974.

Kelly, L.Y. Nursing Practice Acts. *American Journal of Nursing*, Vol. 74, No. 7 (July, 1974), 1310–1319.

Kroll, J., & Mackinzie, T.B. When Psychiatrists are Liable: Risk Management and Violent Patients. *Hospital and Community Psychiatry*, Vol. 34 (January, 1983), 29–36.

Mahon, K.A., & Fowler, M.D. Moral Development and Clinical Decision-making. *Nursing Clinics of North America*, Vol. 14, No. 1 (March, 1979), 3–12.

Mappes, T.A., and Zimbaty, J.S. *Biomedical Ethics*. New York: McGraw-Hill, 1981.

McShea, M.M. Clinical Judgement: An Ethical Issue. *Journal of Psychiatric Nursing and Mental Health Services*, Vol. 16, No. 3 (March, 1978), 52–55.

Mental Health Law Project. *Basic Rights of the Mentally Handicapped*. Washington, D.C.: Mental Health Law Project, 1973.

Muir, Judge R., Jr. Interview: Providing for the Rights and Safety of Patients. *Journal of Psychosocial Nursing and Mental Health Services*, Vol. 24, No. 22 (November, 1986), 29–31.

Muyskens, J.L. No Easy Choice: Resolving Everyday Ethical Dilemmas. *Nursing Life*, Vol. 4, No. 4 (July/August, 1984), 29–32.

Nelson, M.J. Authenticity: Fabric of Ethical Nursing Practice. *Topics in Clinical Nursing*, Vol. 4, No. 1 (April, 1982), 1–6.

Nursing Ethics: What Are Your Personal and Professional Standards? A Survey Report. *Nursing 74*, Vol. 4, No. 9 (September, 1974), 34–44.

Oriol, M.D., & Oriol, R.D. Involuntary Commitment and the Right to Refuse Medication. *Journal of Psychosocial Nursing and Mental Health Services*, Vol. 24, No. 11 (November, 1986), 15–16, 18–20.

Quinn, N., & Somers, A.R. The Patient's Bill of Rights. *Nursing Outlook*, Vol. 22, No. 4 (April, 1974), 240–244.

Rabinow, J. Avoiding Legal Trouble When You and the Doctor Disagree. *Nursing Life*, Vol. 4, No. 4 (July/August, 1984), 41–44.

Rabner, C.J., & Lurie, A. The Case for Psychiatric Hospitalization. *Nursing Digest*, Vol. 3, No. 3 (May/June, 1975), 42–44.

Rocereto, L., & Maleski, C. All About Rights to Medical Records. *Nursing Life*, Vol. 4, No. 4 (July, August, 1984), 50–51.

Rosenhan, D.L. On Being Sane in Insane Places. In B.A. Backer, P. M. Dubbert, & E. Eisenman (Eds.), *Psychiatric/Mental Health Nursing: Contemporary Readings*. New York: D. Van Nostrand Co., 1978, 405–426.

Rothman, D.A., & Rothman, N.L. *The Professional Nurse and the Law*. Boston: Little, Brown, 1977.

Sigman, P. Ethical Choice in Nursing. *Advances in Nursing Science*, Vol. 1, No. 3 (April, 1979), 37–52.

Smith, S.J., & Davis, A.J. Ethical Dilemmas: Conflicts among Rights, Duties and Obligations. *American Journal of Nursing*, Vol. 80, No. 8 (August, 1980), 1462–1466.

Smoyak, S.A. Editorial: Ethical Perspectives. *Journal of Psychosocial Nursing and Mental Health Services*, Vol. 24, No. 11 (November, 1986), 7.

Steele, S.M., & Harmon, V.M. *Values Clarification in Nursing*, 2nd ed. Norwalk, Conn.: Appleton-Century-Crofts, 1983.

Stone, A.A. *Mental Health and Law: A System in Transition*. U.S. Department of Health, Education and Welfare, Pub. No. (ADM) 76–176. Washington, D.C.: U.S. Government Printing Office, 1975.

The Joint Information Service of the American Psychiatric Association and the Mental Health Association. *Preventing Mental Illness: Efforts and Attitudes*. Washington, D.C.: American Psychiatric Association, 1980.

Trotter, C.M.F. I Never Promised You a Rose Garden But I Must Remember to Tell You About the Thorns. *Journal of Psychosocial Nursing and Mental Health Services*, Vol. 23, No. 3 (March, 1985), 15–17.

3

THE THERAPEUTIC ENVIRONMENT

LEARNING OBJECTIVES

On completion of this chapter the reader should be able to:

1. Define **therapeutic environment.**
2. Identify the three significant components that contribute to the creation and maintenance of a therapeutic environment.
3. List specific nursing behaviors that contribute to the development and maintenance of a therapeutic environment.
4. Identify the biological, physical, and psychological influences affecting the creation of a therapeutic environment.
5. State a minimum of four principles governing privacy, safety and protection, and comfort within the therapeutic environment.

INTRODUCTION

Historically, the concept of a therapeutic environment originated in 1959 with Maxwell Jones, who coined the term **therapeutic community.** Jones used the therapeutic community as a treatment modality that created a corrective life experience and nurtured the healthy aspects of personality. The two major premises on which his concept was based were: first, that the whole person, including his living environment, could be used to bring about changes in personality; and second, that manipulation of living conditions, including physical facilities, types of therapy, and interpersonal relationships, would be effective in fostering healthy change.

Contemporary psychiatric care has incorporated some of the basic assumptions of a therapeutic community that Jones advocated, and from this has emerged the concept of a therapeutic environment. Currently, in order to be considered therapeutic, an environment must contain those factors that contribute to, provide for, and promote maximum opportunity for growth and development. To achieve this end, a therapeutic community is designed so that the care providers and the care receivers work together as a cohesive unit in which the staff and clients assume a shared responsibility. In this enterprise, the clients govern themselves while the staff provide essential information and consultation. The focus of attention is on the positive development of existing strengths and resistance resources. A therapeutic community is a learning environment based on reality and behavior modification that is designed, through democratic process, to extinguish behaviors that are deemed unacceptable and, through shaping, to create thoughts and actions that foster successful adaptation to life.

Thus, a **therapeutic environment** is reviewed as a deliberate structured set of living situations and experiences directed toward problem solving, resolution of conflict, and the implementation of stress-decreasing goals. It is a dynamic environment in which the major focus is on health and wellness. A therapeutic environment is organized on the concept of healthy living and interacting. It simulates social experiences and directly involves the client in his own care. The essence of the therapeutic environment is the emotional, social, and psychological atmosphere prevailing within the patient's setting that allows him to focus on the exploration and resolution of existing problems. Nursing assumes an important function in the creation of a therapeutic environment in that the nurse provides for healthy interactions and learning situations that enable the patient to formulate adequate adjustments.

We believe there are three major components that contribute to the formation and maintenance of a therapeutic environment. These are **privacy, safety** and **protection**, and **comfort**. In this chapter we explore each of these components and highlight several specific nursing activities and areas of responsibility. The primary emphasis of this chapter is directed toward residential facilities, although the practice principles that follow can be universally applied to any environment or setting. The nurse should apply the principles of a therapeutic environment to whatever setting in which patient care takes place.

We offer the following principles as guidelines governing the establishment and implementation of a therapeutic environment.

I. Principles applicable to the concept of **privacy** include:
   1. People need a living and working situation that allows them to feel safe from outside intrusions.

2. People have the right to exclude others from certain information.
3. Territoriality is an innate, instinctual behavior reflected by the individual's need for privacy.
4. Past experiences as well as social and cultural expectations influence the degree to which the need for privacy is manifested by each individual.
5. Acknowledgment of the need for privacy conveys respect for personal integrity and worth.
6. Privacy promotes a feeling of security while decreasing feelings of hostility, embarrassment, and dehumanization.
7. Privacy provides an opportunity for the individual to engage in behavior directed toward the relief and release of emotional pressures.
8. Privacy allows an opportunity for self-examination, evaluation, and integration.
9. Interpersonal communication and self-disclosure is facilitated through a respect for maintaining privacy.
10. The potential effectiveness of therapeutic intervention is enhanced when consideration is given to the client's need for privacy.
11. Provision for quiet areas within the environment acknowledges the need for privacy.
12. Confidentiality with respect to verbal and written communication preserves privacy.
13. Physical facilities and environmental conditions can be structured to promote privacy.

II. Principles applicable to the concept of **safety** and **protection** include:

1. Preservation of self and the species is a basic drive motivating behavior.
2. An alien environment threatens preservation and therefore interferes with safety and protection.
3. A feeling of security is enhanced by the degree of alertness and concern displayed.
4. Safety and protection are promoted when democratic, participatory encounters between and among clients and staff are fostered.
5. Lack of consideration for safety invites acting-out behavior.
6. Monitoring the environment for potential hazards is essential to maintenance of safety and protection for self and others.
7. The exercise of external control through limit setting or physical constraint may be necessary to provide safety and

protection when clients demonstrate an inability to maintain self-control.

8. Preparedness for emergency interventions reduces the potential for immobilizing anxiety and self-recrimination.
9. Adherence to established policies, rules, and regulations promotes safety and security.

III. Principles applicable to the concept of **comfort** include:

1. The degree of comfort felt by an individual is influenced by his age and level of activity as well as his physical condition and emotional state.
2. Personal, interpersonal, and environmental comfort is closely associated with the concepts of privacy and safety.
3. When privacy and safety are disrupted or disregarded, physiological and psychological comfort is decreased.
4. Since the mind and the body operate as an integrated whole, comfort measures will have an influence on the total functioning of the individual.
5. Comfort allows the individual freedom to be and to become by increasing coping mechanisms and decreasing the expenditure of psychic energy.
6. Comfort tends to increase the level of hopefulness within the individual and the environment.
7. Comfort mandates attention to details.

PRIVACY: A BASIC NEED

Everybody has a need for privacy. Throughout recorded history people have sought to protect this basic need for themselves, their loved ones, and their immediate community. Anthropologists have vividly described the privacy sought and protected by mankind through past millenniums. As technology developed, people became more interdependent on extended environments to provide them with the means by which they could achieve daily needs. Technology did not change the value of privacy, but rather it challenged people to find ways to meet this persistent need. Yet these are the essential elements of nursing care for individuals who are experiencing emotional and other psychological distresses. So the nurse's attention should be directed toward utilizing the physical environment to develop an atmosphere that promotes as much privacy as possible.

One of the environmental modifications the nurse might consider is the arrangement of furniture in the recreation room, common areas, and visitors' rooms of the hospital units. If the furniture is placed in small, circular or semicircular groupings, it is more like a family room or living room. This type of physical arrangement provides the patient with tangible evidence that his need for privacy is recognized, acknowledged, and accepted. Small groups of patients can talk together without disrupting other groups that might be in the immediate area, and a patient and visitor can have at least some limited privacy.

One or two small rooms should be set aside for individual use. This provides a private area for patients whose therapeutic plan permits them freedom of movement. Away from the general flurry of ward activities, patients can be alone, read, play their radio or musical instruments, or share their experiences with special friends they have selected among other patients, without being interrupted or overheard. These small rooms could also be used by staff members for interviewing, counseling, or "rapping" with the assurance of privacy during therapeutic engagements.

In our culture, bathing and toileting are considered private functions. Most people are accustomed to carrying out these functions alone without assistance or supervision. It can be quite embarrassing when patients have to bathe or shower with other patients or "according to schedule." Modern constructions, both public and private, have incorporated in the architectural design patient rooms with private facilities. However, rarely do the larger and older institutions provide a bath in each patient's room. To minimize the feelings of embarrassment and reluctance to maintain personal hygiene due to such lack of privacy, only a minimum number of personnel should be deployed to assist or supervise during bathing periods. The nurse should schedule bathing and toileting periods after examining the patient's preference and eliciting related feelings from the patient.

Personal possessions, however trivial, take on added significance when a person is hospitalized. For the patient they become a part of identity, contribute to feelings of security, provide a sense of ownership, and serve as a link with the reality of the environment outside the hospital. Disappearance or misplacement of personal items can produce an increase in anxiety, extend frustration, and foster distrust.

Provisions must be made that guarantee the preservation and privacy of the patient's personal effects, as demonstrated in this actual case history.

> Mr. Ragan, a 57-year-old divorced male, was readmitted to a state hospital following an exacerbation of his psychiatric condition diagnosed as schizophrenia, paranoid type. He had stopped taking his medications and was imbibing alcoholic beverages in order to "relax and sleep." His aged mother had died of natural causes approximately 11 months prior to admission and Mr. Ragan continued to reside alone at the parental home. Mr. Ragan had been unemployed and maintained himself with disability benefits from Social Security.
>
> One day Mr. Ragan became intoxicated and fell asleep in a dilapidated easy chair. A fire broke out because of his careless smoking and he was

miraculously saved by the alertness and swiftness of the local firemen. Subsequent to treatment for smoke inhalation at the local hospital, the doctor recommended psychiatric hospitalization and treatment because the patient was confused, guarded, suspicious, and hostile.

Relatives reported that Mr. Ragan had been acting bizarre for some time. He did not leave the house except late at night to purchase alcohol, and he refused to allow anyone to enter his home. After hospitalization, the relatives discovered that the utilities had been turned off because Mr. Ragan had not paid the bills. After the fire the Health Department condemned the dwelling as unfit and unsafe for habitation. The Probate Court awarded Mr. Ragan's sister legal guardianship of his affairs. At the same time, Mr. Ragan's mother's will was probated and the home was bequeathed to the patient.

Several weeks after admission Mr. Ragan was assisted in purchasing a new wardrobe, since his clothing had been destroyed in the fire. Two days later, another patient stole Mr. Ragan's new clothing and absconded from the hospital. This incident intensified Mr. Ragan's suspicions, guardedness, and hostility. He began to accuse the staff of collusion with his sister to keep his money and his inheritance from him. He refused to participate in ward activities and was constantly complaining about his personal dignity being "trampled on" by everyone. He was verbally hostile and made frequent collect calls to his sister in order to ventilate. Mr. Ragan would claim that everything in his life had been taken from him—his wife, mother, home, money, freedom—and insisted on leaving the hospital against medical advice.

This behavior continued for 6 weeks and created a series of disruptions for himself, other patients, and ward activities. When Mr. Ragan was being disruptive, he would isolate himself from everyone by sitting alone in the corner of the room. Because of Mr. Ragan's limited financial benefits, he was awarded a clothing voucher from the county welfare department through the collaborative efforts of the nurse and social worker. The nurse requested a special order for a lock and key to be placed on his bedside closet; she gave Mr. Ragan one key and placed a spare key in the safety of the nursing station in case Mr. Ragan should lose his key. She requested other staff persons to bring in extra hangers they might have at home to give to Mr. Ragan.

When Mr. Ragan and the nurse returned from their shopping trip, there was a noted change in the patient. Smiling, he carefully placed his new clothing, new hat, new shoes, and even gloves in his locker. The nurse reported that Mr. Ragan had offered to buy her lunch and coffee. His facial muscles seemed to relax and his eyes were brighter. Mr. Ragan began to attend group therapy regularly. He became gentle and courteous towards others and took great pride in personal hygiene and appearance. His appetite improved and he began to involve himself in planning for his discharge to a halfway house in the community.

Another consideration for privacy is respect for closed doors. A patient's room is, in a way, his home away from home. Consequently, the patient is entitled to respect, courtesy, and privacy as though he were indeed in his own home. How many people do you know who go to the house next door and enter without knocking and receiving permission to enter? Respect for privacy requires knocking before entering. A healthy respect for privacy does not mean allowing the patient to isolate himself from the therapeutic environment and the usual daily activities of the hospital ward. It does mean respecting the limited physical space a patient has for quiet reflection, periods of rest, or uninterrupted relaxation.

Staff need privacy as much as the patients in order to execute their duties and maximize the benefits of the therapeutic environment. Daily contacts with individuals and groups whose primary problems are psychological require a tremendous expenditure of emotional and physical energy. Thus, an area where staff can periodically retreat for readjusting their perspectives, recuperating their energy, and regaining objectivity is a must. In addition, privacy is needed by staff for engaging in clinical conferences, planning patient care, sharing nursing reports, and discussing relevant and sundry patient problems.

A nursing station is not a private place. It is the center from which the daily activities of the ward are directed, and it is open on a 24-hour basis. Here the nurses and other staff members are accessible to the patients, and frequently several patients at a time approach the staff for various reasons. This flurry of activity surrounding the nursing station makes it a very open and public place. Consequently, it is not an expedient setting for nurse–patient interviews or counseling. Thus, utilizing other offices and private small rooms, as described earlier, allows the nursing station to remain open and freely accessible to the patients at all times.

Medication rooms are areas that require absolute privacy. For years, these rooms have been attached to nursing stations. This arrangement has some potentially undesirable effects. One is the numerous interruptions by staff or patients, which interfere with the level of attention and concentration of the nurse pouring medications. This interference can result in errors in the distribution of patient medication. Since the pouring of medication requires diligent attention, we believe the medication room should be placed in close proximity, but not adjacent to, the nursing station and that it should be situated away from the general flow of ward traffic.

SAFETY AND PROTECTION: A NECESSITY

Provision for patient safety and protection has always been a high priority in the nursing profession. The major emphasis is appropriately on the creation of a physical environment that meets the physiological and psychosocial needs of the patient while protecting him from injury—by self, from others, or from objects. The idea of safety and protection implies a great deal, both from a physical as well as a psychological standpoint. Shatterproof windows, heavy gauge screening, locked doors, and fire-fighting equipment are all important devices used to insure patient safety and protection; however, they are not wholly sufficient. The therapeutic environment can neither exist nor be effective without the provision and consideration of additional factors that influence the safety and protection of the patient.

These factors can be broadly divided into three major categories: **interpersonal, structural,** and **functional**. **Interpersonal factors** are those that arise from within the interactional process between people and include such aspects as behavior, communication patterns, values, and attitudes or roles. **Structural factors** are those that deal with the architectural design and the material objects within the environment. Specific structural aspects might include but are not necessarily limited to equipment, supplies, or identifiable environmental hazards. **Functional factors** relate to the operational mechanism under which the community conducts its affairs. Aspects of environmental living that are subsumed under this category might include institutional policies, the rules and regulations for the units, or the governance mechanisms.

Each of these factors demand that the nurse cultivate a sense of awareness regarding the prevailing environmental atmosphere and its attendant conditions, as well as the assumption of responsibility regarding the implementation of changes conducive to healthy and harmonious living. In order to promote safety and protection and to intervene effectively, the nurse might find the following suggestions helpful:

1. Observe interactional patterns between patients, patients and staff, patients and visitors, staff and visitors.
2. Assess patient behavior to identify signs of mounting tension.
3. Apply precrisis strategies to avert physical or psychological trauma.
4. Orient and instruct patients, personnel, and nonresident transients regarding the governance operations of the unit.
5. Develop and maintain an optimistic positive outlook.
6. Monitor environment for safety hazards, such as defective equipment, inadequate supplies, obstacles, or outdated policies.
7. Foster staff preparedness to deal with emergency situations both physiological and psychological, such as cardiac arrest, diabetic coma, seizures, panic, or suicide attempts.
8. Use ward government meetings as an opportunity to promote

learning and engage in conflict resolution and problem-solving regarding issues involving safety and security.

9. Use adjunctive therapy of physical constraint when appropriate to promote self-control and minimize interpersonal and environmental hazards.
10. Conduct periodic cognitive and affective appraisal of the environment.
11. Promote and encourage open, honest discussion of environmental issues such as smoking, cleanliness, activities, or use of equipment.
12. Emphasize individualized treatment plans that give recognition to existing differences and needs.

Alertness and spontaneity characterize the nurse's approach to meeting the client's need for a secure and protected environment. The nurse has a dual obligation. First, the nurse must act as a role model through the demonstration of concern for both the large and small details of the environment. Second, the nurse must intervene effectively in those situations characterized by disorganization or destructiveness. In such a constantly changing place as a hospital unit, the creation of a safe and protected environment is no easy task. It requires that the nurse exercise vigilance and judgment.

COMFORT: A RIGHT

To be therapeutic, the environment must be comfortable physically and psychologically. To achieve a satisfactory and healthy level of comfortableness, the nurse should create an appealing aesthetic atmosphere, provide for monitoring biological functions, and foster emotional growth and development.

The provision for comfort as part of a therapeutic environment includes measures to satisfactorily monitor biological functioning. Because an individual's primary diagnosis and reason for hospitalization fall in the area of an identifiable psychological problem, the physiological aspects of the total person may be deemphasized. The nurse must keep in mind that treatment and care of any patient, regardless of diagnosis, include the soma and the psyche as an integrated whole. Although she may not need to care for a recognized health deficiency, she should do preventative health care and health teaching. It is important to realize the impact emotional and psychological distress has on physiological functioning. In both schizophrenia and depression, for example, food intake may have a profound effect. Concentration or avoidance of certain foods may produce severe diarrhea or constipation, resulting in electrolyte imbalance, which in turn may produce signs and symptoms similar to known side effects of tranquilizing agents. Until attention is paid to biological monitoring, the nurse has no factual data on which to differentiate possible causes. It is only after the differentiation has been made that the nurse can institute appropriate intervention.

Another example that points out the necessity for monitoring biological functioning is the importance of taking a patient's temperature when there are specific drug combinations and climatic conditions. This is particularly true when Thorazine and Cogentin are given together. Both drugs affect the heat-regulating function of the hypothalamus. In hot, humid weather the patient is susceptible to heat prostration because this combination of drugs prevents adequate perspiration. The only way the nurse can make sure the patient is not experiencing temperature irregularities is by monitoring.

Our biological nature exists in accordance with definitive patterns, but each individual's pattern is different. There is for each person a specific, constant biological rhythm and timing—**biorhythm**. Illness or stress does not necessarily change the rhythm or timing, but it does interfere with its regularity. This interference accounts for some of the increase in the level of anxiety and feelings of discomfort expressed by patients as somatic complaints. Many of these complaints are, in fact, due to the loss of synchronization in the person's biological functioning. To prevent such disruption, it is important for the nurse to learn as much as possible about the normal life pattern of each individual. This knowledge is gained through the assessment process.

The gathering of such factual information should occur immediately or as soon after admission as possible. (See Chapter 26 for assessment and the development of the nursing care plan.) The patient is the prime source for this information; however, if the person is unable to supply data regarding self, then relatives, friends, and acquaintances of the patient should be contacted. Assessment of biological functioning is as vital as the assessment of social, cultural, or psychological functioning in determining and evaluating deviations. Individual biological functioning must be considered when planning nursing care. Some individuals function adequately on 6 hours of sleep, while others require 10 hours. If we believe that nursing care is based on individual needs, then it becomes imperative to adapt usual ward routines to accommodate individual functioning. Thus, consideration should be given to such things as the scheduling of activities. Activities should be at a time when the patient is most alert and receptive. Adaptation to meet individual patient needs does not imply that the unit functions chaotically. Any large system, such as a hospital, has to operate on some type of organized structure, but structure should be flexible and humane rather than rigid, impersonal, and dogmatic in its rules and regulations. There must be built into the system the attitude that the individual comes first and that the preservation of the system takes second place.

The therapeutic environment can promote comfort by fostering emotional growth and development. Since the therapeutic process is one of reeducation, the setting of the unit must incorporate and utilize those features most likely to be found in the majority of social living situations. Inclusion of such features encourages a sense of identity, feelings of security and independence, and provides opportunities for self-actualization and reality orientation. If opportunities for growth and development are to be realized, the nurse must pay special attention to the details involved in any usual living experience. For instance, we are a time-oriented society; but hospitalized individuals, particularly the elderly, tend to lose track of time and may even manifest time disorientation. Some simple, practical aids for the nurse to use in dealing with this problem are clocks, calendars, and daily newspapers. Convenient placement and accessibility to these aids encourage independent functioning. Their use decreases the need for patients to ask the staff the time or the date and decreases the chance that a patient will be labeled confused or disoriented. The decrease in interruptions gives staff more time to communicate with patients on a more in-depth level of therapeutic interaction.

Another environmental factor influencing growth and development concerns the personal possessions of patients. We are a materialistic society and as such, we tend to closely identify who we are with what we have. Personal possessions are seen as an extension of self. Therefore, possessions may play an important part in the development and maintenance of identity. Hospitalization forces people to limit the number and types of possessions they can keep with them. Therefore, those they have take on an even greater significance.

Nursing has paid lip service to the need for the nurse to develop an attitude of acceptance toward the patient. Unfortunately, nursing has sometimes become caught up in hospital bureaucracy. The result is that the patient is subjected to a dehumanizing experience. The idea of a therapeutic environment implies that the health team limit the restrictions imposed on all specific components that comprise the whole person. Personal possessions are one such component. They reflect a person's social, cultural, economic, and religious status. They convey to the observer how and in what manner the individual has established his interdependency within society. When a person is deprived of a significant portion of himself, the health team is also deprived. Assessment and identification of problem areas and the establishment of guidelines for normalcy for a particular individual are impaired because a significant portion of that person is not available for observation, evaluation, and incorporation into the total treatment program.

Personal possessions include a variety of items that have often been viewed in the past as either nonessential, too costly to be safe from light-fingered individuals, superfluous, or potentially hazardous. Items that have been accorded these designations are personal wearing apparel, cosmetics, wedding and engagement rings, costume jewelry, purses, wallets, ties, nostalgic mementoes and souvenirs, a favorite chair, needlework, musical instruments, family pictures, and projects completed in occupational therapy. To insure psychological comfort and facilitate the growth and development processes with respect to personal possessions, the nurse should carefully examine existing hospital policy and work toward offering modifications where the restrictions are excessively limiting.

Another nursing action is to discuss with the patient the meaning various personal items have for him. If it is determined that the significance is great, the nurse should make every attempt to carry out her advocacy role and provide him with the "security blanket" he needs. Other ways to advocate for a therapeutic environment in fostering growth and development might be to encourage participation in ward government; invite the patient to assume a coresponsibility with staff for effecting changes within his environment; set up and maintain ward kitchens to which patients have free access to make a pot of tea, bake a cake, or make some popcorn; provide places for patients to visit with their children; organize groups of patients to concentrate on beautification of hospital grounds; introduce a ward pet; and as many more modifications or adaptations as the nurse can think of—the possibilities are endless.

Additional common aspects of daily living that can be used as opportunities for growth and development include comfort items related to sleeping, bathing, and dressing. For example, in her initial assessment of sleep patterns, the nurse might want to know if the person uses one pillow or two or none. The same would hold true for blankets or extra coverings. Such information recognizes individuality and fosters the patient's awareness of the environment as one that displays care and concern.

With regard to bathing, the nurse can promote comfort by making sure that bathing items generally taken for granted are readily available for patient use. Such daily personal care items might include shampoo, soap, shaving equipment, hair spray, nail clippers and files, aftershave lotion, deodorants, or hand and body lotion. This does not mean that the institution must provide these items, but rather that the nurse assists the patient to meet his own needs. Possible interventions could include helping the patient to purchase the required items;

and encouraging the patient to contact his family to furnish the items or, if there is no family, the nurse might advocate on behalf of the patient and contact appropriate agencies both within and without the care setting, such as the Red Cross, volunteer services, church groups, or welfare offices.

Another aspect of comfort involves wearing apparel. Whenever possible, patients should be encouraged to wear their own clothes. If they do, the nurse should make certain that the clothing is appropriate to the season, intact, and coordinated and that the total appearance of the patient is neat, clean, and presentable. Where the patient must rely on the institution to provide these items, the nurse must insist on advocating in the patient's behalf for correct sizes, sufficient numbers to allow for changing, and up-to-date style and fashion.

Comfort and therapeutic effectiveness is enhanced through the creation of an aesthetic atmosphere. By an aesthetic atmosphere we mean an environment that is not only appealing and pleasing to the senses but also one that is conducive to and supports consideration for the humanity of both patients and staff. Three features of such an environment are color, proportion, and design.

Color schemes influence mood, and mood influences behavior. Therefore, when colors are selected for the unit, the nurse should be an active participant in the selection process. Some factors for the nurse to consider might include the age range of the population, effect of color on feelings, and the purpose or intended use of an area.

Soft, warm, light colors tend to create an atmosphere that aids in promoting a feeling of comfort and well-being. On the other hand, overly bright hues and shades may produce negative effects by exposing an individual to overstimulation. Color or lack of it can make a working or living environment very pleasant and comfortable or very negative and uncomfortable.

Proportion and design are also important in producing an appealing aesthetic atmosphere. By *proportion* we mean the dimensions used, that is, the size and ratio of such things as room space, furniture, draperies, pictures, and other furnishings; while *design* refers to the environmental living plan. Living space in terms of room size is a necessary element for consideration in planning for a therapeutic environment if the freedom to move and to be is to be encouraged and maintained.

In planning for the amount of space needed, thought should be given to the purpose for which the room is to be used, the type and size of furniture and equipment it is to accommodate, as well as the possible maximum number of people it will be required to hold. A light background gives a sharper outline. Smaller furniture increases the size of the room. Cramped quarters for patients and staff tend to produce inhibitory effects and are therefore not conducive to productive functioning or to the development of a feeling of freedom of movement. Where possible, furnishings should be selected on the basis of their size, suitability, and appropriateness for the area in which they will be used.

There are other features that contribute to the creation of an aesthetic environment. One example is the use of tablecloths, attractive china, glassware, and table arrangements in the dining room. Objects pleasing to the eye do much for the promotion of comfort. They also create an atmosphere in which positive expectations are directed toward acceptable social behavior. Other important items are the introduction of such things as pictures, mirrors, plants, carpeting in living areas, and toss pillows. These additions contribute to comfort by making the ward atmosphere more livable and homelike as opposed to the dreary, gloomy, sterile atmosphere that still prevails in many wards. The creation of this kind of "design for living" falls within the province of nursing. The nurse is responsible for using her creativity and perceptiveness to advocate and recommend those features that contribute to the maintenance of an environment that is pleasing, appropriate, and useful.

SUMMARY

This chapter has pointed out some of the significant factors involved in the creation and maintenance of a therapeutic environment. We have identified the major components that must be considered: privacy, safety and protection, and comfort. In each of these categories we have emphasized specific nursing activities that are essential and when utilized and integrated can produce an environment conducive to healthy functioning and can stimulate the patient to assume an active, participatory role in the psychotherapeutic processes of treatment.

SUGGESTED READINGS

Almond, R. *The Healing Community: Dynamics of the Therapeutic Milieu.* New York: Jason Aronson, 1974.

Baer, O.J. Protecting Your Patient's Privacy. *Nursing Life*, Vol. 5, No. 3 (May/June, 1985), 50–53.

Bayer, M. The Multipurpose Room: A Way-Out Outlet for Staff and Clients. *Journal of Psychiatric Nursing and Mental Health Services*, Vol. 18, No. 10 (October, 1980), 35–37.

Block, D. Privacy. In C.E. Carlson and B. Blackwell (Eds.), *Behavioral Concepts and Nursing Intervention (2d ed.).* Philadelphia: Lippincott, 1978.

Boettcher, E.G. Boundary Making. *Journal of Psychosocial Nuring and Mental Health Services,* Vol. 23, No. 8 (August, 1985), 25–30.

Cooper, K.H. Territorial Behavior Among the Institutionalized. *Journal of Psychosocial Nursing and Mental Health Services,* Vol. 22, No. 12 (December, 1984), 6–11.

Corey, L.J., et al. Psychiatric Ward Atmosphere. *Journal of Psychosocial Nursing and Mental Health Services,* Vol. 24, No. 10 (October, 1986), 10–16.

Devine, B.A. Therapeutic Milieu/Milieu Therapy: An Overview. *Journal of Psychiatric Nursing and Mental Health Services,* Vol. 19, No. 3 (March, 1981), 20–23.

Hinds, P.S. Music: A Milieu Factor with Implications for the Nurse-Therapist. *Journal of Psychiatric Nursing and Mental Health Services,* Vol. 18, No. 6 (June, 1980), 28–33.

Hirst, S.P. Understanding the Difficult Patient. *Nursing Management,* Vol. 14, No. 2 (February, 1983), 68–70.

Hogarth, T. Providing a Therapeutic Milieu on an Inpatient Adolescent Unit. *Ohio Nurses Review,* Vol. 60, No. 4 (April, 1985), 7.

Holmes, M., & Werner, J. *Psychiatric Nursing in a Therapeutic Community.* New York: Macmillan, 1967.

Jones, M. Nurses Can Change the Social Systems of Hospitals. *American Journal of Nursing,* Vol. 78, No. 6 (June, 1978), 1012–1014.

Jones, M. *The Therapeutic Community: A Treatment Method in Psychiatry.* New York: Basic Books, 1953.

Kerenberg, O., & Harin, C. Milieu Treatment With Borderline Patients: The Nurse's Role. *Journal of Psychosocial Nursing and Mental Health Services,* Vol. 22, No. 4 (April, 1984), 29–36.

Kukuk, H.M. Safety Precautions: Protecting Your Patients and Yourself. *Nursing '76,* Vol. 6, No. 5 (May, 1976), 45–51.

Kukuk, H.M. Safety Precautions: Protecting Your Patients and Yourself. *Nursing '76,* Vol. 6, No. 6 (June, 1976), 49–52.

Leininger, M. Caring: A Central Focus of Nursing and Health Care Services. *Nursing and Health Care,* Vol. 1, No. 3 (October, 1980), 135–143.

Luce, G.G. Trust Your Body Rhythms. *Psychology Today,* Vol. 8, No. 11 (April, 1975), 52–53.

Maagdenberg, A.M. The "Violent" Patient. *American Journal of Nursing,* Vol. 83, No. 3 (March, 1983), 402–403.

Miller, T.W., & Lee, L.I. Quality Assurance: Focus on Environmental Perceptions of Psychiatric Patients and Nursing Staff. *Journal of Psychiatric Nursing and Mental Health Services,* Vol. 18, No. 12 (December, 1980), 9–13.

Mitchell, R. The Therapeutic Community. In B.A. Backer, P.M. Dubbert, & E. Eisenman (Eds.), *Psychiatric-Mental Health Nursing: Contemporary Readings.* New York: D. Van Nostrand Co., 1978, 377–382.

Murphy, K. Use of Territoriality in Psychotherapy. *Journal of Psychiatric Nursing and Mental Health Services,* Vol. 19, No. 3 (March, 1981), 13–15.

Natalini, J.J. The Human Body as a Biological Clock. *American Journal of Nursing,* Vol. 77, No. 7 (July, 1977), 1130–1132.

Norbeck, J.S. Social Support: A Model for Clinical Research and Application. *Advances in Nursing Science,* Vol. 3, No. 4 (July, 1981), 43–59.

Porter, R., & Watson, P. Environment: The Healing Difference. *Nursing Management*, Vol. 16, No. 6 (June, 1985), 19–24.

Rasinski, K., Rozensky, R., & Pasulka, P. Practical Implications of a Theory of the "Therapeutic Milieu" for Psychiatric Nursing Practice. *Journal of Psychiatric Nursing and Mental Health Services*, Vol. 18, No. 5 (May, 1980), 16–20.

Raunsley, M.M. The Concept of Privacy.' *Advances in Nursing Science*, Vol. 2, No. 2 (January, 1980), 25–31.

Ricci, M.S. An Experiment With Personal-Space Invasion in the Nurse–Patient Relationship and Its Effect on Anxiety. *Issues in Mental Health Nursing*, Vol. 3, No. 3 (July–September, 1981), 203–218.

Robertson, P.A. The Therapeutic Community and the Nurse: A Blurring of Traditional Roles. *Journal of Psychiatric Nursing and Mental Health Services*, Vol. 14, No. 4 (April, 1976), 28–31.

Robinson, L.A. Therapeutic Paradox—To Support Intimacy and Regression or Privacy and Autonomy. *Journal of Psychiatric Nursing and Mental Health Services*, Vol. 17, No. 10 (October, 1979), 19–23.

Ryan, J.L. The Single Room: A Right for Every Patient's Privacy. *Nursing Digest* (September–October, 1975), 46–47.

Stillman, M.J. Territoriality and Personal Space. *American Journal of Nursing*, Vol. 78, No. 10 (October, 1978), 1670–1672.

Whall, A.L. Congruence Between Existing Theories of Family Functioning and Nursing Theories. *Advances in Nursing Science*, Vol. 3, No. 1 (October, 1980), 59–87.

Wilson, H.S. Limiting Intrusion—Social Control of Outsiders in a Healing Community. *Nursing Research*, Vol. 26, No. 2 (March/April, 1977), 103–111.

Warner, S.L. Humor and Self-Disclosure Within the Milieu. *Journal of Psychosocial Nursing and Mental Health Services*, Vol. 22, No. 4 (April, 1984), 17–21.

II

CONCEPTUAL AND THEORETICAL FRAMEWORK FOR NURSING PRACTICE

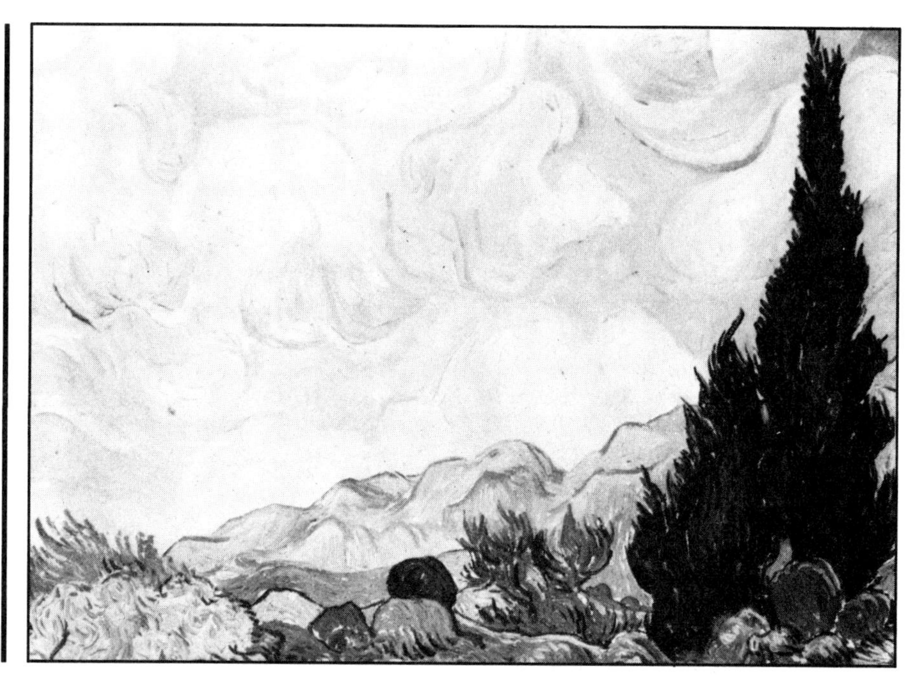

4

SHAPING PROFESSIONAL PRACTICE

Theories, Strategies, Modalities

LEARNING OBJECTIVES

On completion of this chapter the reader should be able to:

1. Define and differentiate among the terms **theory**, **strategy**, and **modality**.
2. Identify the fundamental concepts of the eight theories presented—psychoanalytic, interpersonal, sociocultural, behavioral, cognitive, communicative, humanistic, and existential.
3. Define and distinguish between the strategies of **assertiveness**, **decision-making**, **problem-solving**, and **conflict resolution**.
4. Enumerate the benefits derived from an assertive approach to life and living as they apply to the nurse and to the client.
5. Discuss the manner by which the nurse can employ the strategy of decision-making within her roles of change agent and teacher.
6. Discuss client benefits derived from the use of problem solving.
7. Discuss the manner by which the nurse can facilitate goal attainment through the use of conflict resolution.
8. Identify the seven treatment modalities presented and their differentiating characteristics—behavior modification, group therapy, family therapy, transactional analysis, gestalt therapy, reality therapy, and crisis intervention.

INTRODUCTION

The conceptual framework for the practice of psychiatric–mental health nursing identified in the Introduction is influenced, supported, and operationalized by the theories, strategies, and modalities that have become the foundation of contemporary practice. In this chapter, we will address selected theories, strategies, and modalities that we believe play a significant role in today's practice. We caution the reader that the material contained within this chapter presents only the highlights of each of the complex topics addressed. To increase the depth of knowledge about and understanding of this material, the reader is encouraged to explore additional reference sources contained in the suggested readings at the end of the chapter.

THEORIES

A **theory** is a rational, logical, intellectual, and systematized statement of beliefs that explains a given set of phenomena. A theory provides a mechanism for identifying and viewing the interrelatedness of the fundamental concepts detailed within the theory. It is used as a basis for testing hypotheses to establish their validity. A theory provides the practitioner with a tool for guiding practice toward a predictable outcome.

The major theories presented in this chapter include psychoanalytic, interpersonal, sociocultural, behavioral, cognitive, communicative, humanistic, and existential. Table 4–1 provides a concise, comparative perspective of these selected theories. This overview illustrates the positions of each of these selected theories with respect to such fundamental concepts as the self, the individual's relationship to others, the environment, and the beliefs concerning health and illness.

Psychoanalytic Theory

Psychoanalytic theory is fundamentally concerned with the internal dynamics of the individual personality. Its advent greatly influenced psychiatric practice, and its constructs established one of the first frameworks to explain psychiatric phenomena from a developmental point of view. The basic premise upon which this theory rests is that the individual is influenced by unconscious motivating forces. Operationally this is interpreted to mean that all behavior has meaning and consequently can be understood. In essence, psychoanalytic theory is composed of a group of interrelated theories outlining mental and developmental functioning.

The first theoretical construct deals with differentiating levels of awareness: conscious, preconscious, and unconscious. The **conscious** portion of the mind is described as that segment together with its associated activity or function to which the individual has access and awareness at any given point in time. The conscious portion perceives both internal and external stimuli. The **preconscious** is referred to as that area of the mind containing those repressed mental events, processes, and content that are hidden from awareness but are capable of being brought into conscious focus. The process that facilitates movement from the preconscious to the conscious level is termed **recall**. Recall involves the focusing of attention through the use of such techniques as free association, hypnosis, narcotherapy, and dream analysis.

The **unconscious** portion broadly includes the sum of all psychic material not in the immediate field of the individual's awareness at any given moment. The unconscious serves as a reservoir of all experiences to which the individual has been subjected, and the material contained within cannot be recalled at will. The unconscious is often considered the motivating force of behavior. It seeks conscious expression through symbolic representation as evidenced by dreams, slips of the tongue, impulsive acts, or specific symptoms associated with various clinical conditions.

The second theoretical construct hypothesizes a structuring of the mind. This structure is designated as the id, ego, and superego. The **id** is that portion of the mind that consists of basic, instinctual, primitive drives. The id is inherent in man and operates from an unconscious level in its search for immediate gratification of wants, wishes, desires or needs. Its operation is regulated by the **pleasure principle**. This principle states that the individual seeks fulfillment without consideration of the effect satisfaction of the wish, want, or need will have on the self or on others. The pursuit of gratification is somewhat akin to the idea of "me first and everybody else last."

The **superego** is that portion of the psyche that consists of internalized ideals, norms, values, and attitudes. It represents society within the psyche, that is, the collective conscience or morality that serves as a system of internal control over thoughts, feelings, and actions. It is that segment of the mind to be developed within the personality around the age of two. The superego evolves through the processes of identification and introjection and is mainly unconscious in operation. Its functions include: (1) approval or disapproval of the ego's actions, that is, judgment of an act as being right or wrong; (2) critical self-observations; (3) disciplinary and self-punishing activity; and (4) rewarding of the ego with self-love and self-esteem for the ego's acceptable actions.

The **ego** is that part of the psyche that is the mediator between the individual and reality. In this role of mediator, the ego seeks to exercise rationality and compromise between the instant gratification

TABLE 4–1. A COMPARATIVE PERSPECTIVE OF SELECTED THEORIES

Theory	Man	Relationship to Others	Environment	Health/Illness
Psychoanalytic	Man is viewed as a psychosexual being who functions in accordance with internal determination. Behavior stems from unconscious motivation. Childhood experiences are critical to the development of adult functioning. Past has relevance for present and future functioning.	Acknowledged but not systematically addressed.	Asserts that conditions surrounding the self bear no direct relationship to the character of the self's inner development; rather, the self is concerned with adaptation to the environment in a way that will obtain pleasure and avoid pain.	Health is equated with "normalcy." Illness results from unsuccessful completion or interruption of developmental stages.
Interpersonal	Man is viewed as a self-system that evolves from the reflected appraisal of significant others.	Addresses the influential role specific individuals and significant groups have for the development of personality.	Recognizes a sociocultural context but credits environment as having only a limited, if any, impact on the individual.	Health is equated with effective interpersonal functioning. Both health and illness can be transmitted via specific modes of communication.
Sociocultural	Man is viewed as an entity existing within the scope of his relatedness to others. This view tends to deemphasize individual personal dynamics.	Emphasizes interdependence as a means of satisfying wants and needs and promoting a feeling of well-being.	Stresses the social process as a significant aspect of enculturation.	Health is defined according to the meaning assigned to it within the social and cultural context of a given society. Failure to conform to normative behavior is labeled as illness.
Behavioral	Man is viewed as a biologically complex organism who is subjected to and conditioned by external factors and events; man is a product of his environment.	Conformity to existing norms, mores and modes is expected.	Exerts strong influence and plays an important part in shaping and reinforcing learned behavior.	Health is equated with performance of expected behavior. Illness per se is viewed as a myth; symptoms associated with "illness" represent learned behaviors that continue because the individual experiences some reward through their existence.

Cognitive	Man is viewed as a rational being with the capacity to be self-directive in accordance with his intellectual capabilities.	Emphasis is on the individual's responsiveness via awareness and perception of external stimuli.	Provides for continuity of knowledge and experience.	Health is viewed as an attainable real state. Thought processes determine emotional and behavioral responses to life situations. Illness is not addressed per se; however, the inference can be drawn that illness can be equated to misperceptions of reality resulting in irresponsible behavior.
Communicative	Man is viewed as a speaking-listening agent, an interactional being who is able to persuade and be persuaded by others.	Views social contacting as a mechanism by which the self is identified and enriched.	Acknowledges a mutuality of influence existing between man and the environment.	Health is viewed as a demonstration of congruency between verbal and nonverbal messages. Illness is manifested by the lack of congruence, which produces behavioral deviations.
Humanistic	Man is viewed as an integrated, organized whole who is motivated toward meeting basic human needs.	Interactional activity exists for the purpose of satisfying needs. Mutuality of interdependence and need fulfillment is recognized.	Strongly emphasized. Considered vital in differentiating humans from animals. Underscores the importance of culture in the promotion of man's survival.	Health is viewed as an intrinsic and explicit good and as a significant component of self-actualization. Illness is defined by the individual rather than by societal norms.
Existential	Man is viewed as a responsible being who exists in the here and the now and is closely attuned to both self and others.	Emphasizes genuine and rewarding relationships as essential to self-awareness and self-approval.	Given secondary consideration. Significant only in terms of its meaning and value to the individual.	Health is achieved when rapport exists between self and the environment. Illness is viewed as alienation.

sought by the id and the inhibitory demands imposed by the superego. The ego functions at all levels of awareness, but operates primarily at the conscious level, utilizing the **reality principle**. As such, it is considered to be the executive organ of the mind whose prime function is the perception of reality and adaptation to it. Ego functions develop gradually and are dependent upon physical maturation and experiential factors. Basic functions attributed to the ego include: (1) control and regulation of instinctual drives; (2) maintenance of relationships with the external world; (3) development of object relationships that are mutually satisfying; (4) protection of the ego through the mobilization and use of defensive operations; and (5) the ability to integrate various aspects of its functioning, thus enabling the person to think, feel, and act in an organized and directed manner. The outcome of ego functioning is the emergence of a self-identity. Self-identity includes a defined self-concept. The ego begins to emerge in infancy and is open to change and further development throughout life.

The third major thrust of this theory incorporates a view of personality growth and development that is based on a concept of psychic determinism. This implies that the individual's early personality development plays a significant role in and, in effect, serves as a foundation for all future responses to ensuing life experiences. Accordingly, current life experiences are viewed as reflections of either positive or negative experiences previously encountered. Thus, dynamic patterns of interaction and reaction are formulated and influence all future affective and behavioral responses. For further discussion relevant to personality development embraced by the proponents of psychoanalytic theory, the reader is referred to Chapter 5.

Interpersonal Theory

Interpersonal theory emphasizes relationships—relationships between self and others at any given moment in time. According to interpersonal theory, the individual is motivated by two strong drives—the drive for self-satisfaction and the drive for security. Achievement of both these drives has a direct correlation with the approval and acceptance demonstrated by significant others to and for the self. Thus, the self-system attempts to learn a set of operations or coping mechanisms designed to protect the self from disapproval, overwhelming anxiety, and loneliness.

Interpersonal theory is primarily concerned with the current, ongoing life experiences of the developing personality and is founded on a reality orientation to life and living. Its proponents subscribe to the belief that individuals have a need to be socialized and integrated into society and the environment. The biological changes that accompany growth and maturation act as stimuli for emergent needs. Thus, as the individual matures, there is a gradual progression and refinement in his ability to relate to both objects and people within the environment. This ever increasing ability is evidenced by the cognitive modes of experience Sullivan referred to as **prototaxic**, **parataxic**, and **syntaxic**.

In infancy, the prototaxic mode of experience predominates and is characterized by a lack of differentiation between the self and the environment. Essentially, this experience is primitive and referred to as the **primary process**, in which there is no distinction between thoughts and feelings; that is, a pervasive, undifferentiated oneness exists between self and the environment.

As the individual moves through childhood into the juvenile period, the parataxic mode becomes operational. This mode of experience is characterized by a breaking up of the undifferentiated whole. This means that, as the person undergoes recurrent experiences, these experiences remain unrelated and unconnected. Since the experiences themselves are usually inconsistent in nature, there occurs an illogical and disjointed perception of life events.

With further maturation, the individual manifests the ability to perceive the whole along with recognition of the logical interrelatedness of its parts. The ability to make connections between the past and the present as well as the ability to confirm the perception of the experience as real comprises the syntaxic mode of experience. This implies that the adult, in order to gain an understanding of his environment and his relationship to others within that environment, engages in a process of **consensual validation** to confirm his perceptions. To compare the significant differences of the developmental aspects of interpersonal theory with other theoretical formulations as well as to compare the developmental stages postulated by major theorists, the reader is referred to Chapter 5.

Sociocultural Theory

Sociocultural theory views the development of personality from a multivariant standpoint: man is subjected to a wide range of values that impinge on the performance of his social roles relative to his position within his social network. These multivariant aspects take into consideration familial, socioeconomic, cultural, social, developmental, and environmental conditions.

This theoretical approach proposes a dualistic thrust. Simply stated, this means that sociocultural theory acknowledges that a reciprocal effect or relationship exists between the individual and his external world and between the external world and the individual. This theory supports the belief that a dynamic interchange exists between man and society and that each exerts a sphere of influence to change and be changed. It focuses on the effect social definitions, norms, and values have on the development of human behavior. Effective functioning is a reflection of positive assurance coupled with a feeling of self-worth. The effect of the environment on self is viewed from the individual's perceptual field and in this sense portrays a very personalized and sensitive framework emphasizing individual uniqueness as opposed to categorical stereotyping. Thus, sociocultural theory explains human behavior in terms of the social processes to which the individual is subjected throughout the maturation process and tends to deemphasize the intrapsychic components.

Behavioral Theory

Behavioral theory is founded on the basic premise that all behavior is learned. Within the context of this theory, behavior is defined as all human action. As such, behavior can be observed, recorded, objectively measured, and systematically modified. This theory espouses the idea that human behavior is conditioned by events that occur within the developmental process. These events include the totality of human experience and affect physiological functioning as well as produce changes in the cognitive and affective spheres of functioning. The events themselves produce a response within the individual and through repetition perpetuate the response.

According to behavioral theory, autonomous and self-actualizing man is nonexistent. Behaviorists believe that the individual is controlled or can be manipulated by events within the environment. Furthermore, behavioral theory stipulates that individuals learn to behave in one of two ways—either through respondent or operant conditioning. In **respondent conditioning**, the individual is exposed to a particular event—the event serves as a stimulus—the individual responds. In this situation, an association or connection is made by the individual between the event (stimulus) and the behavior (response). Through repetition the behavior is learned, and the response becomes a habit or a habitual pattern of behaving. In **operant conditioning**, the individual acts upon his environment to produce a response by or within the environment. In this instance, the individual's behavior is the stimulus, and the environment's action or reaction is the response. If the response elicited is consistently similar, the individual's behavior is reinforced or extinguished.

Cognitive Theory

Cognitive theory focuses on man's interaction with his environment and primarily concerns itself with how an individual learns and the manner in which he uses the acquired knowledge in his dealings with the external world.

According to cognitive theory, thought processes progress from a concrete level to a more formal set of operations involving abstract and logical thinking. Thus, the epitome of effective functioning is viewed as the ability to assess critically, problem solve, and act on decisions in a variety of situations.

Cognitive theory, like the psychoanalytic and interpersonal theories, divides the life span into specific stages and identifies specific cognitive processes that occur at each stage. For further information regarding these stages, the reader is referred to Chapter 5.

Communicative Theory

Communicative theory explains the complex intrapersonal and interpersonal exchange of thoughts and feelings between and among people. It accounts for the various independent and intervening variables involved in the intricate methodology used in sending and receiving messages. Communicative theory details a system of practices, conventions, and procedural rules that functions as a means of guiding and organizing a transactional flow.

Communicative theory stipulates that communication occurs within a sociocultural context and that an individual is more responsive if the communication patterns and messages are similar and familiar to the receiver. Communicative theory operates on the premise that the individual uses communication to gain control of his physical and psychological environment. This, then, allows the individual to assert and support self, initiate and expand social contacts, and exert influence over others and the environment. Two important assumptions relative to communicative theory are that: (1) all behavior is some form of communication and conveys some message; and (2) breakdown in communication produces and is responsible for disequilibrium. In Chapter 14, the reader will find a more detailed explanation related to the method, process, and practice of communication.

Humanistic Theory

Humanistic theory focuses on the whole person and stresses the integrative and interactive aspects of man's nature. It supports the interplay among the physical, mental, emotional, social, and cultural dimensions of man's humanness. Humanistic theory is essentially optimistic in outlook and professes the belief that man is intrinsically good. Although its proponents acknowledge that an individual's actions can be influenced by his past, they firmly believe the individual is not bound by his past, and therefore the past does not preclude the individual's ability to change and to grow. Thus, the emphasis of humanistic theory is placed on the individual as a full functioning human being. This means that each individual is recognized not only as a person capable of self-actualization but also as possessing the intrinsic ability to govern and control the direction of the actualizing process. Humanistic theory recognizes uniqueness, freedom of choice, and the right of the individual to set and be accountable for his values.

Existential Theory

Existential theory holds that an individual's life can be humanized and rendered authentic or meaningful if the individual thoughtfully probes each conflict or crisis within the self, makes a choice about action, and then assumes responsibility for the consequences of that choice. Existential theory stresses the individual's current reality and the specific meaning any given experience has to or for the individual. In comparison to other theoretical frameworks, little, if any, attention or credence is placed on or given to the individual's past history. Rather, this theory emphasizes the belief that the person should be closely attuned to self and environment. A corollary to this belief is that the individual is responsible for his behavior and that any alienation from self or others is a direct result of self-imposed inhibition. The thrust of existential theory underscores full acceptance by the individual of the current living situation coupled to the idea that the individual recognizes that the future can hold a better promise and is attainable. Choice, freedom, and responsibility are the keynotes of existential theory, and recognition is given to what man is and wishes to become.

STRATEGIES

By definition, a **strategy** is a system, tactic, method, or scheme of operation. It consists of an enabling set of behaviors that allows an individual to organize and operationalize an appropriate set of selected theoretical constructs within the contextual application or framework of a particular modality. We have identified that current nursing practice makes use of four major strategies in the daily, operational delivery of effective care to clients. These strategies are assertiveness, decision-making, problem solving, and conflict resolution. Within the nursing process, they are used specifically by the nurse to formulate, plan, and implement nursing interventions in client care situations. Use of these strategies can be extended beyond clinical application and can be incorporated into the total living experience of the professional. Just as the nurse can employ these strategies to enhance her living and working conditions, so too can she teach others to use these strategies for maximizing their adapting and coping potential.

Assertiveness

Assertiveness is a relatively new strategy within the nursing field that has gained a great deal of popularity over the past five years. Its roots lie in the behavioral, cognitive, and interpersonal theories. Assertiveness is portrayed through behavior. Assertive behavior calls for the mobilization of internal and external resources in prioritizing needs. It operates under the assumption that self-satisfaction is an appropriate, healthy feeling and that the individual maintains integrity by manifesting the courage of his convictions. Assertiveness is open, honest, direct, nondestructive, appropriate behavior that conveys the expression of real feelings, opinions, beliefs, wishes, wants, and needs. It consists of setting goals, acting on these goals in a clear and concise way, and assuming responsibility for the consequences. Implicit in this strategy is the realization that assertiveness stems from a power base—self-power. This means that the individual is in control of his destiny. Assertiveness permits the individual the exercise of legitimate rights without violation of the rights of others.

Certain benefits accrue to the individual as an outcome of engaging in assertive behavior. These benefits lead to the promotion of a positive self-image with a corresponding increase in self-confidence and the maintenance of more meaningful relationships with others. These benefits include a reduction in insecurity and vulnerability; facilitation of communication and sharing; enhancement of self-respect; affirmation of a more positive self-image; and an increase in overall effective functioning and productivity. As a strategy in psychiatric nursing, assertiveness is used to reduce the potential for anxiety, diffuse and dissipate anger, cope with criticism, postpone impulsive action, resolve conflict, or manage crisis. Common client care situations frequently encountered by nurses where assertiveness might be useful include those in which a client displays negative feelings about self, exhibits a pattern of helplessness, manifests sensitivity to perceived rejection, demonstrates an inability to accept or receive compliments, and remains nonexpressive in fear of hurting someone.

In making clinical application, assertiveness translates into assisting clients to work through their feelings and effectively interrupt set patterns of behavior. Assertiveness tends to deemphasize exploring and identifying reasons for the particular behavior displayed while emphasizing the constructive changes in behavior required to achieve disruption of the old and reinforcement of the new pattern. This therapeutic task is accomplished through the mutual setting of very specific short-term goals directed toward the successful completion of one step at a time. This process permits the patient to experience a sense of mastery and control and makes the overall transition and substitution from unacceptable to acceptable behavior more manageable, less overwhelming, and worth the effort. From the nurse's standpoint, assertiveness prevents the nurse from becoming involved in a power struggle with the patient. Thus, the nurse can adroitly avoid the trap leading to such ineffective and nontherapeutic endeavors as defensiveness, condescension, possible retaliation, or avoidance.

Becoming assertive is a strategy that requires time, effort, and continuous practice. In implementing assertiveness, both the nurse and the client must be able to distinguish assertive behaviors from nonassertive and aggressive behaviors. To help make this distinction clear, it should be kept in mind that assertiveness recognizes the need for self-fulfillment without infringing on the rights of others, while nonassertive behavior is self-negation in action. In nonassertion, the individual denies his right to feel to the extent that his behavior is inadequate, ineffectual, and, in fact, may inhibit him from attaining desired goals. Engaging in aggressive behavior most often places the self in a position of jeopardy while seeking fulfillment of needs. Aggressive behavior is essentially destructive (versus constructive) and tends to place the recipient of aggressive behavior in the position of being dominated, manipulated, or threatened.

Implementing the strategy of assertiveness with self and with the client involves a specific step-by-step procedure that begins with the review of usual coping behaviors and ends with constant repetition of assertive behaviors in varying situations. Steps in this procedure are as follows:

- Review usual coping behavior patterns as applied to different situations, noting outcomes.
- Propose alternative assertive actions and examine potential results.
- Try out the alternative behavior in a simulated or imaginary situation.
- Review effectiveness of behavior.
- Implement assertive behavior in a real situation.
- Identify feelings of well-being, comfort, satisfaction, approval, or sense of accomplishment associated with positive outcome.
- Repeat behavior until change demonstrates consistency in application.

Teaching assertive behavior as a strategy oriented toward helping individuals change may be applied in a number of clinical situations. Its appropriateness for a specific client must be carefully evaluated prior to its use. The nurse-therapist must consider the personal characteristics of the individual; the purpose for which assertiveness is to be employed; the ability of the nurse to display assertiveness in her own behavior; the appropriateness of the setting for demonstrating effective outcome; opportunities for continued reinforcement; the length of time available; the particular method(s) employed; and lastly, the inclusion of follow-up procedures to validate effectiveness of teaching and evaluation of the learning.

Decision-Making

Decision-making is a logical, rational, systematized, cognitive process whose outcome is the selection and execution of a set of behaviors. These behaviors have been deemed by an individual, group, or organization as the most appropriate, correct choice available for a given set of circumstances. Decision-making involves *choice* and is arrived at through a process of deliberative thinking. **Choosing** is motivated by the internal quest for fulfillment of needs and wants and is directed by the individual's knowledge base as well as prevailing attitudes, values, and beliefs. Pursuit of an appropriate choice is contingent upon awareness and understanding. Acquisition of both awareness and understanding demands exploration of self in relationship to self, to others, and to the environment. In other words, the individual, group, or organization must consciously acknowledge and examine those factors that will exert influence on subsequent action.

Choice selection is predicated on need fulfillment. If this is a true assumption, then it can be anticipated that an individual will choose to act in a manner that is congruent with his nature and needs. This congruency is maintained by *primary motivation factors* that mandate behavior or movement toward satisfaction of basic needs. However, when basic needs no longer impel the individual to act, action or choice is then influenced by *secondary motivational factors*. These secondary motivational factors are those learned social needs that allow or enable the individual to function effectively and with satisfaction both intra- and interpersonally. Therefore, rational decision-making cannot take place in a climate that violates an individual's beliefs, values, and attitudes or denies gratification of basic physiological and psycho-sociocultural needs.

As initially stated, decision-making involves two sets of behaviors—those directed toward making the choice and those directed toward implementing the choice. To begin operationalizing the decision-making process requires acknowledgment of existing alternatives. These alternatives are then explored in light of the personal, individual, and collective values, attitudes, and beliefs associated with each potential choice. The next step involves a threefold assessment: consideration of the consequences attributed to each choice; examination of possible risks affecting the integrity of the self-system; and estimation of the likelihood, based on preestablished criteria, that the alternative selected will be successful when implemented. Alternatives are then prioritized based on the closest match to cognitive-affective response projections. This means that an individual will tend to select a choice that reinforces his usual and familiar system of operation. Selection of the alternative depends on completion of the steps just described. Once an alternative has been chosen, implementation becomes the final step. Implementation is governed by the individual's, group's, or organization's acceptance of the alternative selected. Table 4–2 illustrates the decision-making process.

In nursing, decision-making is a strategy the nurse employs within the context of her roles as change agent and teacher. If the implementation of the change agent role is to be successful and if change behavior is to occur as an outcome of the decision-making process, then the nurse must consider two essential components, either of which can be used to alter client decision-making. These components are: (1) the addition of new data to the client's existing knowledge base, that is, the introduction of new beliefs and information into the client's realm of awareness; and (2) making provisions to shift in some degree the level of belief, attitude, or value regarding the subject or situation about which a client decision is needed.

In the teaching role, the nurse provides the client with opportunities to observe the nurse's use of decision-making, thereby serving as a role model that permits learning to occur through the process of identification. Furthermore, the nurse can actively engage the client in the experience of decision-making within the context of the interactive–interventive process. In this instance, the nurse is promoting learning by doing. In such experiential learning, not only does the nurse concern herself with an outcome directed toward formulation of a decision for a specific situation, but she also assists the client with learning and practicing the process itself so that the client will be equipped with a tool that can be of use in future situations that necessitate decision-making. The major benefit to be derived from teaching this process to the client is that the client can come to experience and enjoy more freedom and control over his entire life and living situation.

TABLE 4–2. OPERATIONAL DEFINITION OF THE DECISION-MAKING PROCESS

Step	Process	Outcome
Recognition of alternatives	Identify. Explore.	Knowledge base, values belief, attitudes, and needs clarified.
Assessment of alternatives	Consider overall consequences. Identify personal risk factors. Establish success criteria.	Probability of success increased.
Prioritization of alternatives	Match familiar cognitive, affective responses. Acknowledge need dominance.	Choice selected.
Implementation of choice	Execute chosen behavior.	Decision accepted and need satisfied.

Problem-Solving

The strategy of problem-solving is, first of all, a process that employs a disciplined, systematic and formal framework of operation for the analysis of multiple and complex propositions. Secondly, this process moves through a series of sequential actions and activities that begin with a clear demarcation of an identified concern and progresses to a specific effect—resolution. In essence, problem-solving is a means for surmounting and alleviating identified difficulties that interfere with or create a barrier to the attainment of an objective or goal. This strategy is primarily a unique intellectual technique for resolving cognitive dissonance, that is, bringing order out of chaos.

Operationalizing the problem-solving process entails a blending of creative and reflective thinking with deductive reasoning. **Creative thinking** permits the individual to tap and explore limitless potential, as evidenced through such activities as brainstorming, quota setting, and groupthink. **Reflective thinking** allows the individual to view the problem situation from varying perspectives, taking into account past experiences, current prevailing conditions, and future consequences. Reflective thinking also implies participation in such activities as systematic observation, identification of existing attitudes, and clarification of values. Deductive reasoning concerns itself with drawing inferences from isolated observed phenomena and generalizing both cause and effect. Together, these operations achieve harmony in intellectual functioning that enables the individual to pursue and discover a workable solution.

Although various authorities allude to the fact that some individuals engage in the problem-solving process by beginning in the middle and working toward the ends or by starting at the end and working toward the beginning or, in fact, engaging in any variant form conceivable, we believe that the problem-solving process is sequential in nature and follows a logical progression. Thus, we see the problem-solving process as including six major operations. These six operations are depicted in Table 4–3. First, an individual, group, or community becomes aware that some difficulty or unmet need exists. Implicit in this awareness are three critical aspects: (1) isolation, identification, and description of the specific concern; (2) recognition of the possibility for change; and (3) motivation to undertake resolution. The second operation is directed toward exploration of the parameters pertinent to the identified concern. In this step, data collection and analysis are pursued to clarify the exact nature and extent of the problem. The result of this operation is the development of a data base from which inferences and judgments can be made. These inferences and judgments are employed in the third operation of the process, which involves reaching a set of conclusions based on the knowledge

TABLE 4–3. OPERATIONAL DEFINITION OF THE PROBLEM-SOLVING PROCESS

Step	Call to Action	Process	Outcome
Problem awareness	Recognize need to change.	Isolate. Describe.	Problem identified.
Exploration	Establish data base.	Collect data. Analyse data.	Inferences drawn. Judgments made.
Alternative solutions	Establish evaluation criteria.	Generate options. Formulate proposal.	Alternatives identified.
Selection	Prioritize list.	Review choices. Identify consequences. Clarity beliefs, values, and attitudes.	Final choice made. Plan of action decided.
Implementation	Affirm response to demand for change.	Activate plan: who, what, how, and how long?	Response made.
Evaluation	Assess outcome. Observe effect.	Obtain feedback.	Problem resolved or reconsidered.

derived from the observations, investigations, and dissection of the data obtained in the first two steps of the process. The outcome of this third operation is the generation and formulation of potential, workable alternatives or solutions to the identified problem. Concurrent with the designation of potential alternatives is the establishment of outcome criteria by which the feasibility and acceptability of the resolution can be evaluated.

The fourth operation is concerned with decision-making. It is at this point that choices are made between the alternatives. The end result is the selection of the single most appropriate alternative needed to meet the demands posed by a given set of circumstances. The fifth step calls for putting the designated solution into action, that is, implementation of the chosen alternative. The designated plan sets the parameters for responsibility and accountability. The sixth and last operation of the process entails evaluation. In this step, the action taken is assessed according to the previously determined criteria to test and to supply feedback as to whether or not the solution chosen did effect, in actuality, resolution of the problem.

In nursing, the use of this problem-solving strategy emphasizes the collaborative nature of the process. Collaborative effort implies that the nurse actively engages with the client in the pursuit of problem resolution. Problem-solving is usually introduced when the client evidences an inability to employ or a total failure to institute his usual methods of coping. As a strategy, problem-solving can be used to alter alienated self-concept and maladaptive life-styles that lead to disequilibrium. Thus, the most outstanding benefit to be derived from involvement in this process is the restoration of human integrity and equilibrium. Use of this strategy strives to strike a balance by allowing the client an opportunity to adjust to circumstances; reduce hindrances and barriers to goal attainment; restore sense of control over life situations; and assume responsibility for action.

Another benefit to be derived from the use of this strategy is that the client may come to realize that the process itself can be used not only from a corrective but also from a preventative standpoint. The client can learn to anticipate situations that may give rise to potential problems. This recognition coupled with the use of the strategy can prevent the potential from becoming actual. Thus, engagement in the problem-solving process permits the mind to expand, be creative, and unlock internal resources for movement toward change and self-actualization.

Conflict Resolution

Conflict resolution is a strategy for dispelling discord and for restoring harmony. The strategy of conflict resolution is a systematic process that promotes goal attainment while preserving self-esteem, personal dignity, and respect for self and others. Conflict resolution deemphasizes incompatibilities and facilitates tension management by reducing the need to engage in power struggles. Thus, as an intra- and interpersonal technique, it heightens compatibility and preserves homeostasis. It is a stratgegy that has potential for increasing motivation, imagery, and creative resourcefulness that can make constructive use of the previously mentioned strategies of assertiveness, decision-making, and problem-solving. The outcome of its use should be a heightened level of energy, since the satisfaction experienced from being in charge and in control of self fosters pleasurable effects. These effects, in turn, create an ambiance that allows for personal growth and development toward increased automony, awareness, and understanding of self and others, as well as movement toward self-actualization. Furthermore, conflict resolution has the potential for reducing residual negative behaviors or feelings, such as defensiveness, resistance, assaultiveness, frustration, resentment, hostility, or anger. Lastly, conflict resolution acts as a positive stimulus for promoting responsibility and accountability.

When conflict is perceived by an individual or by a group, two alternative options exist. There can be a conscious denial of the per-

TABLE 4–4. AN OVERVIEW OF CONFLICT RESOLUTION

Behavioral Patterns	Tactic	Nature of Tactic	Outcome Implication
Win-Lose	Competition	Adversarial Egocentric	Dominance Control
	Accommodation	Submissive	Cooperation
Lose-Lose	Compromise	Adversarial	Frustration Anger
Win-Win	Collaboration	Transactional	Harmony Collegiality

ception through suppression, or there can be an attempt to institute goal-directed behaviors that will bring about resolution. Three behavioral patterns have been documented in the literature as outcomes of conflict resolution activity. These outcomes are win-lose, lose-lose, and win-win.

Table 4–4 illustrates an overview of conflict resolution. The table includes the behavioral pattern, the tactics associated with each behavior, the underlying nature of the tactic, outcome implications, factors influencing choice of behavioral patterns, and the end result or status of the conflict.

Win-Lose. In a win-lose outcome, whether or not the conflict originates within the self or originates between and among people, you have, as the terms imply, a winner and a loser. This means that one goal, one value, one need, or one force emerges as dominant over the other. A win-lose outcome is by its very nature adversarial and egocentric. This type of outcome may tend to leave scars—the scars of guilt, anger, resentment, loss of personal worth, integrity, or self-esteem—and may give rise to more conflicts than they resolve.

Competition is the primary tactic associated with a win-lose outcome. This tactic implies dominance and control in which there is single-minded pursuit of the identified goal without recognition of the effect on self or others. Competition in and of itself is not negative or unhealthy and, in fact, can be productive in conflict resolution. From a positive standpoint, competition as a tactic offers a challenge to do the best one can. Undeniably, there exist conflict situations in which competition can and should be the tactic of choice. One must be very careful, however, in selecting this tactic because, more often than not,

Factors Influencing Choice	Status of Conflict
Situations requiring immediate action	Temporary resolution
Recognition of a "greater good" and preservation of harmony	Partial resolution with potential for victimization of loser
Societal attitudes and norms	No resolution
Major issues Unlimited time Prevalence of safety and security	Satisfactory resolution through consensus

the negative aspects of competition prevail. The option to choose this tactic is situation-dependent. Situations in which competition could be a successful tactic are those in which time is a factor and those in which an emergency or crisis exists. These two types of situations demand immediate action and do not allow for exploration, clarification, or validation. Use of a win-lose outcome in situations other than those identified may very well lead to continued conflict.

Another tactic that results in a win-lose outcome is that of accommodation. **Accommodation** is a tactic of reconciliation through acquiescence. It is most often selected when an individual consciously or unconsciously recognizes that there is a "greater good" to be achieved. Accommodation is most frequently employed when cooperation is viewed as being more desirable than self-assertion.

Like competition, accommodation involves both a positive and negative aspect. Seen from a positive perspective, the loser is "turned on" and "tuned in" to the needs of others and is willing to forego gratification of needs, wants, or desires out of deference. Within this perspective, the preservation of harmony becomes the overriding directive for behavior. On the other hand, the habitual use of accommodation as a tactic to bring about resolution of conflict may produce many serious consequences, particularly to the self. Since submission characterizes this tactic and since abrogation of self-assertion allows another ascendancy, control is always in the hands of the winner. The loser forfeits his chance to make clear his issues, concerns, and opinions. There is limited opportunity for either exploration or clarification. Because the loser gives in, alternatives are seldom considered and common ground is never established or shared. Self-sacrificing, concessive behavior leads to victimization and ultimate alteration of one's standards and values. The decision to use accommodation is determined by either of two conditions. If the individual cannot operate from a power base to effect change, or if the individual values intrapsychic tranquility and the preservation of a harmonious interpersonal relationship more than the conflict issue, accommodation is an appropriate tactic of choice.

Lose-Lose. A lose-lose outcome guarantees no winners. It is an adversarial outcome in which each person, while being aware of the needs of others, attempts to gain mastery, but fails. In lose-lose conflict resolution, the outcome is generally destructive—destructive in the sense that personal goals cannot be achieved and the relationship between the participants cannot be strengthened and advanced. In fact, open, honest communication between participants is seriously inhibited and often relegated to the superficial and mundane.

The tactic employed that results in a lose-lose outcome is that of compromise. **Compromise** is a "giving-in" tactic that is reached through mutual concession that allows for only partial fulfillment of individual goals. It is a tactic that is frequently employed but probably the least productive. In our society, we have been taught to value "give and take," that is, compromise. Compromise has been cloaked in the guise of each person "getting something." Unfortunately, what each person gets is not necessarily what he really wants. Hence, in compromise, both end up as losers. What compromise does achieve is a more rapid solution but not necessarily a more satisfying solution. In actuality, because both parties hold back and hedge, neither one has full opportunity to explore or clarify and, thus, no one benefits. Ultimately, creative problem-solving is jeopardized.

Win-Win. When major issues are involved, when time is not a factor, or when an individual is functioning from within a position of safety and security, probably the most successful and most productive conflict resolution outcome is that of win-win. As the name implies, everyone wins; that is, each and every participant in the encounter derives gratification and satisfaction of his unique needs, wants, or desires.

A win-win outcome is achieved when self-assertion is tempered with a cooperative spirit. To arrive at such an outcome requires the expenditure of time, effort, and energy. Thus, each conflict resolution situation becomes a transactional encounter in which effective communication is the vehicle through which empathic, mutual understanding is sought. In these encounters, barriers in the form of misunderstandings, irrelevancies, differing viewpoints, false assumptions, territoriality, and defensiveness are dealt with, while harmony, helpfulness, and collegiality are keynoted. This outcome has virtually no negative aspects, since maximum potential has been used to achieve self-satisfaction and self-actualization. Because mutual understanding rather than self-interest is the desired goal and because behavior is directed toward generating the greatest number of options available, the interpersonal relationships that exist are enhanced by the sharing.

The specific tactic that can be used to arrive at a win-win outcome is that of collaboration. **Collaboration** is cooperative effort involving both cognitive and affective components. From a cognitive standpoint, cooperative effort demands the use of a problem-solving approach in which creative and innovative options are not only encouraged, but solicited. From an affective standpoint, collaboration refers to the establishment of consensus without personal sacrifice and the loss of self-esteem, thereby preserving psychological comfort and maintaining rapport between and among participants.

As the nurse makes a conscious decision to become actively involved in conflict resolution, it is important to keep in mind which outcome—win-lose, lose-lose, or win-win—will meet the needs of client or professional. Therefore, selection of the outcome becomes the first step in the process of conflict resolution. The second consideration must be directed toward selecting the appropriate tactic. The third step in the process involves implementation, while the fourth concerns itself with the aftermath in which evaluation of outcome is mandated. The nurse must bear in mind that no one outcome is applicable in all situations and the habitual use of a single outcome may very well create more conflict than it resolves.

MODALITIES

A **modality** is a method or technique of treatment that utilizes a specific set of operations based on a distinctive set of theoretical constructs. A modality involves a process directed toward facilitating change; that is, it provides an effective means of enabling an individual or group to move toward a definitive therapeutic goal. It is a system of psychic treatment that depends primarily on a verbal or behavioral interchange between the care giver and the care receiver(s).

Current therapeutic practice allows for a wide range of approaches. However, each approach provides the practitioner with a set of procedures and techniques for assisting those who are alienated, distressed, frustrated, or unclear about present and future goals to move toward involvement, acceptance, and satisfaction with respect to self and others. Each modality, irrespective of basic assumptions, principles, or theoretical framework, has an overall goal—the provision of new learning experiences designed to reduce strong negative and self-defeating emotions and to enhance realistic problem-solving activities.

The seven treatment modalities discussed in this chapter are: behavior modification; group therapy; family therapy; transactional analysis; gestalt therapy; reality therapy; and crisis intervention. Table 4–5 is a comparative overview of these therapies. It provides a definition of each modality, information regarding the clientele best served, specific therapeutic goals, the theoretical basis on which each is founded, along with the basic principles espoused, therapeutic process employed, and specific techniques used.

Behavior Modification

The concepts underlying behavior modification can be traced to the psychological and learning laboratories of the late 19th and early 20th centuries. The practice of behavior modification as a widespread treatment modality, however, did not achieve recognition or approach outstanding significance until the early 1960s. Behavior modification is, as its name implies, a therapeutic process designed to produce changes in behavior. Its initial use was predicated on the belief that the classic psychoanalytic, social, and interpersonal approaches to treatment were and are inappropriate and ineffective. In support of this declaration, behaviorists point out that the symptoms observed are not related to a fundamental disease process. They maintain that the observable psychiatric symptoms are in and of themselves the problem, so that treatment of underlying causation becomes a futile and wasted effort. This perspective forms the foundation of application of theory to practice. The outcome is that behavior modification as a treatment modality places emphasis on symptom relief by environmental control as opposed to intrapsychic or biochemical manipulation. Currently, clinical use of behavior modification employs three major techniques. These techniques are systematic desensitization, operant conditioning, and aversion. Choice of technique is usually guided by the type of behaviors presented by the client, the environment in which the client resides, and the approach favored by the therapist.

In **systematic desensitization**, the primary goal is to change associations. Specifically this technique is designed to alleviate the perceptual sensations of anxiety and fear. Initially, in implementing this technique, the individual is involved in relaxation training for the purpose of producing a sense of well-being. Once this state of psychological comfortableness is achieved, the client is asked to identify anxiety-producing stimuli. These stimuli are prioritized according to the level of anxiety evoked. Desensitization is begun by having the client generate psychic imagery associated with the least traumatic stimulus. The scene created is discussed until the anxiety or fear is no longer felt. The client learns to associate the relaxed and comfortable state with the previously traumatic stimulus. This process is continued until all the stimulus imagery has been explored and the client becomes anxiety free. The outcome of this technique is that when the client is confronted with the real life situation, he will no longer respond to the stimulus with anxiety or fear. The objective of systematic desensitization is to replace unpleasant sensations with positive or pleasant sensations.

In **operant conditioning**, the sequence of stimulus response is reversed. That is, this technique requires that the individual display a particular positive or acceptable response first. Once the response is made, the individual receives a reward. This reward is the stimulus for encouraging repetition of the desired behavior and serves as reinforcement for facilitating the repetition. In this procedure, negative behaviors are automatically extinguished because they do not earn sought rewards. The benefit to be derived from this approach is that the individual learns that he can exercise control over his environment in a way that will attract positive reinforcement not only within the designated treatment setting but also within the broader context of his total social environment.

With **aversion**, the type of reinforcement changes from a positive or pleasant stimulus to a negative or unpleasant stimulus. This technique is usually employed to extinguish socially unacceptable or exaggerated behaviors through the application of negative stimuli that are interpreted by the client as punishment. In essence, aversion therapy attempts to make the client aware of and sensitive to the undesirability of presenting behaviors (symptoms). Thus, every time the client displays the undesirable behavior, the therapist applies punishing stimuli. Again, the learning is accomplished through association and reinforcement. The assumption on which this technique is based is that problematic behavior is originally carried out by the client for the purpose of need gratification, no matter how maladaptive that behavior might be. Application of the aversive stimuli forces the client to resort to alternative behavior to obtain the desired gratification.

Aversion therapy is much less widely used than desensitization and operant conditioning and is often employed as a therapy of last

TABLE 4–5. A COMPARISON OF MAJOR TREATMENT MODALITIES

Modality	Definition	Application	Goal
Behavior modification	A mode of treatment designed to alter previously learned responses to specific environmental or interpersonal stimuli.	Used with a wide range of clinical conditions that demonstrate observable problem behaviors interfering with the individual's or group's optimum level of functioning.	To alter problematic behavior.
Group therapy	A structured or semi-structured process of therapeutic intervention in which the behavioral and emotional reactions of the individual members toward each other and toward the leader are acknowledged and understood as projections of individual, interpersonal distress.	Applicable to a wide variety of client needs, especially when dealing with the needs for support; task accomplishment; socialization; learning behavior; change; and effective human relations and insight.	To develop a cooperative mutuality for achieving a reduction in stress, an increase in individual and collective awareness, and a constructive and integrative pattern of behaving within a protected environment.

Theoretical Framework	Principles	Therapeutic Process	Strategies and Techniques
Grounded in associationistic learning theory that involves operant and respondent conditioning utilizing a stimulus-response-reinforcement approach.	1. All behavior is learned. 2. Behavior occurs in response to stimulus. 3. Environment influences behavior. 4. Reinforcement of desirable behavior can be used to change behavior. 5. Change in behavior leads to change in thinking and feeling.	Manipulation and control of variables to either reinforce desired behaviors or extinguish undesired behaviors.	1. Systematic desensitization. 2. Muscular relaxation. 3. Operant conditioning. 4. Aversion. 5. Imagery.
Classical psychoanalytic theory and social learning theory form the basis for group therapy. To this foundation are added theories related to group process, dynamics and structure; communication; interpersonal relationships; and conflict and its resolution.	1. Primary intervention is with the group rather than with the individual. 2. Clear communication promotes effective group interaction. 3. Disturbed perceptions can be corrected through consensual validation. 4. Socially ineffective behaviors can be modified or changed through peer pressure. 5. Learning of new behaviors can be reinforced through positive feedback from group members. 6. Feedback is a mechanism by which group participants can gauge their interpersonal, social, and behavioral effectiveness.	Multiple social interaction between and among members whose activity is directed toward the realization of an identified goal for the purpose of undergoing change.	1. Exploration. 2. Clarification. 3. Validation. 4. Feedback. 5. Evaluation. 6. Role playing. 7. Brainstorming. 8. Values clarification. 9. Conflict resolution. 10. Problem-solving.

(*continued*)

TABLE 4–5. CONTINUED

Modality	Definition	Application	Goal
Family therapy	A treatment modality designed to bring about change in communication and interactive patterns between and among members.	Determined by specific clinical situations; most appropriate for those living situations in which conflict is predominant in producing disruption within the family system.	To reorganize the family structure, particularly with respect to patterns of communication and family relationships. To maintain balance and promote wellness.
Transactional analysis	A treatment modality that makes use of cognitive and emotive aspects of self in identifying the interactional and communicational patterns existing between self and others.	Particularly useful with groups, although it can be used in individual psychotherapy; effective in marriage and family counseling; management and industry; and in such special problems as alcoholism, criminal behavior, mental retardation, and schizophrenia.	To examine life situations for the purpose of increasing self-awareness.

Theoretical Framework	Principles	Therapeutic Process	Strategies and Techniques
Draws primarily on the evolving theories related to family systems; also incorporates a blending of theories related to interpersonal, communication, learning, and group processes.	1. A family is a primary unit and operates as a closed system. 2. The family serves as an intermediary between the individual members and society. 3. Families operate within designated limits, restricting the expression of individual behavior within the group. 4. Families attempt to maintain homeostasis.	Social engineering within a natural heterogeneous group.	1. Role playing. 2. Role clarification. 3. Exploration. 4. Validation. 5. Clarification. 6. Feedback. 7. Evaluation. 8. Conflict resolution. 9. Problem-solving. 10. Contracting.
Incorporates a blending of theories and concepts extrapolated from psychoanalytic theory as well as the theories associated with social intercourse, communication, and learning.	1. Ego states develop sequentially and are subject to modification throughout life. 2. A transaction is the unit of social action between people. 3. Learning to change transactions leads to improved communication. 4. Healthy functioning is reflected by adaptability and flexibility. 5. Recognition is a basic human need. 6. Intimacy in relationships is influenced through interest and a common frame of reference. 7. Unconscious feelings interfere with problem solving and ability to relate to others.	A teaching-learning experience involving analysis of the structural and communication patterns employed.	1. Contracting. 2. Stroking. 3. Stimulating. 4. Problem-solving. 5. Decision-making. 6. Game analysis. 7. Script analysis.

(*continued*)

TABLE 4–5. CONTINUED

Modality	Definition	Application	Goal
Transactional analysis (*continued*)			
Gestalt therapy	A treatment modality designed to assist clients in dealing with the how and what of their behavior.	Practiced in a group setting, although emphasis is placed on the individual within the setting as opposed to the total group. As originally conceived, was applied to clients exhibiting neurotic and psychosomatic symptomatology.	To promote self-acceptance through increased self-awareness.
Reality therapy	A treatment modality that deals directly with the client's here and now in assisting him to fulfill his conscious needs.	Can be used with any client whose behavior has been deemed irresponsible, that is, ineffective or socially unacceptable.	To fulfill the two basic needs for love and self-worth. To recognize personal life goals. To assume responsibility for self. To recognize alternatives.

Theoretical Framework	Principles	Therapeutic Process	Strategies and Techniques
	8. Evaluation of transactions promotes self-awareness and effectiveness of performance. 9. Continual sensory input is needed to maintain physical and psychosocial equilibrium.		
Has its foundation in Gestalt psychology and employs an existential philosophical outlook.	1. An individual must be able to exercise freedom of choice. 2. It is only by knowing the present that one can understand the past and plan for the future. 3. Any barrier to goal fulfillment leaves a residual of unfinished business. 4. Accumulation of unfinished business predisposes to breakdown. 5. All men possess the same basic biological and psychological needs. 6. Need fulfillment is necessary if the totality of self is to be experienced. 7. Involvement is a key to satisfactory human interaction.	Completion of gestalts with resultant restoration of homeostasis.	1. Desensitization. 2. Overexaggeration of feelings. 3. Sensorimotor and psychological exercises. 4. Role reversal. 5. Reality testing. 6. Assertiveness.
A blending of several basic theories including developmental, social learning, and communicative.	1. Human beings have two outstanding basic needs: the need to love and be loved and the need to feel worthwhile to self and others.	Focuses on current behavior and stimulates involvement, acceptance, and caring.	1. Decision-making. 2. Problem-solving. 3. Confrontation. 4. Contracting. 5. Limit setting. 6. Validation. 7. Clarification.

(*continued*)

TABLE 4–5. CONTINUED

Modality	Definition	Application	Goal
Reality therapy *(continued)*			
Crisis intervention	A short-term, self-limiting treatment modality that focuses on the concrete facts of an identified current life situation, the client's efforts to bring about change and the effective resolution of crisis.	Can be used in any client care situation where an individual's or group's usual pattern of functioning can no longer be of assistance in handling specific predictable or unpredictable life events.	To restore functioning to a level that existed prior to onset of crisis. To promote personal growth through improved functioning above that demonstrated in the precrisis period. To avert catastrophe.

Theoretical Framework	Principles	Therapeutic Process	Strategies and Techniques
	2. Man is self-determining and has the ability to be self-actualized. 3. Involvement with others is critical to maturation. 4. Behavior depends on decisions rather than conditions. 5. The individual is held responsible and accountable for self-defeating behavior or for making a commitment to change. 6. Responsibility is synonymous with mental health and irresponsibility with mental illness.		
Derived from systems, personality and crisis theories.	1. Everyone has potential for growth. 2. Life experiences involving stress and trauma can be occasions for future growth. 3. Crisis presents a time-limited opportunity for action. 4. Crisis produces disequilibrium. 5. Crisis produces an alteration of an individual's expectation of self with respect to others. 6. Crisis intervention requires support, protection and enhancement of the client's self-image. 7. Learning alternative coping mechanisms facilitates self-reliance and growth. 8. The therapist assumes an active and directive role in the therapeutic process.	A directional encounter leading to adaptation, resolution, and reconstruction.	1. Decision-making. 2. Problem-solving. 3. Active listening. 4. Role playing. 5. Bargaining. 6. Anticipatory planning. 7. Advocacy.

resort. This is in part due to the fact that the whole concept of punishment and associated pain, both psychic and physical, is one that is not generally accepted within our society's system of values.

As a treatment modality, behavior modification can be used to bring about a quick, effective, and meaningful change in behavior. Since change is rapid, the individual can experience a sense of mastery or control over self that facilitates an increase in dignity, self-respect, and self-worth. And, too, if distancing behaviors and the negative feedback associated with them can be reduced, altered, or extinguished, the individual's social horizons and freedom to be and to choose will be enhanced.

The use of a behavior-modification approach does not negate or infringe upon the establishment of an interactive–interventive approach to client care. In fact, the experience of rapid change can strengthen the bond of trust between the client and the nurse, as the client sees and begins to experience the positive effects of change.

Group Therapy

As a treatment modality, group therapy is designed to serve a selected number of clients by involving them in a cognitive and emotional experience that can be instrumental in helping the participants toward some type of new learning or change. Historically, group therapy is not a new modality and was known to and used by the early Greeks. However, the movement to utilize group process did not begin in this country until the early 1900s with the work of Joseph Pratt. Then during the early part of the 20th century others, such as Slavson, Yalom, Lewin, Cartwright, Zander, Wolf, and Moreno, contributed to the development of a scientific and clinical approach to small group process. Group therapy as an interventive technique did not become widespread until early in the 1960s. Today, it is a universally recognized and used modality employed in a variety of treatment settings.

Generally, a therapeutic group consists of between four to ten clients with one or two therapists as designated leaders. Frequency of sessions is governed by the stated objective and the needs of the clients and may range from one to three meetings per week lasting anywhere from 30 to 90 minutes. Types of therapeutic groups are characterized according to population composition of the members; group process emphasized; leadership style demonstrated; theoretical framework employed; type of interaction fostered between and among members and therapist; and specific goals sought. Regardless of the type of group, two major functions emerge to give the group direction. The first is to work on or accomplish a specified task, while the second is to satisfy the psychological, emotional, social, and physiological needs of its members. For a more extensive discussion of group structure, process, and dynamics and the nursing role in group therapy, the reader is referred to Chapters 16, 17, and 18.

Family Therapy

The early 1950s saw the emergence of family therapy as a new, viable treatment modality. The common belief fundamental to the practice of family therapy is that the family system, not the individual member, is the focus of therapeutic concern. The purpose of family therapy is self-rehabilitation within the context of family structure. The goal is exploration, clarification, and reorganization of family patterns relevant to communication and interpersonal functioning. Critical to the concept of restructuring is the presenting need for education toward the facilitation of healthy behavior between and among family members.

Family therapy differs from other forms of group therapy in that, in family therapy, the group is a natural, primary unit of society. It is heterogeneous in nature and is often composed of members from differing generations. Furthermore, within this unit, roles and role functioning have been identified so that maintenance and task functions have already been set. Thus, the unit or ongoing system of the family strives toward wholeness and continuation within that system, outside the therapy session. Another major distinction between group and family therapy is that when group members leave the therapy session they disband, each member going his separate way and returning to the environment from whence he came. In family therapy, however, the group remains intact; the changes that occur are changes within the group, and reinforcement for continuance comes from the internal support and maintenance of the homeostatic balance inherent within the family group.

One of the major benefits to be derived as an outcome of family therapy is a shared awareness within its members that roles and role functioning can be flexible. For example, leadership does not necessarily have to reside in and remain with the parenting figures. Leadership can be assumed by any member of the unit, depending on the situation, the strengths and weaknesses of members with respect to the situation, and the possession of expertise by members relative to the situation. Another benefit to be derived from family therapy is interruption in the transmission of pathogenic conflict and maladaptive coping responses from generation to generation.

Since the nurse must convey to the family group that the origin of the identified problem does not reside in a single member but is shared and perpetuated by all its members, the nurse's own personality plays a key role in the therapeutic process. In implementing her therapeutic role, the nurse needs to be fully aware of her system of operation along with the values, attitudes, and beliefs governing it. She must recognize her responsibility to demonstrate wellness as well as the need to demonstrate professional competency and growth as a person. Furthermore, the demand for an active, open, and honest approach in therapy requires that the nurse possess self-knowledge. This knowledge of self allows the nurse to maintain the flexibility, neutrality, and objectivity that are the key components of therapeutic effectiveness with family groups.

Transactional Analysis

Transactional analysis came into being through the efforts of Eric Berne, who in the early 1960s put forth the premise that the human personality gave evidence of being divided into three ego states. He subsequently entitled these three ego states the **parent**, the **adult**, and the **child**. He described each state in detail and proposed that each one possessed distinct functions along with a characteristic pattern and language of communication. The basic premise underlying the therapeutic process is that the client must come to an awareness of how he functions and be able to identify which ego state is operational at any given moment in time.

As originally conceived, transactional analysis was a treatment modality designed to be used primarily in group therapy. Its current use, however, is not limited to the confines of treatment programs. This modality focuses on the transactions between and among people. In the therapeutic process, emphasis is placed on the analysis of the person's life in relationship to the type of "scripting" employed, that is, becoming in touch with the unconscious plan for living formulated and decided on in early childhood. This analysis is used to assist the client in differentiating what he thinks, feels, and does as a parent, adult, and child. Also identified are the types of games (that is, ulterior transactions engaged in) that tend to reinforce maladaptive response patterns.

Transactional analysis is a direct and active form of therapy in which the therapist assumes a vigorous role in the teaching-learning process. The primary objective is to increase the client's awareness of ego functioning and for the client to be able to exert control over the use of each ego state within a given transaction. The teaching-learning process is guided by the basic assumption that an individual can consciously change his mode of operation and thereby influence his relationship with others.

In using a transactional approach to client care, the nurse deliberately engages the client in an active exploration of his life and living experiences for the purpose of making sense or finding meaning. As the client becomes aware of his functioning, the nurse assists him to formulate decisions regarding which aspects of functioning he wishes to retain or discard. Once the client decides, the nurse works with him to devise a plan that will implement the change as well as identify the means for evaluating progress. The major goal of nursing intervention is to establish a climate of trust in which the client can arrive at a more satisfied, loving and lovable self.

Gestalt Therapy

In the mid-1950s Frederick (Fritz) Perls introduced Gestalt therapy. The major premise underlying this treatment approach is that man is considered a total organism who functions as a whole rather than as a dichotomous entity of mind and body. In Gestalt therapy, the emphasis is on the present (here and now) ongoing life situation involving the interactional processing between self and others.

An outgrowth of the basic premise and the cornerstone of therapeutic intervention is the idea that people can deal adequately with their own life problems if they know what these problems are and can bring all their abilities into coordinated action to solve them. Therefore, this treatment modality is directed toward assisting the client to bring into conscious awareness desensitized sensorimotor-affective modes of operation. Thus, Gestalt therapy is getting in touch with self. Self-awareness is achieved by becoming cognizant of sensations, acknowledging corresponding behaviors, and identifying existing feelings. Proponents of this therapy postulate that enhancement of total awareness results in self-acceptance.

Since awareness of and responsibility for behavior are the two major issues of the therapeutic process, the primary task of the therapist is to help the client overcome the barriers that block awareness. To arrive at self-awareness, the client, with the assistance of the therapist, learns to deal with unfinished business by focusing on the "what and how" of behavior rather than the "why." The role of the therapist then becomes that of observer, commentator, and occasional guide, so that the client, in essence, carries on his own therapy. It is important to note that in Gestalt therapy, the therapist does not engage in problem solving with the client but rather works to assist the client to reestablish life conditions under which he can use his own problem-solving abilities.

Gestalt therapy can be reflected in the nursing process. For example, data collection is carried out when the nurse identifies those areas of the client's life and living experience that are open, incomplete, or unfinished. Once these open gestalts have been determined, the nurse can then move toward assessment by identifying the unrecognized or unexpressed needs that impinge upon and prevent the forward movement of the client in achieving life goals and successful relationships. The objective of nursing intervention is to direct the client's efforts toward closure or resolution of the identified concern. Effectiveness of the intervention is determined by the client's demonstrating self-awareness to the extent that he is able to assume responsibility for self and implement alternative coping devices.

The interactional process from a Gestalt viewpoint involves openness and honesty in dealing with self, others, and the environment. These qualities are manifested in various ways. First, the therapeutic relationship acknowledges the individuality and uniqueness of the participants while at the same time recognizing the commonalities associated with their humanness. Furthermore, no value judgments are attached to acknowledged differences. Second, the relationship involves acceptance of responsibility for self in all its aspects. This means that the participants maintain their own integrity and respect the integrity of the other. Third, each participant enters and engages in the interactional process with the expectation that full advantage and use will be made of all personal, interpersonal, and situational resources available. Lastly, sharing is by choice and not design. However, it must be pointed out that it is the responsibility of the nurse to share, for by sharing self the nurse demonstrates to the client that openness and honesty are valuable aspects of communication and interpersonal functioning.

Reality Therapy

This treatment modality was first introduced by William Glasser in the early 1960s. Glasser's treatment process is based on the concept that education is the key to effective human functioning. In his approach, Glasser disregards the traditional concept of mental health and mental illness and instead discusses and focuses on human behavior—responsibility versus irresponsibility as the major concept of social wellness.

Reality therapy stresses that identity, particularly identity with respect to accepting self and one's social role, is the most significant outcome of the treatment process. This outcome is related to the individual's ability and potential for fulfilling what Glasser identifies as the two most basic human needs, the need to love and be loved and the need to feel worthwhile. To achieve these goals the therapist must provide an interactional–interventive atmosphere that reflects warmth, understanding, and concern. Essentially, the client's problems are held to be a result of his inability to accept responsibility for his own behavior. Glasser defines this fundamental concept of responsibility as the capacity to satisfy one's needs without infringing on the ability of others to gratify their needs. Within this structure, the therapist begins by identifying with the client immediate and long-term life goals. The interaction process focuses almost exclusively on the behavior of the client as he moves toward goal attainment. Furthermore, in this quest for fulfillment emphasis is placed on the individual's value system and consequent moral outlook without the therapist attempting to indicate the rightness or wrongness of the particular value judgments made. The purpose of such exploration is to assist the client to identify meaning within the context of his life situation so that the resultant responsible behavior is always in line with what is right and good for the individual while meeting basic needs.

The nurse's role is to assist the client in the examination of his life and to aid him in making constructive decisions regarding those aspects or areas of functioning that have been identified as irresponsible. The nurse works with the client to develop a plan designed to bring about changes in behavior. The focus of therapeutic intervention within this plan is encouragement in and adoption of a success identity as opposed to a critical, self-deprecatory failure identity. Since rationalizations and intellectualizations about behavior are not acceptable excuses for behavior, confrontation is a tactic that is frequently employed as part of the interventive process. As a result of this process of self-examination, the individual develops a mature ego identity that is able to constructively change behavior and, in this process of change, resolve those symptoms that heretofore prevented involvement and social acceptance.

Crisis Intervention

Crisis intervention is a short-term treatment modality employed to reestablish client equilibrium. It is used for those individuals seeking assistance with the resolution of an immediate problem. It is a treatment of eminent need. The entire treatment process is time-limited, ranging from a few days to no longer than six weeks. It is a modality for primary prevention, since the chief purpose is the prevention of maladaption and the restoration of equilibrium.

The therapeutic process involves active collaborative effort on the part of the participants in the problem-solving process. Toward this end, the procedure involved in crisis intervention encompasses the following steps. First, the therapist displays toward the client the attitudes of personal worth, integrity, open-mindedness, and advocacy in order to establish rapport and facilitate communication. Second, the therapist engages the client in exploring and assessing the parameters surrounding the problem with a view toward accurate identification. Third, the therapist determines the areas of strength the client comes with as well as those potential resources the client can call upon for support. In the fourth step, the coparticipants formulate a plan of action directed toward successful resolution of the crisis event. Fifth, the therapist assists the client to mobilize and translate the plan into action. The sixth step is closure, that is, actual resolution of the crisis. Follow-up is the last step of the procedure. In this step, the therapist reinforces the learning that has taken place as the client has regained control and resumed self-direction. Follow-up allows the client to consciously inspect and articulate the process employed in the search for resolution.

In this section of the text we have presented the concept of crisis intervention as a specific treatment modality. We have made no attempt to explore and discuss here the phenomenon of crisis as part of an individual's life and living experience. To understand the concept of crisis and its significance, the reader is referred to Chapter 8, where this concept is presented.

SUMMARY

Theories set the stage for practice and guide the selection of both strategy and modality. Selection is based on two factors: the presenting need of the client as identified through nursing diagnosis; and the knowledge, understanding, and skill the nurse has acquired. Likewise, these two factors also influence the application of strategies within a selected modality.

This chapter has attempted to set the stage for contemporary practice. We have presented an overview of the theoretical concepts that form the basis for each modality, and we have identified four common nursing strategies that can be used within the interactive–interventive process with clients. We believe that the identified strategies can be used with any of the treatment modalities. The reader must keep in mind that congruence has to exist between and among theory, modality, and strategy. Furthermore, application is not haphazard, but is a systematic, rational, planned operation that flows from the nursing process.

SUGGESTED READINGS

Ackerman, N. W. *The Dynamics of Family Life*. New York: Basic Books, 1958.

Alberti, R. E., & Emmonds, M. L. *Your Perfect Right*. 2nd ed. San Luis Obispo, Calif.: Impact, 1974.

American Psychiatric Association Commission on Psychiatric Therapies, Karasu, T. B., Chairman. *The Psychiatric Therapies*. Washington, D.C.: American Psychiatric Association, 1984.

Bakdash, D. P. Becoming an Assertive Nurse. *American Journal of Nursing*, Vol. 78, No. 10 (October, 1978), 1710–1712.

Bandura, A. *Social Learning Theory*. Englewood Cliffs. N.J.: Prentice-Hall, 1977.

Benson, H. *The Relaxation Response*. New York: Morrow, Inc., 1975.

Berger, M. S., et al., (Eds.). *Management for Nurses: A Multi-disciplinary Approach*. 2nd ed. St. Louis: C. V. Mosby, 1980.

Bergman, L. H. A Cognitive Behavioral Approach to Transactional Analysis. *Transactional Analysis Journal*, Vol. 11, No. 2 (April, 1981), 147–149.

Berne, E. *Games People Play: The Psychology of Human Relationships*. New York: Grove Press, 1964.

Bowen, M. *Family Therapy in Clinical Practice*. New York: Jason Aronson, 1978.

Bowman, Sister C., & Spadoni, A. J. Assertion Therapy: The Nurse and Psychiatric Patient in an Acute, Short-Term Hospital Setting. *Journal of Psychiatric Nursing and Mental Health Services*, Vol. 19, No. 5 (May, 1981), 7–21.

Carter, J. W. Assertiveness and Post-Divorce Adjustment in Women. *Issues in Mental Health Nursing*, Vol. 3, No. 4 (October-December, 1981), 365–380.

Chenevert, M. *Special Techniques in Assertiveness Training for Women in the Health Professions*. St. Louis: C. V. Mosby, 1978.

Curtis, D. B., Mazza, J. M., & Runnebohm, S. *Communication for Problem Solving*. New York: Wiley, 1979.

Elder, J. *Transactional Analysis in Health Care*. Menlo Park, Calif.: Addison-Wesley, 1978.

Erickson, G. D., & Hogan, T. P. (Eds.). *Family Therapy: An Introduction to Theory and Technique*. New York: Jason Aronson, 1976.

Ewing, D. W. Discovering Your Problem Solving Style. *Psychology Today*, Vol. 11, No. 7 (December, 1977), 68–73, 138.

Fagan, J., & Shepherd, I. L. (Eds.). *Gestalt Therapy Now*. New York: Harper & Row, 1970.

Filley, A. *Interpersonal Conflict Resolution*. Glenview, Ill.: Scott, Foresman Co., 1975.

Fishel, A. H., & Jefferson, C. B. Assertiveness Training for Hospitalized, Emotionally Disturbed Women. *Journal of Psychosocial Nursing and Mental Health Services*, Vol. 21, No. 11 (November, 1983), 22–27.

Ford, J. G., Trygstad-Durland, L. N., & Nelms, B. C. *Applied Decision Making for Nurses*. St. Louis: C. V. Mosby, 1979.

Friedman, M., & Shmukler, D. A Model of Family Development and Functioning in a T. A. Framework. *Transactional Analysis Journal*, Vol. 13, No. 2 (April, 1983), 90–93.

Gerace, L. Phenomenon of Early Engagement in Family Therapy. *Journal of Psychiatric Nursing and Mental Health Services*, Vol. 19, No. 4 (April, 1981), 25–28.

Gilmour, J. R. Psychophysiological Evidence for the Existence of Ego States. *Transactional Analysis Journal*, Vol. 11, No. 3 (July, 1981), 207–212.

Glasser, W. *The Identity Society*. New York: Harper & Row, 1972.

Glasser, W. *Reality Therapy*. New York: Harper & Row, 1965.

Glende, N. H. The Essence and Illusion of Hope. *Transactional Analysis Journal*, Vol. 11, No. 2 (April, 1981), 110–121.

Gunderson, S. S. Advocacy and Family Therapy. *Journal of Psychiatric Nursing and Mental Health Services*, Vol. 18, No. 9 (September, 1980), 24–28.

Harper, R. A. *The New Psychotherapies*. Englewood Cliffs, N.J.: Prentice-Hall, 1975.

Harris, T. A. *I'm OK—You're OK*. New York: Harper & Row, 1969.

Hatcher, C., & Himelstein, P. (Eds.). *The Handbook of Gestalt Therapy*. New York: Jason Aronson, 1976.

Hauser, M. J. Assertiveness Techniques Origins and Uses. *Journal of Psychiat-*

ric Nursing and Mental Health Services, Vol. 17, No. 12 (December, 1979), 15–17.

Herman, S. J. *Becoming Assertive: A Guide for Nurses*. New York: D. Van Nostrand Co., 1978.

Hill, W. F. *Learning: A Survey of Psychological Interpretations*. 2nd ed. Scranton, PA: Chandler Co., 1971.

Hutchings, H., & Colburn, L. An Assertiveness Training Program for Nurses. *Nursing Outlook*, Vol. 27, No. 6 (June, 1979), 394–397.

Jacobson, E. *Progressive Relaxation*. 3rd rev. ed. Chicago: University of Chicago Press, 1974.

James, M. *Techniques in Transactional Analysis*. Reading. Mass.: Addison-Wesley Co., 1977.

James, M., & Savary, L. *A New Self*. Menlo Park, Calif.: Addison-Wesley Co., 1977.

Jenkins, H. M. Improving Clinical Decision Making in Nursing. *Journal of Nursing Education*, Vol. 24, No. 6 (June, 1985), 242–343.

Jenkins, L. M. The Concept of Assertion: From Theory to Practice. *Issues in Mental Health Nursing*, Vol. 4, No. 1 (January-March, 1982), 51–64.

Kazdin, A. E. Token Economies: The Rich Rewards of Rewards. *Psychology Today*, Vol. 10, No. 6 (November, 1976), 98, 101–102, 105, 114.

Kramer, M., & Schmalenberg, C. E. Conflict: The Cutting Edge of Growth. *Journal of Nursing Administration*, Vol. 6, No. 10 (October, 1976), 19–25.

Krizinofski, M. T. Evolution of the Communication Model of Therapy. In *Current Perspectives in Psychiatric Nursing: Issues and Trends*, edited by C. R. Kneisl & H. S. Wilson. St. Louis: C. V. Mosby, 1976.

Kutash, I. B., et al. *Handbook on Stress and Anxiety*. San Francisco: Jossey-Bass, 1980.

Lakein, A. *How to Get Control of Your Time and Your Life*. New York: Signet, 1973.

Mallory, G. A. Turn Conflict Into Cooperation. *Nursing 85*, Vol. 15, No. 3 (March, 1985), 81–83.

Masserman, J. H., (Ed.). *Current Psychiatric Therapies*. Orlando, Fla.: Grune & Stratton, Inc.

McDonald, T. S. Facing Conflicts. *Nursing Life*, Vol. 4, No. 3 (May/June, 1984), 24–27.

McKenzie, M. E. Decisions: How You Reach Them Makes the Difference. *Nursing Management*, Vol. 16, No. 6 (June, 1985), 48–49.

Moniz, D. Putting Assertiveness Techniques into Practice. *American Journal of Nursing*, Vol. 78, No. 10 (October, 1978), 1713.

Montmeny, R. Perception. *Journal of Psychiatric Nursing and Mental Health Services*, Vol. 18, No. 6 (June, 1980), 22–27.

Morgan, S. A., & Macey, M. J. Three Assessment Tools for Family Therapy. *Journal of Psychiatric Nursing and Mental Health Services*, Vol. 16, No. 3 (March, 1978), 39–42.

Numerof, R. E. Assertiveness Training. *American Journal of Nursing*, Vol. 80, No. 10 (October, 1980), 1796–1799.

O'Hearne, J. Good Grief. *Transactional Analysis Journal*, Vol. 11, No. 1 (January, 1981), 85–87.

Okun, B. F. *Effective Helping: Interviewing and Counseling Techniques*. North Scituate, Mass.: Duxbury Press, 1976.

O'Neill, G. W., & Gardner, R., Jr. Behavior Therapy: An Overview. *Hospital and Community Psychiatry*, Vol. 34, No. 8 (August, 1983), 709–715.

Perls, F. S. *Gestalt Therapy Verbatim*. LaFayette, Calif.: Real People Press, 1969.

Perls, F., Hefferline, R. F., & Goodman, P. *Gestalt Therapy: Excitement and Growth in Human Personality*. New York: Dell Co., 1951.

Phelan, L. A. Crisis Intervention: Partnership in Problem Solving. *Journal of Psychiatric Nursing*, Vol. 17, No. 9 (September, 1979), 22–27.

Porter, N. Caring for Connectedness: Transactions of Trust. *Transactional Analysis Journal*, Vol. 11, No. 2 (April, 1981), 134–137.

Programmed Instruction. Assertiveness in Nursing: Part I. *American Journal of Nursing*, Vol. 83, No. 3 (March, 1983), 417–434.

Programmed Instruction. Assertiveness in Nursing: Part II. *American Journal of Nursing*, Vol. 83, No. 6 (June, 1983), 911–928.

Putt, A. M. A Biofeedback Service by Nurses. *American Journal of Nursing*, Vol. 79, No. 1 (January, 1979), 88–89.

Raudsepp, E. More Creative Gamesmanship. *Psychology Today*, Vol. 14, No. 2 (July, 1980), 71–75, 88.

Raudsepp, E., & Hough, G. P., Jr. Jumping to Solutions. *Psychology Today*, Vol. 11, No. 7 (December, 1977), 75–76, 78, 80, 130–132, 135–136.

Rose, S. D. *Group Therapy: A Behavioral Approach*. Englewood Cliffs, N.J.: Prentice-Hall, 1977.

Rush, A. J. Cognitive Therapy of Depression. Rationale, Techniques and Efficacy. *Psychiatric Clinics of North America*, Vol. 6, No. 1 (March, 1983), 105–127.

Satir, V. *Conjoint Family Therapy*. Palo Alto, Calif.: Science and Behavior Books, 1967.

Shmukler, D., & Friedman, M. Clinical Implications of the Family Systems Model. *Transactional Analysis Journal*, Vol. 13, No. 2 (April, 1983), 94–96.

Sullivan, H. S. *The Interpersonal Theory of Psychiatry*. H. S. Perry & M. L. Gowel (Eds.). New York: W. W. Norton Co., 1954.

Todd, S. S. Coping With Conflict: Know Which Technique To Call Into Play. *Nursing Life*, Vol. 5, No. 3 (May/June, 1985), 41–43.

Valinoti, E. Mrs. Bradley Knew It All—and Couldn't Keep it to Herself. *Nursing Life*, Vol. 1, No. 2 (January/February, 1984), 54–55.

Wahll, A. L. Nursing Theory and the Assessment of Families. *Journal of Psychiatric Nursing and Mental Health Services*, Vol. 19, No. 1 (January, 1981), 30–36.

Ware, P. Personality Adaptations: Doors To Therapy. *Transactional Analysis Journal*, Vol. 13, No. 1 (January, 1983), 11–19.

Wathney, S. Paradoxical Interventions in Transactional Analysis and Gestalt Therapy. *Transactional Analysis Journal*, Vol. 12, No. 3 (July, 1982), 185–189.

White, J. (Ed.) *Relax (How You Can Feel Better, Reduce Stress and Overcome Tensions)*. New York: Dell Publishing Co., 1976.

Wilson, G., & Davison, G. C. Behavior Therapy: A Road to Self-Control. *Psychology Today*, Vol. 9, No. 5 (October, 1975), 54, 58–60.

Winston, S. *Getting Organized: The Easy Way To Put Your Life in Order*. New York: W. W. Norton, 1978.

Wyss, D. *Psychoanalytic Schools from the Beginning to the Present*. New York: Jason Aronson, 1973.
Yalom, I. D. *The Theory and Practice of Group Psychotherapy*. New York: Basic Books, 1970.
Zuk, G. H. *Family Therapy*. New York: Behavioral Publications, 1971.
Zuk, G. *Family Therapy: A Triadic-Based Approach*. New York: Behavioral Publications, 1971.

5

A COMPARISON OF DEVELOPMENTAL THEORIES

A Frame of Reference

LEARNING OBJECTIVES

On completion of this chapter the reader should be able to:

1. Identify the major contributions made by Freud, Sullivan, Erikson, and Piaget to developmental theory.
2. Recognize the stages of normal growth and development.
3. Identify the stages of development conceived by Freud, Sullivan, Erikson, and Piaget.
4. Understand the significance of developmental theory in the practice of psychiatric nursing.
5. Assess the developmental level of a client using the theories presented.

INTRODUCTION

A person is a complex social creature. A person is a composite of all he is, all that he thinks, feels, and does both consciously and unconsciously. He is the product of his experiences, which he has integrated through the five basic senses—sight, hearing, touch, taste and smell.

He is like all others, and yet he remains distinctly individual. A person functions from his personal framework, and all aspects of his totality—mind, body and spirit—work in unison to produce and maintain equilibrium. Hence, there are interrelationships among the physical, intellectual, social, spiritual, and emotional components of the self.

The individual is engaged in an ongoing interactional process with his environment, which facilitates movement toward continued growth and development. His total functioning is an outcome of his developmental process—the quantitative and qualitative ways in which the individual changes over time. His personality with its intrinsic dignity is a reflection of his composite nature and as such reveals his instincts, needs, desires, physical talents and attributes, feelings, beliefs, and values. He manifests the characteristics of his personality through his verbal and nonverbal communication and through his behavioral patterns.

A working knowledge of fundamental concepts and theories of human development is essential if the nurse is to arrive at an understanding of normal human functioning and ultimately interpret a person's behavior in light of the developmental process. This knowledge gives the nurse a frame of reference upon which to begin to assess where the patient is within his life experience. The nurse's application of this knowledge results in the delivery of competent and comprehensive nursing care.

Psychiatric nursing predicates its practice on the assumption of an eclectic approach that combines the psychoanalytic, interpersonal, and sociocultural theories with learning theory. We have briefly summarized the contributions made by Freud, Sullivan, Erikson, and Piaget to assist the student to establish a frame of reference and to rapidly review some major concepts relevant to each of these developmental theories.

MAJOR THEORIES

Within the field of human development there are a multiplicity of diverse and controversial theories. For simplification, these theories may be broadly divided into four major schools of thought: the psychoanalytic, the interpersonal, the sociocultural, and the cognitive.

Analytic theory and the first systematic theories of development came from the research and writings of Sigmund Freud. From this initial thrust the analytic school of thought was expanded, and the first Freudians—Jung, Adler, Rank, Meyer, and Ferencze—made significant contributions. Each of these theorists expanded the basic Freudian theories by adding different dimensions and placing varying degrees of emphasis on the growth and developmental process. Basically, analytic theory views man and his development as an intrapsychic experience related to the satisfaction and gratification of basic needs and drives.

From this foundation came the Neo-Freudian groups, which integrated the psychic process with interpersonal transactions. With the advent of interpersonal theory, whose advocates include Sullivan, Horney, and Fromm, there was gradual movement away from viewing the unconscious as the prime motivator of human behavior. In essence, interpersonal theory focuses on the kind of relationship an individual establishes and maintains with a "significant other."

Subsequently, social theory, an outgrowth and expansion of interpersonal theory, was advanced through the efforts of such people as Eric Erikson and Kurt Lewin. The chief concept underlying social theory is the humanistic, realistic, and conscious development of the individual's personality as a direct outcome of a group interactional process.

Each of these schools of thought contributed ideas of personality development in terms of an individual's biophysical, psychological, and social growth. Within this theoretical framework, however, little emphasis was placed on the cognitive development of the individual. Concurrently, but not relatedly, behavioral psychologists such as Hull, Skinner, and Piaget advanced theories of the development of cognitive styles and motor skill ability in relationship to the development of learning theory. Cognitive theory focuses on the interplay between the person's genetic endowment and the external environmental influences surrounding him. Man's development is viewed as primarily an intellectual process that shapes, modifies, and contributes to growth through learning, adaptation, assimilation, and accommodation. Cognitive theory states that communicative and problem-solving behavior, especially the use of language and logical thought processes, are learned human characteristics.

Table 5–1 contains a brief description of the major theories and contributions made by Freud, Sullivan, Erikson, and Piaget. Table 5–2 illustrates the stages of development postulated by each of these theorists.

In comparing Freud's, Sullivan's, Erikson's, and Piaget's conceptualizations about the developmental process, it can be noted that although they differ regarding time span, specific aspects of development, and emphasis within a particular stage, each theory accounts for a complete process. Thus, regardless of which theory the nurse uses as her frame of reference, certain outcomes are expected and should occur in the developmental process. In other words, each individual must move through a series of operations—physical, mental, emotional, and social—that lead to maturation, even though the rate

TABLE 5–1. A COMPARISON OF THE MAJOR THEORETICAL CONTRIBUTIONS OF FREUD, SULLIVAN, ERIKSON, AND PIAGET

Sigmund Freud (1856–1939)	Harry Stack Sullivan (1892–1949)	Eric Erikson (1902–)	Jean Paul Piaget (1896–1980)
1. First to identify and classify developmental stages.	1. First to focus on the interactional process between mother and child.	1. First to include adulthood as a stage of growth and focus on the formation of personal identity as a key concept.	1. First to be concerned with the development of cognition.
2. Theory focused on the concept of libidinal energy and instinctual drives as the forces that motivate behavior.	2. Theory focused on the concept of anxiety as the dynamic force in the developmental process.	2. Theory combines Freud's biological or heredity factors with Sullivan's social factors.	2. The theory concentrates on the development of intellectual capabilities with little reference to emotional or social development.
3. Developed the concept that the mind operates on three levels—the unconscious, the preconscious, and the conscious. Emphasis placed on intrapsychic behavior.	3. Used Freud's concept of the unconscious and conscious mind. Emphasis placed on observable behavior.	3. Used Freud's concept of the divisions of the mind. Emphasis placed on the individual's relationship as influenced by family, peers and society.	3. Emphasized the processes of assimilation, adaptation, and accommodation with respect to the development of reasoning, language, intelligence, and the concepts of nature, time, space, and causality.
4. Experience is always viewed in relation to unconscious material and reconstruction of the past.	4. Experience is viewed as an interactional process existing between self and others, which depends on previous experience.	4. Experience is viewed as a continuous growth process characterized by a degree of attainment between two extremes within each developmental level.	4. Experience is viewed as a building-block process for the expansion of intrinsic capabilities.

5. The mind has a structural division—the id, the ego, and the superego.	5. Experience is divided into three cognitive modes—prototaxic, parataxic, and syntaxic.	5. The extended social experience is the primary framework in learning.	5. Development is influenced by individual differences and social influences; focus is on the mind rather than on the self.
6. Developed theories while working with pathological adults, primarily neurotics.	6. Developed theories while working with pathological adults, primarily schizophrenics.	6. Developed theories while working with children and emphasized both health and illness in the personality.	6. Developed theories while working with normal, healthy children.
7. Believed that no behavioral change can be effected without understanding the content and meaning of the individual's unconscious.	7. Believed that change occurs only when improved interpersonal relationships are combined with an understanding of the basic good-bad influences.	7. Believed that behavioral change occurs only when the individual achieves integration of attitudes, libido, and social roles to form a stronger ego identity.	7. Believed that change occurs as an outcome of the socialization process.
8. Focused on emotional development.	8. Focused on emotional and interpersonal development.	8. Focused on emotional, interpersonal, and spiritual development.	8. Focused on intellectual and psychomotor skill development.

TABLE 5–2. A COMPARISON OF THE DEVELOPMENT STAGES POSTULATED BY FREUD, SULLIVAN, ERICKSON, AND PIAGET

Freud	Sullivan	Erikson	Piaget
I. Oral (0–18 months) a. The mouth is a source of satisfaction. b. Two phases: 1. Passive Only interests are satisfying hunger and **sucking**. Completely helpless, **security** is the greatest need. Narcissistic and egocentric; operates on **pleasure principle**. Omnipotent feelings are prevalent. 2. Active Biting is a mode of pleasure. Continuous experimentation and associations. Sensory discriminations. Differentiation between mental images and reality. Differentiation of others and discovery of self.	I. Infancy (0–18 months) a. The mouth is a source of satisfaction. b. Mouth—takes in (sucking), cuts off (biting), and pushes out (spitting) objects introduced by others. c. Crying, babbling, and cooing are modes of communication used by the infant to call attention of adults to self. d. **Satisfaction** response (**pleasure principle**) Infant's biological needs are met and a mutual feeling of comfort and fulfillment is experienced by mother and child. (Mother gives and child takes.) e. **Empathic observation** Capacity to perceive feelings of others as his own immediate feelings in the situation. f. **Autistic invention** State of symbol activity in which the infant feels he is master of all he surveys. g. Experimentation, exploration, and manipulation are methods used to acquaint self with environment.	I. Oral-sensory stage (0–12 months) a. The mouth is a source of satisfaction and a means of dealing with anxiety-producing situations. b. Focus is on the development of the **basic attitudes of trust vs. mistrust**. c. Attitudes are formed through mother's reaction to infant needs.	I. Senscrimotor stage (0–12 months) a. Emphasis is on **preverbal intellectual development**. b. Learns relationships with external objects. c. Focus is on physical development with gradual increase in ability to think and use language.

II. Anal stage (1½–3 years) a. Primary activity is on learning muscular control associated with urination and defecation (**toilet training period**). b. Exhibits more self-control; walks, talks, dresses, and undresses. c. **Negativism**—assertion of independence. d. Introduction of **reality principle, ego development**. e. Superego begins to develop. f. Engages in **parallel play**.	II. Childhood (1½–6 years) a. Begins with the capacity for communicating through speech and ends with a beginning need for association with peers. b. Uses **language** as a tool to communicate wishes and needs. c. Anus is power tool used to give or withhold a part of self to control significant people in environment. d. Emergence and integration of **self-concept** and **reflected appraisal of significant persons**. e. Awareness that postponing or delaying gratification of own wishes may bring satisfaction. f. Begins to find limits in experimentation, exploration, and manipulation. g. More aggressive. h. Uses parallel play and curiosity to explore environment. i. Uses exhibitionism and masturbatory activity to become acquainted with self and others. j. Demonstrates a beginning ability to think abstractly.	II. Anal-muscular stage (1–3 years) a. Learns the extent to which the environment can be influenced by direct manipulation. b. Focuses on the development of the **basic attitudes of autonomy vs. shame and doubt**. c. Exerts self-control and will power.	II. Preoperational stage (2–7 years) a. Learns to use **symbols and language**. b. Learns to **imitate** and play. c. Displays **egocentricity**. d. Engages in **animistic thinking** (endows objects with power and ability).

(*continued*)

TABLE 5–2. CONTINUED

Freud	Sullivan	Erikson	Piaget
III. Phallic stage (3–6 years) a. **Libidinal energy** is focused on the **genitals**. b. Learns **sexual identity**. c. **Superego** becomes **internalized**. d. **Sibling rivalry** and manipulation of parents occur. e. Intellectual and motor facilities are refined. f. Increased socialization and **associative play**.		III. Genital-locomotor stage (3–6 years) a. Learns the extent to which being **assertive** will influence the environment. b. Focus is on the development of the **basic attitudes of initiative vs. guilt**. c. Explores the world with senses, thoughts, and imagination. d. Activities demonstrate direction and purpose. e. Engages in first real social contacts through **cooperative play**. f. **Develops conscience**.	
IV. Latency (6–12 years) a. **Quiet stage** in which sexual development lies dormant, emotional tension eases. b. **Normal homosexual phase** For boys, gangs. For girls, cliques. c. Increased intellectual capacity. d. Starts school. e. **Identifies with teachers and peers**.	III. Juvenile stage (6–9 years) a. Learns to form satisfactory relationships with peers. b. **Peer norms** prevail over family norms. c. Engages in **competition, experimentation, exploration** and **manipulation**. d. Able to **cooperate** and **compromise**. e. Demonstrates capacity to love.	IV. Latency (6–12 years) a. Learns to utilize energy to create, develop, and manipulate. b. Focus is on the development of **basic attitudes of industry vs. inferiority**. c. Able to initiate and complete tasks. d. Understands rules and regulations. e. Displays **competence** and **productivity**.	III. Concrete operations stage (7–11 years) a. Deals with visible concrete objects and relationships. b. Increased intellectual and conceptual development—employs **logic** and **reasoning**. c. More socialized and rule conscious.

f. Weakening of home ties. g. Recognizes authority figures outside home, age of **hero worship**.	f. Distinguishes fantasy from reality. g. Exerts internal control over behavior. IV. Preadolescence (9–12 years) a. Learns to relate to a friend of the same sex—**chum relationship**. b. Concerned with group success and derives satisfaction from group accomplishment. c. Shows signs of **rebellion**—restlessness, hostility, irritability. d. Assumes less responsibility for own actions. e. Moves from egocentricity to a more full social state. f. Uses experimentation, exploration, manipulation. g. Seeks consensual validation from peers.		
V. Genital stage (12–early adulthood) a. Appearance of secondary sex characteristics, **reawakening of sex drives**. b. Increased concern over physical appearance. c. Strives toward **independence**. d. Development of **sexual maturity**.	V. Early adolescence (12–14 years) a. Experiences physiological changes. b. Uses rebellion to gain independence. c. Fantasizes, overidentifies with heroes. d. Discovers and begins relationships with opposite sex.	V. Puberty and adolescence (12–18 years) a. Demonstrates an ability to **integrate life experiences**. b. Focus is on the development of the **basic attitudes of identity vs. role diffusion**. c. Seeks partner of the opposite sex.	IV. Formal operations stage (11–15 years) a. Develops **true abstract thought**. b. Formulates hypothesis and applies logical tests. c. **Conceptual independence**.

(*continued*)

TABLE 5–2. CONTINUED

Freud	Sullivan	Erikson	Piaget
e. **Identity crisis**. f. Identification of love object of opposite sex. g. Intellectual maturity. h. Plans future.	e. Demonstrates **heightened levels of anxiety** in most interpersonal relationships.	d. Begins to establish identity and place in society.	
	VI. Late adolescence (14–21 years) a. Establishes an **enduring intimate relationship** with one member of the opposite sex. b. Self-concept becomes stabilized. c. Attains physical maturity. d. Develops ability to use **logic** and **abstract concepts**.	VI. Young adulthood (18–25 years) a. Primarily concerned with developing an **intimate relationship** with another adult. b. Focus is on the development of the **basic attitudes of intimacy and solidarity vs. isolation**.	
	VII. Adulthood (21 years +) a. Assumes **responsibility** relevant to station in life. b. **Maintains balance and involvement** between self, family, and community. c. Further develops **creativity**. d. **Reaffirms values** in life.	VII. Adulthood (25–45 years) a. Primarily concerned with establishing and maintaining a family. b. Focus is on the development of the **basic attitudes of generativity vs. stagnation**. c. Displays a marked degree of creativity. d. Adjusts to circumstances of middle age. e. **Reevaluates life's accomplishments and goals**.	

VIII. Maturity (older than 45 years)

a. **Acceptance of life-style** as meaningful and fulfilling.
b. Focus is on the development of **basic attitudes of ego integrity vs. despair**.
c. Remains optimistic and continues to grow.
d. Adjusts to limitations.
e. Adjusts to retirement.
f. Adjusts to reoganized family patterns.
g. Adjusts to losses.
h. Accepts death with serenity.

of movement may be different for each individual. All stages need to be completed if the individual is to progress. Illness or deviation occurs when progression is inhibited, interrupted, or terminated. Successful progression through and completion of the developmental process requires that the individual be able to:

1. Express needs and feelings.
2. Learn to count on others for part of his need gratification and fulfillment.
3. Recognize people and objects as being external to self.
4. Develop an ego identity.
5. Accept delayed gratification.
6. Develop, refine, and coordinate physical skills.
7. Establish, integrate, and utilize a set of values.
8. Function independently, dependently, and interdependently as appropriate.
9. Use cooperation and compromise in dealing with others.
10. Pursue intellectual and aesthetic activities.
11. Develop an intimate relationship.
12. Establish a work role.
13. Adapt to changing roles and needs.
14. Attain self-actualization.

SUMMARY

Effective nursing care stems from the nurse's application of a basic principle fundamental to the developmental process, which is, that *all behavior has meaning, can be understood, and is relative to an individual's culture, specific situation, and time frame.* The field of psychiatric nursing relies heavily on the use of this principle and the various theories regarding normal human development. Armed with this knowledge, the nurse is in a position to recognize disruptions and dysfunction within the developmental pattern, identify missing steps within the growth process and, as a result, emphasize the healthy aspects while including within the plan of care those corrective experiences that may be necessary to foster further growth and promote continued development.

SUGGESTED READINGS

Arnold, H. M. Snow White and the Seven Dwarfs: A Symbolic Account of Human Development. *Perspectives in Psychiatric Care,* Vol. 17, No. 5 (September/October, 1979), 218–222, 236.

Brandt, M. A. Consider The Patient Part of a Family. *Nursing Forum*, Vol. 21, No. 3 (1984), 19–23.

Chapman, A. H. *Harry Stack Sullivan: His Life and His Work*. New York: G. P. Putnam's Sons, 1976.

Dacey, J. S. *Adult Development*. Glenview, Ill.: Scott, Foresman and Company, 1982.

Dashiff, C. J. Coaching Developmental Differentiation. *Topics in Clinical Nursing*, Vol. 1, No. 3 (October, 1979), 11–20.

DeMaio, D., DeMaio-Esteves, M., & Shuzman, E. Technological Society: Its Impact on Youth. *Topics in Clinical Nursing*, Vol. 5, No. 1 (April, 1983), 55–65.

Dodson, P. *How to Parent*. New York: New American Library, 1971.

Dressen, S. E. Autonomy: A Continuing Developmental Task. *American Journal of Nursing*, Vol. 78, No. 8 (August, 1978), 1344–1346.

Erikson, E. *Childhood and Society*. 2nd ed. New York: W. W. Norton, 1963.

Englehardt, K. Piaget: A Prescriptive Theory for Parents. *Nursing Digest* (November-December, 1974), 22–26.

Fox, K. Adolescent Ambivalence: A Therapeutic Issue. *Journal of Psychiatric Nursing and Mental Health Services*, Vol. 18, No. 9 (September, 1980), 29–33.

Fraiberg, S. H. *The Magic Years*. New York: Charles Scribner's Sons, 1959.

Fraiberg, S. H. *Clinical Studies in Infant Mental Health*. New York: Basic Books, 1980.

Ginott, H. *Between Parent and Child*. New York: Macmillan, 1969.

Ginott, H. *Between Parent and Teenager*. New York: Macmillan, 1969.

Giuffra, M. J. Demystifying Adolescent Behavior. *American Journal of Nursing*, Vol. 75, No. 10 (October, 1975), 1724–1727.

Goodman, P. *Growing Up Absurd*. New York: Vintage Books, 1960.

Hofstedt, S., & Wolfarth, G. The Child As a Psychobiological Being—Implications for Health Care. *Topics in Clinical Nursing*, Vol. 3, No. 4 (January, 1982), 29–34.

Johnston, M., Kayne, M., & Mittleider, K. Putting More Pep in Parenting. *American Journal of Nursing*, Vol. 77, No. 6 (June, 1977), 994–995.

Kestenberg, J. S. *Children and Parents: Psychoanalytic Studies in Development*. New York: Jason Aronson, 1975.

Kopp, S. *Mirror, Mask and Shadow: The Risk and Rewards of Self-Acceptance*. New York: Bantam Books, 1982.

Levinson, D. *The Seasons of a Man's Life*. New York: E. P. Dutton, 1974.

Lidz. T. *The Person: His Development Throughout the Life Cycle*. New York: Basic Books, 1968.

Maier, H. (Ed.) *Three Theories of Child Development*. New York: Harper & Row, 1965.

Malmquist, C. P. *Handbook of Adolescence*. New York: Jason Aronson, 1985.

McClelland, D. C., et al. Making It to Maturity. *Psychology Today*, Vol. 12, No. 1 (June, 1978), 42–43, 45–50, 52–53, 114.

Mead, M., & Wolfenstein, M. (Eds.) *Childhood in Contemporary Cultures*. Chicago: University of Chicago Press, 1963.

Menninger Foundation. *Menninger Perspective*, Vol. 16, No. 1 (1985), 5–30.

Murray, R., & Zentner, J. *Nursing Assessment and Health Promotion Through the Life Span*. Englewood Cliffs, N.J.: Prentice-Hall, 1975.

Neill, A. S. *Summerhill*. New York: Hart, 1964.

Papalia, D. E., & Olds, S. W. *Human Development*. New York: McGraw-Hill, 1978.

Peplau, H. Mid-Life Crises. *American Journal of Nursing*, Vol. 75, No. 10 (October, 1975), 1761–1765.

Pontious, S. L. Practical Piaget: Helping Children Understand. *American Journal of Nursing*, Vol. 82, No. 1 (January, 1981), 114–117.

Pressey, S. L., & Kuhlen, R. G. *Psychological Development Through the Life Span*. New York: Harper & Row, 1957.

Richmond, P. G. *An Introduction to Piaget*. New York: Basic Books, 1971.

Roberts, S. L. Piaget's Theory Reapplied to the Critically Ill. *Advances in Nursing Science*, Vol. 2, No. 2 (January, 1980), 61–78.

Roman, M., & Railey, P. E. *The Indelible Family*. New York: Rawson, Waide, 1980.

Rubin, Z. Does Personality Really Change after 20? *Psychology Today*, Vol. 15, No. 5 (May, 1981), 18–24.

Sarnoff, C. *Latency*. New York: Jason Aronson, 1976.

Selekman, J. The Development of Body Image in the Child: A Learned Response. *Topics in Clinical Nursing*, Vol. 5, No. 1 (April, 1983), 12–21.

Sherwen, L. N. Separation: The Forgotten Phenomenon of Child Development. *Topics in Clinical Nursing*, Vol. 5, No. 1 (April, 1983), 1–11.

Spock, B. *Baby and Child Care*. New York: Pocket, 1976.

Streff, M. B. Examining Family Growth and Development: A Theoretical Model. *Advances in Nursing Science*, Vol. 3, No. 4 (July, 1981), 61–69.

Sullivan, H. S. *The Interpersonal Theory of Psychiatry*. H. S. Perry, & M. L. Gowel (Eds.) New York: W. W. Norton, 1954.

Talbot, T. (Ed.) *The World of the Child: Clinical and Cultural Studies from Birth to Adolescence*. New York: Jason Aronson, 1974.

Teung, A. *Growth and Development: A Self-Mastery Approach*. Norwalk, Conn.: Appleton-Century-Crofts, 1982.

Walke, M. A. K. When a Patient Needs to Unburden His Feelings. *American Journal of Nursing*, Vol. 77, No. 7 (July, 1977), 1164–1166.

6

MENTAL MECHANISMS

Automatic Coping Devices

LEARNING OBJECTIVES

On completion of this chapter the reader should be able to:

1. Define the term **mental mechanism.**
2. Explain how a mental mechanism is used.
3. List the purpose and function of each mechanism.
4. Identify and differentiate between each of the mental mechanisms cited.
5. Give an example to illustrate the use of each mechanism.

Mental mechanisms are intrapsychic devices that serve as the first line of ego protection and defense. They are adjustment and coping techniques that provide the individual with a "ready-made" constructive means for maintaining emotional equilibrium. Defense operations are universal. They are used by all people in the conduction of their day-to-day lives and are indispensable to adjustment.

Mental mechanisms are those specific psychological maneuvers existing primarily outside of and beyond conscious awareness. They may be described as stereotyped, repetitive, and rigid means of adaptation, healthy or unhealthy. The primary functions of these coping devices are to: (1) facilitate the resolution of emotional conflict; (2) provide relief from stress; (3) cushion emotional pain; and (4) avoid or alleviate anxiety. In essence, their principal role is to protect and maintain the individual's self-esteem and ego identity from the continuous blows of reality. In other words, use of the defense mechanisms furnishes the individual with a "safety valve," a consciously acceptable outward set of responses that permits the individual to redirect, absorb, or neutralize unbearable internal pressures. Thus, the use of mental mechanisms facilitates acceptable compromise and minimizes self-alienation, producing a state of relative comfort and self-acceptance.

Each psychic distress may activate the use of defense operations. Such activity engenders a discharge of psychic energy. Under normal and usual circumstances, the discharge of psychic energy serves to conserve the individual's time and effort. However, if the demand is too great, that is, if the individual's system experiences overload, then the individual cannot pursue problem-solving and decision-making activity. As a result, the individual is apt to experience self-deception, distortions in reality, interference with interpersonal relationships, limitations in ability to work productively, and increased movement toward ego disintegration. Therefore, excessive reliance on and inappropriate use of these mechanisms may lead to the development of pathological symptomatology within the individual. Assessment of whether or not their presence and use falls within the parameters of normalcy is contingent upon three factors: first, the manner in which they are employed; second, how effective they are in promoting psychological comfort; and third, whether or not their overall use promotes or inhibits the maintenance of psychological integrity and functioning.

In Table 6–1, we identify, define, interpret, and provide examples for some of the more common ego defenses. In studying this chart, the nurse will note that the defense mechanisms tend to overlap and that there is a close interrelationship between them, particularly with regard to purpose and function. The examples used to illustrate each of the mechanisms point out specific instances in which these mechanisms become operational. However, the nurse must keep in mind that in a reality situation, mental mechanisms seldom operate in total isolation, one from another, but rather tend to be used in combination. The outline form of Table 6–1 fulfills a dual purpose. First, it provides the reader with a format that allows for comparison and contrast of distinctive features, particularly in light of the problem of overlap. Second, it provides the reader with an easy, concise, accessible reference to use in nursing practice.

SUMMARY

Through observation of behavior, the nurse becomes aware of the existence of and the manner in which these mechanisms are opera-

TABLE 6–1. THE DEFENSE MECHANISMS

Mechanism	Definition	Interpretation	Examples
Compensation	A mechanism by which the individual seeks to make up for or offset deficiencies, either real or imagined.	It is a disguising mechanism and involves an attempt to meet self-imposed standards, thereby preserving self-respect. It is a means of overcoming failure or frustration in some sphere of activity by over-emphasizing another.	An undersized young man becomes a bantamweight prizefighter. An unattractive and unpopular girl cultivates intellectual abilities and is on the honor roll at school.
Conversion	A mechanism through which elements of intrapsychic conflict are disguised and expressed symbolically through physical symptoms.	It is a symbolic mechanism used to rechannel and externalize unbearable feelings in terms of motor or sensory manifestations.	A young mother, when told she is going to have twins, becomes blind. Mr. Jones develops laryngitis the evening before he is scheduled to give a speech at a business lunch.
Denial	A mechanism by which the ego refuses to perceive or face emotional conflict.	It is an avoidance and protecting mechanism that permits the individual either to disregard or transform the implication or consequences of a thought, act, or situation. It enables the individual to remain unaware of unpleasant reality as if it did not exist.	A patient with a cerebral vascular accident refuses to attend physical therapy, saying, "There's nothing wrong; all I need is rest." A comment often heard from patients in a psychiatric unit: "I have no problem; I don't need to talk with you."
Displacement	A mechanism through which emotional feeling is transferred, deflected, and redirected from one idea, person, or object to another.	It is a mechanism of substitution and redirection that allows an individual to discharge pent-up emotional feelings, particularly hostility, toward a convenient or less threatening target.	The boss berates Mr. Smith for a mistake. That evening Mr. Smith yells at his wife because dinner is 10 minutes late. Jane does not make the cheerleading team at school, and when she comes home tears down all the football posters in her room.
Dissociation	A mechanism through which the effective emotional significance is separated and detached from an idea, situation, object, or relationship.	It is a compartmentalizing mechanism that allows an individual to isolate from awareness those segments of behavior, thoughts, or feelings that generally comprise his normal or usual personality or behavior pattern.	Jim grins and smiles as he relates the details about his automobile accident. Some clinical examples include somnambulism (sleep walking), traumatic amnesia, or fugue states.

(*continued*)

TABLE 6–1. CONTINUED

Mechanism	Definition	Interpretation	Examples
Identification	A mechanism by which an individual patterns himself to resemble the personality and traits of an admired other.	It is a disguising mechanism used as an attempt to preserve the ego ideal. Its use contributes to ego development but does not replace the person's own ego.	An adolescent girl adopts the mannerisms and style of dress of a particular recording star. A young man chooses to become a draftsman just like his father.
Introjection	A mechanism through which loved or hated attitudes, wishes, ideals, values, objects, or persons are symbolically incorporated into self.	It is a denying and disguising mechanism in which the ego structure is changed to keep the individual free from threat.	While playing, 5-year-old Tommy says to his pal Joey, "Don't get dirty; it's not nice." A patient claims to be Jesus Christ.
Projection	A mechanism through which the individual rejects aspects of self by imputing to others motives and emotional feelings that are unacceptable to self.	It is a denying and blaming mechanism in which there is refusal on the part of the individual to acknowledge undesirable or instinctual aspects of self. It is used to protect the ego from experiencing painful emotions and situations and attempts to preserve the individual's sense of harmony with reality.	Archie Bunker calls Edith a "ding bat." A secretary says. "All the girls in the office are jealous of my position and want to take over my job."
Rationalization	A mechanism through which the ego justifies or attempts to modify otherwise unacceptable impulses, needs, feelings, behavior, or motives into those which are consciously tolerable and acceptable.	It is a disguising and self-deceptive mechanism used to increase self-esteem and to obtain and retain social approval and acceptance.	Mrs. Ferris, who can't afford to buy a new dress, says to her friend Stella, "I'd love to have the dress in that window, but I don't think the color suits me." While at a party, Mr. Peters says, "I'll have one more drink. I don't have far to go."

Reaction formation	A mechanism through which an individual assumes attitudes, motives, or needs that are opposite to consciously disowned ones.	It is a disguising and protective mechanism in which emphasis is placed on an opposing attitude, belief, or value in order to prevent the emergence of painful undesirable or unacceptable behavioral responses to an individual or situation.	A young mother who is unaware of her hostile feelings toward her child becomes overprotective toward the child. Mr. Brown is extremely polite and courteous toward his mother-in-law, whom he intensely dislikes.
Regression	A mechanism through which an individual retreats to an earlier and subjectively more comfortable level of adjustment.	It is a denying mechanism that allows the individual to withdraw from reality, resolve conflictual situations, and reduce anxiety by returning to a state in which unmet dependency needs can be handled.	A 4-year-old begins to suck his thumb and wet the bed shortly after the birth of a sibling. Doris, 18, flies into a temper tantrum when she can't have her own way.
Repression	A mechanism in which there is automatic and involuntary submerging of unpleasant or painful thoughts, feelings, and impulses into the unconscious.	It is the primary forgetting and protective mechanism used by the ego to preserve its boundaries. All other mechanisms reinforce it. Repressed material is not subject to conscious recall.	Mr. Willis can't remember attempting to commit suicide. Mary, an unmarried, pregnant 20-year-old, can't remember the name of the baby's father.
Sublimation	A mechanism through which instinctual drives that are consciously intolerable or that are blacked and unattainable are then directed into channels that are personally and socially acceptable.	It is a disguising mechanism that serves to channel libidinal energy into constructive, ego-rewarding activities. It is the most efficient, healthy, and creative of the defensive mechanisms.	A man who has strong competitive or aggressive drives channels his energy into building up a successful business. A young unmarried woman derives satisfaction from taking care of neighborhood children.
Substitution	A mechanism through which a goal, emotion, drive, attitude, or need that is consciously unacceptable is replaced by one that is more acceptable.	It is a replacement mechanism that allows the individual to disguise and divert unobtainable aims into more realistic ones, thereby reducing frustration and promoting satisfaction.	A rejected boyfriend "rushes" into marriage on the rebound. A student who is prevented by a sudden change in family economic status from entering medical school elects to pursue a career in nursing.

(*continued*)

TABLE 6–1. CONTINUED

Mechanism	Definition	Interpretation	Examples
Suppression	A mechanism in which there is a deliberate, intentional exclusion of thoughts, feelings, or experiences from the conscious mind.	It is a voluntary forgetting and postponing mechanism that allows the individual to preserve the status quo and protect self-esteem It is the conscious counterpart of repression and is considered by many not to be a true defense mechanism.	Mr. Gordon carries the bills in his pocket before remembering to mail in the payments. During finals week, Lucy says, "I'll watch just one T.V. program before I study."
Symbolization	A mechanism through which an external object becomes an outward representation of an internal idea, wish, attitude, or feeling.	It is a disguising, compensatory mechanism that is used as a vehicle for emotional self-expression. Generally, it is used as an alternative for verbal expression of a feeling.	Carey remarks to her friend, "You have a heart of gold." A boy sends his girlfriend a dozen red roses.
Undoing	A mechanism through which an individual endeavors to actually or symbolically erase a previous consciously intolerable action or experience.	It is an atoning and restoring mechanism in which the individual attempts to prevent rejection or punishment, thereby alleviating guilt and anxiety.	A mother who has just punished her child unjustly decides to bake the child's favorite cookies. A young woman who possesses strong moral convictions against premarital sex engages in sexual activity with her fiancé. Immediately afterward she visits a church and lights candles.

tional within an individual. Observation and scrutiny of the presenting behavior make the identification of mental mechanisms a reality. In reading and thinking about these examples, it should become apparent to the nurse that the experiences or situations portrayed may reflect parts of her own behavior. This awareness should not be surprising, since the mental mechanisms are the supports of daily functioning that we use to handle stress, crisis, and disturbing human emotions. These mechanisms are vitally important to understand because they do assist us in fostering growth and maturation. In addition, since they are a normal part of our own daily patterns of behavior, understanding their operation can help us as nurses to develop a more perceptive therapeutic self.

SUGGESTED READINGS

Bell, J. M. Stressful Life Events and Coping Methods in Mental-Illness and Wellness Behaviors. *Nursing Research*, Vol. 26, No. 2 (March/April, 1977), 136–140.

Elliott, S. M. Denial as an Effective Mechanism To Allay Anxiety Following a Stressful Event. *Journal of Psychiatric Nursing and Mental Health Services*, Vol. 18, No. 10 (October, 1980), 11–15.

English, S. O., & Pearson, T. H. J. *Emotional Problems of Living*. 3rd ed. New York: W. W. Norton, 1963.

Freud, A. *The Ego and Mechanisms of Defense*. New York: International Universities Press, 1946.

Galeman, D. Positive Denial: The Case for Not Facing Reality. *Psychology Today*, Vol. 13, No. 6 (November, 1979), 44–60.

Garland, L. R. M., & Bush, C. T. *Coping Behaviors and Nursing*. Reston, Va.: Reston, 1982.

Hagerty, B. K. Denial Isn't All Bad. *Nursing '80*, Vol. 10, No. 10 (October, 1980), 58–60.

Laughlin, H. *The Ego and Its Defenses*. New York: Appleton-Century-Crofts, 1970.

Shenfield, M. E. The Developmental Course of Defense Mechanisms in Later Life. *International Journal of Aging and Human Development*, Vol. 19, No. 1 (1984–1985), 55–71.

Tatro, S. E. Regression: A Defense Mechanism For The Dying Older Adult. *Journal of Gerontological Nursing*, Vol. 8, No. 1 (January, 1982), 20–22.

White, R. A., & Gilliland, R. M. *Elements of Psychopathology: The Mechanism of Defense*. New York: Grune & Stratton, 1975.

7

BASIC CONCEPTS

An Overview

LEARNING OBJECTIVES

On completion of this chapter the reader should be able to:

1. Define and distinguish among **anxiety**, **conflict**, **frustration**, and **hostility**.
2. Identify the causes of each of these feeling states.
3. Recognize the resultant physiological, psychological, and behavioral effects of these feelings.

INTRODUCTION

There exists a body of knowledge that lends itself to organization and gives direction to practice. This knowledge is in the form of concepts. A **concept** is the statement of an abstract idea in operation form. A concept is used, in part, to explain behavioral phenomena, to provide structure, and to facilitate the collection of additional data in order to obtain more complete, reliable, and valid information.

We have elected to present and discuss four major concepts that nurses frequently experience within themselves and observe within others. These concepts are anxiety, conflict, frustration, and hostility. Each one embraces affective and situational aspects of functioning that influence equilibrium by either adding to or detracting from a person's perception about self.

These concepts take on significance as the nurse initiates the assessment process. To assist the nurse to understand and identify where a person might be with respect to healthy functioning, we have constructed the schematic representations shown in Figures 7–1 through 7–4. These schematic representations illustrate the concepts as they are said to exist and operate within the individual. We believe that if the nurse is cognizant of how these concepts affect the individual and influence his functioning, she is then in a better position to engage in the interactive–interventive process.

ANXIETY

Anxiety is a feeling state in which the individual experiences a pervasive, occasionally vague, intense sensation of apprehension or impending disaster. As such, it is a universal and unavoidable phenomenon intrinsic to man's existence. Furthermore, anxiety is a form of energy that arises out of an intrapsychic threat to an individual's self-concept and security operations. Its presence can only be inferred from behavior, since it is primarily a subjective and hidden experience.

The sensation of anxiety is felt in varying degrees of intensity. The intensity to which anxiety is experienced is proportionate to the meaning that the anxiety-stimulating situation has for the person concerned. Stated in a different way, this means that as the perceived threat to self is increased, the level of anxiety also intensifies. Thus, as the level of intensity increases, so does the individual's sense of helplessness and defenselessness. Most references indicate that differentiation can be made among at least four levels of anxiety. These are commonly referred to as **mild**, **moderate**, **severe**, and **panic**.

Mild anxiety is a heightened state of alertness and anticipation. It has been found to be a necessary and vital component of daily living. At this level, the individual is receptive and attuned to changing stimuli and is motivated toward engaging in the problem-solving process. Thus, mild anxiety is primarily associated with an expanded ability to perceive and learn. In this instance anxiety acts as an enhancer of effective functioning that allows for variation, accommodation, and increased adaptation to the environment by the individual. Common behavioral indicators said to be representative of mild anxiety include: increased awareness; attending and questioning; restlessness; expanded sensory perception; and the increased use and changing patterns of the automatic behavioral coping mechanisms such as walking, sleeping, eating, smoking, and drinking. Corresponding physiological changes associated with a mild level of anxiety are usually minimal and are rarely perceived by the individual as distressing.

Moderate anxiety is an exaggerated state of alertness and anticipation. Its presence inhibits effective functioning. In the previous paragraph we alluded to the fact that in mild anxiety an individual's ability to focus attention on immediate events is enhanced. This enables the individual to pursue voluntarily and consciously and deal effectively with causative factors involved in anxiety-producing stimuli. In contrast, moderate anxiety reduces the individual's ability to recognize factors influencing his heightened state of apprehension to the extent that he may fail to initiate appropriate problem solving. This disturbance in adaptation occurs as a result of the individual's experiencing a narrowing of his perceptual field and a limitation in his power of concentration. Even though there is a loss of ability to function effectively on his own, the individual retains the ability to attend and expand his perceptual field and operationalize problem-solving behaviors with assistance and direction. Some behavioral indications commensurate with a moderate level of anxiety may include: decreased comprehension; inadequate or incomplete responses; increased muscular tension or tremor; voice tremors or change in pitch or tone; increased rate of verbalization; and alterations in physiological functioning.

Severe anxiety is an extreme, intense sensation of overwhelming discomfort. At this level, the individual displays a marked inability to function. Severe anxiety greatly reduces the individual's perceptual field and cognitive functioning. This interference prevents intake and processing of data that are usually employed in seeking reduction or resolution of stress-producing stimuli. This sensory and cognitive disruption is made evident by either the individual's preoccupation with many extraneous details or his fixation and concentration on one aspect or part of the whole. Because of this deficit in functioning, the individual is unable to pursue problem-solving. Intervention at this level of anxiety mandates that the nurse employ techniques or strategies to reduce the level of anxiety to a more manageable and comfortable state for the client. Observable behavioral indications associated with severe anxiety include: purposeless activity; inappropriate and inconsistent verbal responses; tachycardia and hyperventilation; decreased ability to hear and see; and a marked increase in sensitivity to pain.

Panic is experienced by the individual as a sense of impending doom. In this extreme state, the individual is overwhelmed to the point of immobilization and is subject to a high level of vulnerability; that is, there is a complete loss of control over self and the environment. In panic the individual experiences physiological and psychological shutdown, producing system collapse and ego disintegration. Intervention is imperative, otherwise the client will cease to be. Common manifestations of panic include behaviors that are frantic, desperate, and ineffective. Some observable behavioral indications of a panic state include: complete immobility or severely exaggerated and purposeless activity; complete or nearly complete loss of sensory perception; disregard for environmental hazards; inability to engage in cognitive exercises; or a potential for suicide or homicide.

As anxiety mounts, increased deviance in physical and psychological functioning is noted, together with a decreasing ability to mobilize defenses and coping mechanisms to resolve problems produced by stress. Figure 7–1 portrays the causes that produce the altered feeling state of anxiety, which results in perceived threats to the self-system and biological integrity of the individual. It also indicates how the

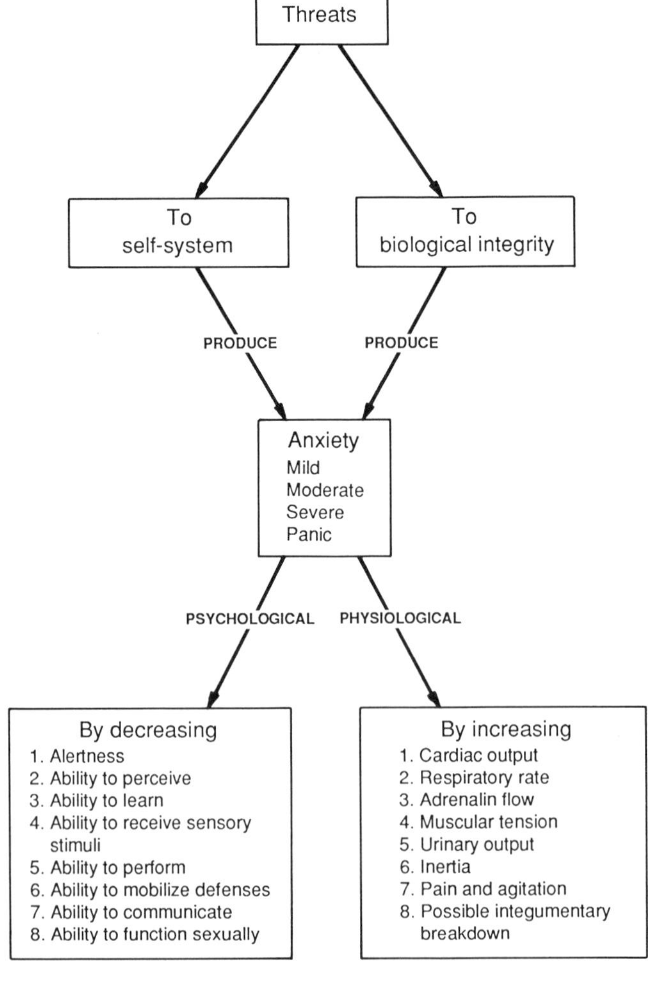

Figure 7–1. Anxiety and Its Consequences

individual responds psychologically and physiologically to the force of anxiety as a mobilizing or immobilizing agent. For further discussion about the concept of anxiety and specific nursing intervention directed toward anxiety reduction and assisting the client to deal with this feeling, the reader is referred to Chapter 21.

CONFLICT

Conflict is a state of disagreement that produces dissatisfaction when a clash between two equally strong and opposing forces occurs. The conflict results in disequilibrium until such time that a satisfactory outcome can be achieved. Conflict is intrapsychic or interpersonal discord. Conflict is tension produced by incompatibility. The incompatibility arises when the individual finds himself in situations that demand definitive action with regard to choice in decision-making. Conflict is competition: competition with self, other people, institutions, organizations, existing value systems, or particular actions or activities that are needed to arrive at a desired goal. Conflict, like many other feelings, behaviors, or thoughts, is not in and of itself necessarily bad. It may even be beneficial in that it prevents the individual or group from stagnation. Conflict can allow for examination of genuine differences in both interests and beliefs, or it can promote change within an individual or system. Furthermore, there appears to be a general consensus regarding the primary factors that seem to be operational in determining the outcome of conflict. These factors include: (1) the issue, (2) power, (3) needs, and (4) communication.

Underlying every conflict is a central issue. The **issue** is the major agenda item around which the conflict revolves. Pinpointing the issue is essential for identifying potential solutions. In effect, identifying the central issue is akin to the first step in the problem-solving process. When the issue remains vague or when there are many focal points, conflict escalates, becomes more complex, or may never be resolved.

The second factor that affects resolution is that of power. **Power** is a mechanism of control influencing human action. It is used to produce an effect—to make a difference. More specifically, it is employed in resource management in order to achieve satisfaction of a desired goal. The resources (such as physical strength, intelligence, emotions, finances, social involvements) can be internal to the self, originate within others, exist within the physical environment, or be part of the sociocultural context of life. In successful resolution of conflict, the power is directed toward the issue and not toward manipulation or coercion of the participants involved in the conflict.

Need is the third factor operational in conflict. By definition, a **need** is a dominant requirement that demands satisfaction in an effort to restore, maintain, or enhance the well-being of an individual, group, or society. In conflict, not only must the predominant need be recognized, but also it must be gratified. If needs are ignored, conflict resolution is inhibited and may result in a negative outcome. Sensitivity and responsivity to the needs of others humanizes the resolution process.

The last factor, **communication**, concerns the type and pattern of dialogue that takes place either on an intrapsychic or interpersonal level. Openness and honesty promote objectivity. Objectivity, in turn, lends clarity to the issue, legitimacy to the power, and provides an opportunity to creatively address and satisfy the presenting need.

Conflict becomes problematic when it prevents the person or group from achieving satisfaction in whatever undertaking is pursued. To date there is no single, universally accepted definition of exactly what conflict is. However, most authorities seem to be in agreement about two facts: first, that conflict is linked to the incompatibility of goals, and second, that it is also linked to the incompatibility of means to attain identified goals.

Although there may not be an exact definition of conflict, much work has been done that focuses on the dynamics associated with this concept. For example, five stages have been identified that enable an individual to analyze the presence of conflict. Stage 1 is evidenced when an individual or group of people is confronted with an issue that demands some decision or action. There are four general characteristics associated with this initial conflict situation in Stage 1. The first of these is what has been termed the **iceberg phenomenon**. It has been identified as the iceberg phenomenon simply because the initial issue is not the real or prevailing problem or concern. What the person or group is trying to cope with lies hidden beneath the surface. The second characteristic is related to a unifying effect that the issue produces within the individual or group. By **unifying effect** is meant the marshalling of forces or resources to cope with the presenting problem. A third characteristic has been termed **rising expectations**. This characteristic begins as movement toward resolution occurs. In terms of conflict resolution, it means that as progression is made toward resolution, the individual or group encounters a whole new set of unanticipated problems or potential conflicts. The fourth characteristic is that the conflict issue may have certain **moral overtones**. This characteristic touches on the very essence of the self in terms of the value systems and beliefs held by the individual or group and lends justification and legitimacy to a given course of action.

In Stage 2 the individual or group begins to explore the circumstances around which the conflict has developed. It is essentially a data-gathering state that leads to the refinement and clarification of the issue(s). Stage 3 occurs when the intensity of the tension increases to the point where decision-making is obviously needed and the call for action is demanded. In this third stage the original issue itself becomes overwhelmingly dominant. Its dominance increases the internal intrapsychic or group momentum. Elements of aggression are discerned, alternatives are sought, consequences evaluated, compromises emerge, and in this process the issue achieves significant polarization.

Stage 4 evidences the cyclical nature of conflict. This means that after polarization occurs, it seems that either the individual or group finds it necessary to maintain that high intensity of feeling initially demonstrated toward the polarized issue; then the original issue is looked at again and becomes generalized once more. In the last stage resolution is achieved.

In summary, conflict may be defined as any or all kinds of opposite, competitive, or antagonistic interaction. It occurs and is based on scarcity of power, resources, social position, or differing value structures. Resolution is mandated because if the conflict situation is left alone, the conflict itself may grow larger and become more serious, resulting in increasing dysfunction and discomfort for the person or the group. Conflict involves effective communication. Conflict often can be prevented by communication that is open and free-flowing, that is, communication in which barriers and misunderstandings have been reduced. Resolution involves a willingness to listen, to share, and to examine all relevant data surrounding the issue in question. Figure 7–2 is a schematic representation of the dysfunctional outcome of conflict where satisfactory resolution has not been achieved.

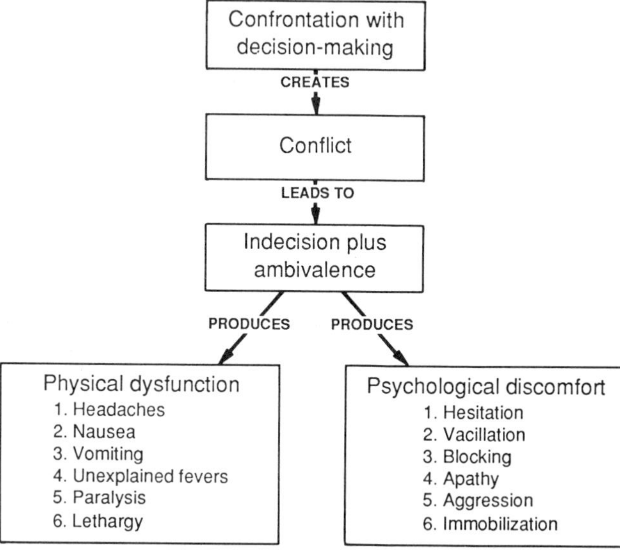

Figure 7–2. Dynamics of Unresolved Conflict

FRUSTRATION

Frustration is a feeling state in which the individual experiences interference in the ability to achieve a specific goal, attain satisfaction of a need, or solve a problem. It is a threat to the individual's feelings of adequacy and security. It is felt as a loss of ability to control self, others, or the environment. As such, it is a universally common and almost inevitable outcome associated with routine events of daily living. Frustration is a primitive feeling that is negatively charged. This means that the discharge of energy usually evokes a display of aggressive behavior. It has been identified as the first emotional component that triggers anger and subsequent rage.

Frustration can be experienced in varying degrees of intensity from minor to major and tends to be cumulative in its effects. **Minor frustration** is identified as an irritation or pinprick that occurs as a normal part of everyday living. Some examples of minor frustration commonly experienced by each of us at one time or another might be: encountering heavier than usual traffic just when rushing to keep a scheduled appointment; getting a run in a new pair of hose, your last pair, while dressing to go out for the evening; or just having your car washed when it rains. These types of experiences arouse sensations that range from annoyance to outright anger. The intensity of the feeling engendered by the experience is governed by the importance the obstruction encountered has with respect to the desired goal. **Major frustration** usually is felt as and equated with disruptive events that dramatically affect or alter the individual's pattern of life. These alterations may be experienced as changes in behavior, values, beliefs, moods, attitudes, and general outlook on life. Examples used to demonstrate this heightened level of frustration might include: economic reversals that prevent continued pursuit of a desired career choice; burnout in a work-related situation; or inability of a community health worker to provide identified needed human services because of budgetary constraints within the agency.

As mentioned previously, frustrations tend to be cumulative in effect. Each succeeding experience leading to frustration tends to take on additional significance so that the energy level begins to build. Once the pressure of this pent-up energy reaches a point where it can no longer be contained, termination results in an explosive incident. Triggering of this explosion is usually activated by a seemingly trivial event—like the straw that broke the camel's back.

All frustration may not be detrimental. In some cases minimal frustration, like mild anxiety, may serve to build tension that can be used by the individual to facilitate goal attainment. The increased tension level produced by the frustration allows the individual to focus his attention more firmly on a particular goal. Consequently, irrelevant and distracting data are pushed into the background along with lesser or secondary goals. Thus, the individual is able to experience intensified striving toward his ultimate aim.

The sources of frustration are not the goal, need, or problem per se, but rather the barriers encountered by the individual. These barriers may be either internal or external. **Internal barriers** include the individual's personality characteristics or specific ego strengths and weaknesses, the lack of specific coping abilities, or the inability to manipulate the number of available alternatives. **External barriers** would include such factors as environmental or situational conditions, overriding authority imposed by others, or the exigencies imposed by a specific system of operation. Hence, all people experience "frustrating situations" as a part of daily life. During such situations the individual is generally aware of other feelings that are the effect of the frustration. Unlike severe anxiety, frustration can allow the individual to utilize his abilities to select one or more alternative choices of action when the person has problem-solving skills and uses these skills as impetus for change. In some instances, we see individuals who choose to procrastinate rather than make definitive choices to resolve the sources of frustration. In other instances, we see individuals who respond to frustration by engaging in aggressive acting out, either verbally or physically.

Each individual reacts to frustration in his own unique, inimicable way, according to learned patterns of behavior established in early childhood. Therefore, reactions to frustration vary from one individual to another, although they usually involve either aggressive or withdrawn behavior. Feelings engendered by frustration include fear, anger, anxiety, hate, resentment, or disappointment. These feelings may occur separately or in any combination. Both the behavior displayed and the emotions evoked by frustration are influenced by the significance of the identified goal and by the ability of the individual to cope with and adapt to interference with goal attainment. In Figure 7–3, we have portrayed the major sources and obstacles associated with the concept of frustration.

HOSTILITY

Hostility is a feeling state in which the individual, consciously or unconsciously, experiences a sense of helplessness or hopelessness with persons or objects and directs negative attitudes or actions toward them. Hostility is equated with enmity, that is, it is open antagonism directed against one or many individuals. It is generally considered to be a long-lasting, pervasive, affective response and motivating force, which, once established, tends to persist without the need of repeated

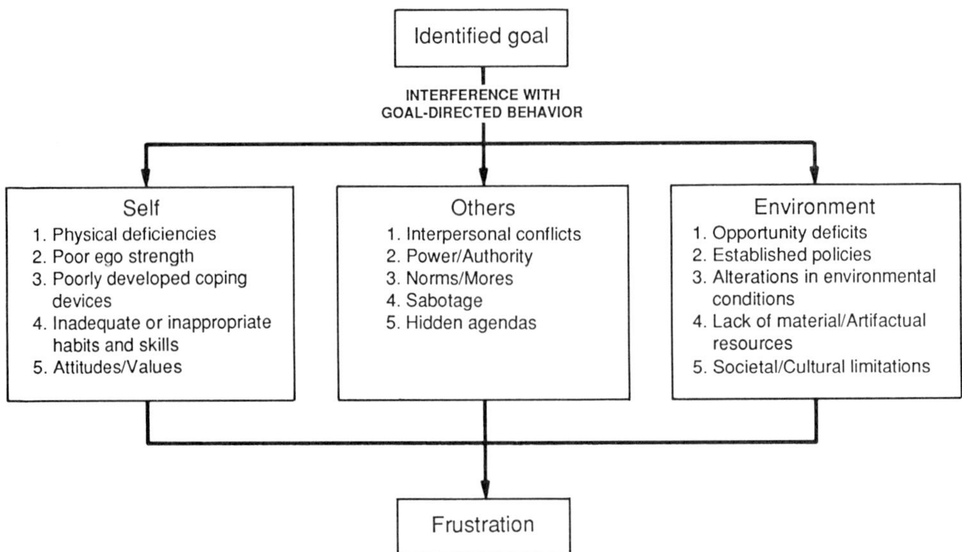

Figure 7–3. Development of Frustration

stimulus reinforcement. Figure 7–4 schematically shows the basic construct of hostility, its causes, resultant feelings, and expressions of overt and covert behaviors, as well as the source and direction of the hostility.

Hostility is always destructive in intent and accompanied by an intense feeling of anger. Hostility directed against the self inflicts pain on the individual and on significant others, but may not necessarily distress society at large. However, when hostility is expressed in the form of direct acting-out behavior, it has societal impact in that it generates violence, crime, and senseless destruction. Hostility, like anxiety, can be transmitted from one person to another, one group to another, one generation to another. Hostility has its seat in disturbances encountered and inadequately resolved within the normal maturation process. In effect, hostility is the result of repeated frustrations during which the individual experiences intensified feelings of inadequacy, inferiority, and the belief that he is being used. Such intensified experiences result in clearly defined acting out as well as in covert signs of negativism. Like anxiety, conflict, and frustration, hostility is experienced in varying degrees of intensity and produces a wide range of behaviors. As a feeling state, it is one of the most prevalent and diffuse of human emotions.

Overt hostility is an open manifestation of attack behavior. As such, it is one of the easiest of human emotions to observe, identify, and handle with the individual. It may be demonstrated by verbal, physical, or attitudinal expressions or actions. Some behaviors that typify overt hostility include, insults, intimidation, abusive language, discrimination, rioting, and suicide or homicide.

Covert hostility is a subtle, hidden form of attack behavior. As

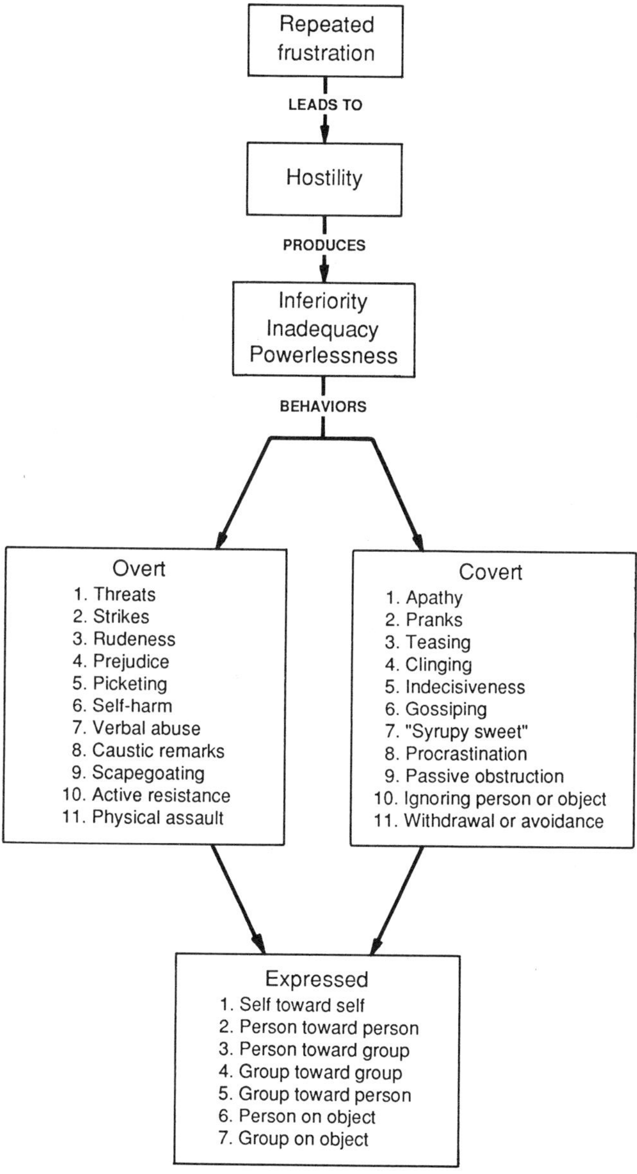

Figure 7–4. The Dynamics of Hostility

such, it is a much less easily discernible and recognizable manifestation, since its presence is often masked by apparent friendliness, joviality, or witticisms which tend to make the listener or the recipient uncomfortable without their fully realizing the source of the discomfort. Behaviors that exemplify the subtleness with which covert hostility can be and usually is expressed include self-deprecating joking, teasing, forgetting and blocking, sexism, racism, or paternalism.

SUMMARY

In the above discussion we have pointed out that each of these concepts—anxiety, conflict, frustration, and hostility—is recognized as a universal phenomenon experienced by both individuals and groups. Of these four, hostility stands alone as the most destructive and disruptive, since it alone does not have potential for altering and motivating the individual or group toward goal attainment and satisfaction. Knowledge of cause, effect, and outcome will enable the nurse to recognize the presence of these feeling states and thereby participate more skillfully with the client in the interactive–interventive process.

SUGGESTED READINGS

Burd, S. F., & Marshall, M. A. *Some Clinical Approaches To Psychiatric Nursing*. New York: Macmillan, 1963.

Burrows, G. D., & Davies, B. (Eds.) *Handbook of Studies on Anxiety*. Amsterdam: Elsevier/North Holland Biomedical Press, 1980.

Cooper, J. Conflict: How To Avoid It and What To Do When You Can't. *Nursing '79*, Vol. 9, No. 1 (January, 1979), 89–91.

DiFabio, S. Nurses' Reactions to Restraining Patients. *American Journal of Nursing*, Vol. 81, No. 5 (May, 1981), 973–975.

Fishman, S. M., & Sheehan, D. V. Anxiety and Panic: Their Cause and Treatment. *Psychology Today*, Vol. 19, No. 4 (April, 1985), 26–32.

Flynn, G. E. Hostility in a Mad, Mad World. *Perspectives in Psychiatric Care*, Vol. 7, No. 4 (1969), 152–158.

Harmin, M . *Better Than Aspirin: How To Get Rid of Emotions That Give You a Pain in the Neck*. Niles, Ill.: Argus Communications, 1976.

Kerr, N. J. Anxiety: Theoretical Considerations. *Perspectives in Psychiatric Care*, Vol. 16, No. 1 (January/February, 1978), 36–40, 46.

Kielinen, C. E. Conflict Resolution: Communication—Good; Withdrawal—Bad. *Journal of Nursing Education*, Vol. 17, No. 5 (May, 1978), 12–15.

Kiening, Sister M. M. Hostility. In Behavioral Concepts and Nursing Intervention, 2nd ed. C. E. Carlson & B. Blackwell (Eds.) Philadelphia: Lippincott, 1978.

Kimmel, M. E. The Age of Anxiety: General Societal Impact and Particular Effects on Criminality. *Journal of Psychiatric Nursing and Mental Health Services*, Vol. 15, No. 11 (November, 1977), 27–30.
Klein, D. F., & Rabkin, J. G. (Eds.) *Anxiety: New Research and Changing Concepts*. New York: Raven Press, 1981.
Knowles, R. D. Handling Depression by Identifying Anger. *American Journal of Nursing*, Vol. 81, No. 5 (May, 1981), 968.
Knowles, R. D. Managing Anxiety. *American Journal of Nursing*, Vol. 81, No. 1 (January, 1981), 110–111.
Kristic, J. Anxiety Levels of Hospitalized Psychiatric Patients throughout Total Hospitalization. *Journal of Psychiatric Nursing and Mental Health Services*, Vol. 17, No. 7 (July, 1979), 33–42.
Lanza, M. L. Origins of Aggression. *Journal of Psychosocial Nursing and Mental Health Services*, Vol. 21, No. 6 (June, 1983), 11–16.
Leininger, M. M. Conflict and Conflict Resolutions: Theories and Processes Relevant to the Health Professions. *American Nurse*, Vol. 6 (December, 1974), 17–22.
Madow, L., MD. *Anger*. New York: Charles Scribner's Sons, 1972.
Mariano, C. The Dynamnics of Conflict. *Journal of Nursing Education*, Vol. 17, No. 5 (May, 1978), 7–11.
May, R. *The Meaning of Anxiety*. New York: Ronald Press, 1950.
Meissner, J. E. Semantic Differential Scales for Assessing Patient's Feelings. *Nursing '80*, Vol. 10, No. 2 (February, 1980), 70–71.
Mortiz, D. A. Understanding Anger. *American Journal of Nursing*, Vol. 78, No. 1 (January, 1978), 81–83.
Penningrath, P. E. Control of Violence in a Mental Health Setting. *American Journal of Nursing*, Vol. 75, No. 4 (April, 1975), 606–609.
Rickels, N. K., & Finkle, B. C. Anxiety: Yours and Your Patients'. *Nursing '73*, Vol. 3, No. 3 (March, 1973), 23–26.
Saul, L. J., Wrobel B. *Psychodynamics of Hostility*. New York: Jason Aronson, 1976.
Schwartzman, S. T. Anxiety and Depression in the Stroke Patient: A Nursing Challenge. *Journal of Psychiatric Nursing and Mental Health Services*, Vol. 14, No. 7 (July, 1978), 13–17.
Sobel, D. E. Human Violence. *American Journal of Nursing*, Vol. 76, No. 1 (January, 1976), 69–72.
Stearns, F. R. *Anger: Psychology, Physiology, Pathology*. Springfield, Ill.: Cha. C Thomas, 1972.
Tavris, C. Feeling Angry? Letting Off steam May Not Help. *Nursing Life*, Vol. 4, No. 5 (September/October, 1984), 58–61.
Topper, V. O. Improving Your Laugh Life. *Nursing Life*, Vol. 5, No. 2 (March/April, 1985), 58–61.
Veninga, R. Defensive Behavior: Causes, Effects and Cures. *Nursing Digest*, Vol. 3, No. 3 (May/June, 1975), 58–59.
Walker, C. E. *Learn To Relax*. Englewood Cliffs, N.J.: Prentice-Hall, 1975.
Watson, J. The Quasi-Rational Element in Conflict: A Review of Selected Conflict Literature. *Nursing Research*, Vol. 25, No. 1 (January/February, 1976), 19–23.

8

STRESS AND CRISIS IN LIVING

Definition and Dynamics

LEARNING OBJECTIVES

On completion of this chapter the reader should be able to:

1. Define **stressor**, **stress**, and **crisis**.
2. Describe the concept of stress as a universal phenomenon.
3. Discuss the effects of stress.
4. Identify the three stages of the stress syndrome.
5. Distinguish between stress and crisis.
6. Differentiate between predictable and unpredictable crisis.
7. Discuss the part stress and crisis play in the developmental process.
8. Identify nursing care goals for clients experiencing stress or crisis.

INTRODUCTION

Stress and **crisis** are phenomena encountered by all living organisms. The entire process of growth and development is a progressive series of adaptations in which stress plays a significant role. Throughout the life span there are periods of heightened growth and activity followed by periods of rest and integration. This pattern becomes visible at birth, continues throughout one's life span, and terminates only in death.

Therefore, in developing an understanding of people as living, growing, maturing, and whole beings, the nurse must know the part these two phenomena play within the total construct of a person's development. Both or either can and do shape life. Stress or crisis can lead to a person's fulfillment or to stagnation and breakdown. The choice of direction is governed by the adaptive responses employed. If the management strategies bring about reduction, resolution, or solution, the amount of adaptive energy is used constructively, and equilibrium is restored. If the individual fails to acknowledge the presence of a stressor and, consequently, makes no conscious effort to ameliorate the effects, the adaptive energy required to maintain the integrity of the system is expended fruitlessly.

STRESS

Living organisms are subjected to a multitude of stimuli that prompt reactions. These stimuli are called **stressors** and the resultant effect is **stress**. A stressor, then, is any agent, condition, situation, goal, feeling, thought, or behavior that demands an increase in vital activity within the autonomic or central nervous system of the individual.

Stressors create pressure. The pressure varies in degree of intensity and kind. There is pressure to mature, to choose, to learn, to develop skills, to perform, to love, to share, to develop values, and to make judgments or decisions. Pressure produces strain. Strain can be equated to stress. For example, stress may be akin to an automobile an individual maneuvers throughout his life; the gas pedal and the brake are analogous to the individual's coping devices. The amount of perceived or real pressure causes the individual to manipulate the gas pedal and the brake. The degree to which the automobile gets out of control is the difference between function and dysfunction.

In addition to the concept of stress as a result of pressure or force, it can also be viewed as a mismatch between the person and his environment. When environmental demands are such that they tax or exceed the adaptive capacities or resources of the individual, or when environmental opportunities constrain or inhibit satisfaction of individual needs, the effect produced is stress.

Stress produces change. The change that results involves the entire organism. It is a complex phenomena that recognizes the interplay and relationship between body and mind. The change may be either healthy and useful or unhealthy and destructive. Healthy change responses facilitate tension reduction and lead to personal growth. This maturational outcome fosters the development of an increased capacity for more flexible, adaptive responses and the potential for identifying additional alternatives. The unhealthy and destructive effects of stress lead to change that is maladaptive. Maladaption prevents stress reduction. Moreover, maladaptive responses may be irreversible. Reversability depends on the degree of damage sustained.

The response to felt stress was first identified by Selye, who named it the **stress syndrome** or the **general adaptation syndrome**. This syndrome is divided into three stages: alarm reaction, resistance, and exhaustion. In the first stage, **alarm reaction**, physiological and psychosocial defensive forces and operations are mobilized for action. The second stage, **resistance**, is the use of these defenses to deal with the felt stress. This stage begins when the immediate, mobilized defenses fail to alleviate the stressor. It continues over an extended period of time during which the person attempts to coexist through adaptation with the stressor and the resultant stress. The third and final stage, **exhaustion**, is the aftermath of coping. It is during this stage that the person displays a marked diminution in ability to continue adaptation and begins to manifest a need for rest, recuperation, and integration. If this need is not met, death results. The general adaptation syndrome applies to each and every encounter in which stress is experienced. Thus, the phenomenological pattern of response remains constant, although the specific outcome differs according to the individual's ability to manage the stress.

A diversity of complex human responses to stress have been reported in the literature. These responses or effects can be categorized under five major headings: physiological, social, affective, behavioral, and cognitive. Table 8–1 contains a partial listing of those effects that have been identified as manifestations of stress.

In addition to the various effects cited in Table 8–1, there is research evidence to support the concept that the prolongation of stress over time can and does produce significant physiological or psychosocial changes that lead to a disruption in homeostasis. This imbalance in the internal environment results in the development of specific symptoms, syndromes, and identifiable disease entities. Included in this group of maladaptive responses are amenorrhea, bronchial asthma, chest and back pain, coronary heart disease, diarrhea, frequent urination, dyspepsia, faintness and dizziness, headaches and migraines, sexual dysfunction, anxiety reactions, psychotic reactions, somatiform disorders, insomnia, skin rashes, ulcers, and generalized weakness.

Since confrontation with any alteration in living has potential for being designated as a stressor and consequently creating a stressful situation, stress avoidance is an impossible task. Thus, the nurse's main purpose in designing effective intervention is not directed toward eradication of stress, but rather toward assisting the client to attain tranquility and, if possible, reducing the number of stressors.

TABLE 8–1. MANIFESTATIONS OF STRESS

Physiological	Social	Affective
Difficulty breathing	Absenteeism	Anxiety
Dilation of pupils	Antagonism	Apathy
Dryness of the mouth	Dependency	Aggression
Hot and cold spells	Disorganization	Boredom
Increased blood and urine catecholamines and corticosteroids	Job dissatisfaction	Frustration
Increased blood glucose levels	Decreased work productivity	Irritability
Increased heart rate and blood pressure	Frequent job changes	Lability of mood
Numbness and tingling in extremities	Decreased or ineffective communication	Worthlessness
Loss of appetite	Interpersonal distancing	Depression
Muscular tension	Limited group involvement	Loneliness
		Guilt
		Shame

Behavioral	Cognitive
Fatigue	Indecision
Violence	Obsession
Negativism	Impaired memory, perception, concentration, and judgment
Excitation	Diminished imagination, incentive, and creativeness
Disorganization	Loss of objectivity
Restlessness	Mental blocks
Nonproductiveness	Denial or rejection of criticism
Tremulousness	
Compulsiveness	
Impulsiveness	
Substance abuse	
Accident proneness	
Impaired speech	
Nervous laughter	
Giggling	
Overeating	

That is, the nurse helps the client learn to recognize potential stress events, to accept those events as a reality in living, and to live within that reality with the least amount of trauma and residual dysfunction possible. This latter aspect is accomplished through the educational process, in which the nurse teaches effective coping skills used in stress management, such as relaxation exercises and biofeedback techniques.

In summary, stress is a persistent and pervasive problem in our society. The intensity and duration of the stress may seriously disrupt and alter homeostasis. Restoration of equilibrium requires adaptation. Stress management is the search for tranquility in an era of disruption and disquietude and, as such, presents a challenge to nursing ingenuity. Since response to stress is unique, the nurse must keep in mind that the nature of the client's response pattern determines the nature and direction of the intervention.

CRISIS

Crisis is a form of severe stress that is perceived and interpreted by the individual as traumatic. A crisis is a reaction to a life problem for which an individual's primary and secondary coping mechanisms fail to bring about successful adaptation and hence resolution of the problem. **Primary coping mechanisms** refer to those patterns of response that have been used by the person to protect and maintain equilibrium. They are habitual, adjustive, learned strategies that have, when used, allowed the individual to experience relief. **Secondary coping mechanisms** are those coping strategies that have not had a usual and customary place in the individual's life style. Secondary coping mechanisms arise through the innovative and creative manipulation of alternatives and are employed when the primary coping mechanisms fail to achieve resolution.

Crisis differs from stress in that it is time-limited (usually no longer than 6 weeks) and is precipitated by new or sudden situations. It usually stems from two major sources: first, a stressful event involving a fundamental loss or deprivation that is perceived as threatening to the individual's self-concept and personal integrity; and second, a crushing threat, either real or imagined, to the physical or psychological well-being of the person. Crisis leaves the individual with an overwhelming feeling of devastation and futility. In other words, the individual finds himself in a state of disequilibrium. Thus, during crisis the individual frequently loses his ability to mobilize his capacity to resolve problems and seek alternative measures. This immobilization can be a temporary loss or a more pronounced dysfunction lasting for the duration of the crisis.

A state of crisis is said to exist when the assessment of the life event and the individual's response to it reveal the following characteristics. First, the individual displays many of the usual symptoms associated with stress. In effect, there are significant disruptions in the person's affective, cognitive, behavorial, social, and physiological responses. These disruptions produce a sense of extreme discomfort. Second, the attitude exhibited is one of defeat. This attitude is made known through subjective statements that convey a sense of total inadequacy, helplessness, and hopelessness. The individual portrays to the observer a picture of complete disorganization. Third, the individual's behavior corresponds with the expressed and demonstrated attitudes and feelings. The two most prevalent behaviors displayed are agitation and withdrawal. The agitation is revealed through the nonproductive activity used in the attempt to discharge the extreme tension. For example, an individual might drive too fast and ignore all precautionary, safety rules and regulations; act out aggressively, usually physically, with limited or no provocation; engage in futile, repetitive action such as pacing; or resort to the ingestion of substances such as alcohol or drugs. Withdrawal, a retreat from the felt pain, is manifested as social isolation. For example, the person may resort to sitting and staring off into space; sleeping for long periods; or losing consciousness via a drunken stupor.

Crisis can be divided into two major types, predictable and unpredictable. In the literature, terms synonymous with predictable crisis include **maturational**, **developmental**, and **internal**, while those applied to unpredictable crisis are **situational**, **accidental**, or **external**. **Predictable crises** are those that have been identified as commonly occurring in the lives of all people and, as such, are viewed as universal stressors. **Unpredictable crises** are those triggered by unexpected traumatic events over which people have little or no control.

Predictable crises occur as an individual moves and progresses through the developmental and maturational process, since these periods of growth produce biological and social role transformation. Some examples of predictable crises are the moment of birth, entering school, adolescence, marriage, menopause, and retirement. During this type of crisis, the individual experiences a period of internal disequilibrium and disorganized behavior concomitant with cognitive and affective disruptions that may have an adverse effect on roles and relationships. The onset is gradual as the individual moves through a period of change or transition. Mood swings, as well as variations in the person's usual pattern of behavior, especially with respect to roles and relationships, occur through this period of internal disequilibrium. Resolution is also gradual as the individual begins to experiment with new feelings, roles, and behaviors in his search for a comfortable fit until he arrives at a new level of mastery and maturity.

If the individual is not able to experience or achieve successful adaptation, negative resolution or maladaption results, giving rise to a developmental lag or symptom formation.

In contrast, unpredictable crises are unanticipated, hazardous life events. These situational crises surface when an individual is confronted with a sudden disruptive life experience that can arise from within the self, the family, or the environment. The outcome is a traumatic interruption in the person's pattern of living that thrusts him precipitously into a state of disequilibrium, disorganization, and chaos, thus leaving him totally unprepared to deal effectively with the disruptive event. Some situations that might occur in an individual's life experience and give rise to an unpredictable crisis are sudden illness, loss of a job, loss of a loved one, separation or divorce, severe financial reversals, change in body image because of an accident, abortion, and rape. Figure 8–1 is a schematic representation tracing the onset of trauma and responses that lead to crisis. This illustration summarizes for the reader the concept of crisis.

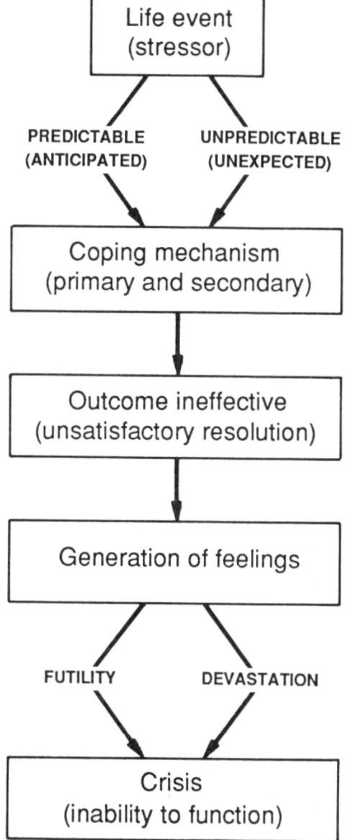

Figure 8–1. Onset and Development of Crisis

NURSING IMPLICATIONS

In stress management, nursing intervention is directed toward three levels of preventative care: primary, secondary, and tertiary. In **primary preventative care** intervention is aimed at the continuation and maintenance of wellness; nursing activity is essentially educational in nature. There are three aspects to this interventive approach. First, the nurse can teach the client to recognize potential stressors and therefore to anticipate the presence of stress. Second, the nurse can teach the client specific coping skills, such as decision-making, problem-solving, and assertiveness, which he can use to reduce the impact of stress. And, finally, the nurse can educate the client to recognize the need to redesign or change the physical, interpersonal, biological, and mental–emotional environments of his day-to-day living situation, thereby reducing the number of stressors.

In **secondary preventative care**, the nurse's intervention involves assisting the client to recognize typical response patterns and accompanying feelings. Once these are recognized, the nurse can then move to helping the client identify what alterations or adaptations may be needed in his life or within himself to increase or enhance his present coping devices as well as his feelings of satisfaction and well-being. The goal of this interventive endeavor is stabilization and promotion of equilibrium so that the stress response remains under the control of the individual.

Tertiary preventative care requires that the nurse direct her energies toward helping the client to modify existing adaptive responses that have become ineffective in coping with the stress or developing new ways of dealing with stress. The aim of intervention is to create a substantial reduction in maladaptive response patterns, while at the same time preserving and fostering the client's self-esteem and self-worth.

In implementing the nursing process in crisis intervention, the nurse must keep in mind that although crisis events demonstrate a certain amount of commonality, regardless of type or source, recognition of individual uniqueness is paramount. This means that the client and his predicament must be viewed within a broad contextual framework. For intervention to be effective and have relevance for the client, the nurse has to be aware that the meaning and interpretation of situations vary according to the individual's perception, intellectual ability and functioning, values, beliefs, and attitudinal sets as well as sociocultural and economic status. Once awareness of individuality is acknowledged, the nurse is in a position to engage the client in assessing the particular reactions surrounding the event and in exploring potential support systems available and acceptable to him. It is critical to effectiveness that the nurse direct interventive efforts toward maintaining a practical, reality-oriented approach in dealing with the here and now. This is important since the nurse's primary purpose is to aid the individual in coping with the critical life problem in some positive way. To achieve this outcome, the nurse presents to the client a view of therapeutic self, portraying sympathetic and empathetic attention by employing active listening, offering support and providing useful information. Not only does the nurse place emphasis on effecting resolution of the immediate crisis, she also makes use of this opportunity to engage the client in educational activity aimed toward improvement of or making additions to his repertoire of coping skills. It should be noted that crisis cannot be eliminated, but its frequency and severity can be reduced. Therefore, in assisting the client in crisis, the key therapeutic issues are prevention of breakdown and the restoration of tranquility.

Stress management and crisis intervention are significant issues in practice, since both stress and crisis are common, recurring human phenomena. For specific interventive strategies, the reader is directed to Chapter 23.

SUMMARY

Stressors are encountered in all aspects of living throughout the life span. Stress and crisis are response phenomena to stressors. Both phenomena can produce alterations in and interruption of a person's usual pattern of living. The outcome depends primarily on the adaptive responses the individual is able to employ. The goal of nursing intervention is fourfold: reduction, as far as possible, of the number of stressors encountered; amelioration of the effects, that is, the impact; restoration of equilibrium; and nurturance of growth potential.

SUGGESTED READINGS

Aguilera D. C., & Messick, J. M. *Crisis Intervention: Theory and Methodology*, 4th ed. St. Louis: C. V. Mosby, 1982.

Brownell, M. Jr. The Concept of Crisis: Its Utility for Nursing. *Advances in Nursing Science*, Vol. 6, No. 4 (July, 1984), 10–21.

Campbell, F. & Singer, G. *Stress, Drugs and Health: Recent Brain-Behavior Research*. Sydney: Pergamon, 1983.

Clark, T. P. Counseling Victims of Rape. *American Journal of Nursing*, Vol. 76, No. 12 (December, 1976), 1964–1966.

Cooper, C. L. (Ed.). *Stress Research: Issues for the Eighties*. Chichester: Wiley, 1983.

Copp, L. A. Research About Stress—Stress About Research. *In Responding to Stress: Community Mental Health in the 80's*. New York: National League for Nursing, Pub. No. 52-1870, 1981, 31–39.

Cox, T. *Stress*. Baltimore: University Park Press, 1978.

Dohrenwend, B. S., & Dohrenwend, B. P. (Eds.). *Stressful Life Events: Their Nature and Effects*. New York: Wiley, 1974.

Friedman, M., & Rosenman, R. H. *Type A Behavior and Your Heart*. New York: Fawcett Publications, 1971.

Garfield, C. A. (Ed.). *Stress and Survival: The Emotional Realities of Life-Threatening Illness*. St. Louis: C. V. Mosby, 1979.

Geissler, E. M. Crisis: What It Is and Is Not. *Advances in Nursing Sciences*, Vol. 6, No. 4 (July, 1984), 1–9.

Graber, R. F. When Divorce Crisis Is the Diagnosis. *The Journal of Practical Family Medicine*, Vol. 11, No. 6 (March 15, 1977), 90–91, 95–123.

Greer, F. L. Toward a Developmental View of Adult Crises: A Re-Examination of Crisis Theory. *Journal of Humanistic Psychology*, Vol. 20, No. 4 (Fall, 1980), 17–27.

Hargreaves, A. G. Coping with Disaster. *American Journal of Nursing*, Vol. 80, No. 4 (April, 1980), 683.

Hoff, L. A. *People in Crises: Understanding and Helping*. Menlo Park, Calif.: Addison-Wesley, 1978.

Hyman, R. B., & Wong, P. Stressful Life Events and Illness Onset. *Research in Nursing and Health*, Vol. 5, No. 3 (September, 1982), 155–163.

Infante, M. S. (Ed.). *Crisis Theory: A Framework for Nursing Practice*. Reston, Va.: Reston, 1982.

Kaplan, H. B. (Ed.). *Psychosocial Stress: Trends in Theory and Research*. New York: Academic Press, 1983.

Kutash, I. L., Schlesinger, L. B., et al. *Handbook on Stress and Anxiety*. San Francisco: Jossey-Bass, 1980.

McCamy, J. C., & Presley, J. *Human Life Styling: Keeping Whole in the 20th Century*. New York: Harper & Row, 1975.

McQuade, W., & Aikman, A. *Stress: What It is, What It Can Do To Your Health, How To Fight Back*. New York: Bantam Books, Inc., 1975.

Murphy, S. A. After Mount St. Helens Disaster Stress Research. *Journal of Psychosocial Nursing and Mental Health Services*, Vol. 22, No. 7 (July, 1984), 9–18.

O'Flynn-Comiskey, A. I. Stress, the Type A Individual. *American Journal of Nursing*, Vol. 79, No. 11 (November, 1979), 1956–57.

Ohio Symposium on Stress Management. *Proceedings of the First and Second Symposia, 1978–1980*. Columbus, Ohio: Ohio Psychology Publishing, 1981.

Palmer, F. B. Adolescent Perception of Stressful Life Events. *Responding to Stress: Community Mental Health in the 80's*. New York: National League for Nursing, Pub. No. 52-1870, 1981, 38–53.

Reichie, M. J. Psychological Stress in the Intensive Care Unit. *Nursing Digest*, Vol. 3, No. 3 (May/June, 1975), 12–15.

Saranson, I. G., & Spielberger, C. D. *Stress and Anxiety*, Vols. I and II. Washington, D.C.: Hemisphere Corp., 1975.

Selye, H. *Stress Without Distress*. Philadelphia: J. B. Lippincott Co., 1974.

Selye, H. *The Stress of Life*. Rev. ed. New York: McGraw-Hill, 1978.

Sheehy, G. *Passages: Predictable Crisis of Adult Life*. New York: E. P. Dutton, 1974.

Sifneos, P. E. *Short-Term Psychotherapy and Emotional Crisis*. Cambridge, Mass.: Harvard University Press, 1972.

Simmons, S. Stress During the Mid-Life Years. *Responding to Stress: Community Mental Health in the 80's*. New York: National League for Nursing, Pub. No. 52-1870, 1981, 24–30.

Stephenson, C. A. Stress in Critically Ill Patients. *American Journal of Nursing*, Vol. 77, No. 11 (November, 1977), 1806–1809.

9

INTERPERSONAL RELATIONSHIPS

A Frame of Reference

LEARNING OBJECTIVES

On completion of this chapter the reader should be able to:

1. Define **individual** and **group interpersonal relationships**.
2. Differentiate between individual and group relationships.
3. Explain individual and group relationships within the context of the process of human development.

INTRODUCTION

If one holds the belief that a person is a social being, then it becomes quite evident that it is necessary to address the types and kinds of relationships that exist between and among people. The concept of the person as a social being clearly points to the fact that people *need* people. Relationships, then, are both an expression of this need and a means for gratification of this need.

Viewed from a slightly different perspective, human relationships are essential for survival and provide the means of maintaining a satisfying life. From birth to death, people are engaged in relationships with few or many in order to meet physical, psychological, spiritual, and sociocultural needs. Human transactions provide opportunities for personal growth, increase confidence through self-acceptance, and make use of beneficial cooperativeness and collaboration through shared responsibilities with others. Thus, the kinds of relationships that people form throughout the life span plays a significant part in the development of a healthy, whole self.

DEFINITION OF TERMS

Relationship is defined as the existence of a connection or association between and among people. An **interpersonal relationship** is that relationship established between a person and those with whom he comes in contact, either on a one-to-one basis or in groups.

Individual Relationships

There are various types of individual interpersonal relationships. First, there is the close, intimate contact with a "significant other." In this type of relationship, the significant other is that person with whom there has been established a reciprocal investment and on whom the individual relies for gratification of his interpersonal needs for *affection, recognition,* and *control.* In other words, this close, intimate relationship involves a great deal of investment and responsibility on the part of at least one of the individuals. This type of relationship is usually found between a parent and a child or a husband and a wife. It may also extend beyond the home to a relationship developed between close friends, a student and his teacher, a clergyman and his parishioner, or a nurse and her patient.

A second type of individual interpersonal relationship is one that is formed for specific goal-oriented purposes and supplementary need gratification. Specific goal-oriented purposes include such things as maintenance of lines of communication among family members, achievement of family concerns, carrying out cultural traditions, and maintaining satisfactory work situations. Supplementary need gratification includes such things as meeting the basic human need for *identification, belonging,* and *security.* This type of individual interpersonal relationship might be with a peer, a blood relation, an extended-family member, an employer, or a co-worker.

A third type is one in which there are daily contacts between and among individuals whose significance may not be essential for daily living experiences and yet whose contact is necessary to further goal-directed activity. This type of individual interpersonal relationship is one that might be established with the check-out girl in the grocery store, with the mailman, or with the next-door neighbor. These particular relationships tend to *preserve harmony* and *provide the "extras" in life.*

Group Relationships

Transactions within groups satisfy a person's need for *establishing* and *maintaining his interdependency* within the social, cultural, and economic environments. As we have advanced in our technological development, so too have our interdependent needs expanded within these environs. History reveals, with each era, shifts in the priorities of needs that affect interpersonal relationships—to man, with one or several others, and with our environment. The 20th century is an era of complex interdependent relationships. This complexity is manifested through the types of group relationships that individuals form.

Group relationships are divided into three major categories—primary, secondary, and tertiary. The rationale for this categorization is based on the individual's need to set priorities in his search for fulfillment.

A **primary group** can be defined as a unit composed of close-knit, mutually interdependent, and reciprocal memberships. In other words, the primary group is any small group to which an individual belongs because of a vested interest, specialized activity, or fulfillment of need gratification. Familial, peer, or religious groups are examples of primary groups. It is in conjunction with the primary group that the individual establishes the norms, mores, and roles for his particular position in life. It is through his continuous involvement with this type of group relationship that the individual finds validation for his ideas, thoughts, actions, and feelings. A primary group relationship provides the members with group security and a means of identity; a basis for role expectations and functioning; and a sense of belonging and acceptance.

Secondary groups are those formed for the purpose of enrichment and refinement of the individual's total living experience. The kinds of interdependent relationships formed within this category manifest a moderate degree of intimacy. The individual retains freedom to move in and out of secondary groups as his priorities change. This freedom of movement is unique to secondary groups and is another characteristic that distinguishes them from primary groups. A work group, a social club, an art class, or a professional organization exemplify this secondary group category. Secondary group relationships are formed because they serve as a necessary and significant vehicle for the individual to meet his social, cultural, and financial needs.

Tertiary groups are those in which there exists between members a limited degree of intimacy and involvement. Membership is based on the necessity for gratifying immediate needs. The relationships formed within the group are not designed to be continuous. They are based on priorities that, most likely but not exclusively, have been established by the individual within his primary or secondary groups.

Participating in a fund-raising campaign, becoming a member of a committee, joining a vacation tour group, or taking part in a community action group is identified as a tertiary type of interpersonal group relationship.

DEVELOPMENT AND PROGRESSION OF INTERPERSONAL RELATIONSHIPS

Interpersonal relationships are learned experiences. They begin with birth and continue to deepen throughout the individual's life. Closely linked with the development of interpersonal relationships is the development of an individual's ability to communicate. For example, at birth an infant cries to announce his presence and to make known his needs. During infancy, the cry is the primary mechanism of communication between the infant and his world. The kind of response the infant receives from the mother or mother-substitute sets up a series of expectations on the part of the infant. These expectations may become habitual and lead to a specific pattern for the development of future interpersonal relationships.

In developing an interpersonal relationship there is a need for *clarity and directness*. A young child uses simple, direct language in interpersonal relationships that leaves little room for misinterpretation. Later interpersonal relationships are affected by the introduction of language complexities. The meanings of specific words and phrases take on varying colorations and connotations, resulting in a gap between the sender and the receiver. This gap makes messages unclear and needs unheard. The individual at this point must constantly strive toward sustaining an interpersonal relationship by varying responses until the communication is clear and the message is heard and understood.

The development of interpersonal relationships is influenced by two other components found within the communication process: honesty and openness. Honesty in communication signifies genuineness and authenticity and is based on the concepts of trust and truth. Honesty implies that the individual says what he means, what he thinks, and what he feels without fear of censure or retaliation. It does not mean that one spouts off impulsively without careful consideration and the exercise of discretional judgment. Brutal expressions of honesty are destructive and harmful, while honesty tempered with warmth, affection, and a desire to be helpful is constructive and facilitates interpersonal bonding.

In early childhood, simple, direct communication reflects this honesty. However, as the child grows, the continuation of this kind of forthright communication is often modified by the restraints society imposes for diplomacy and tact. These limitations are often confusing to the child. As a result he relinquishes a portion of his ability to be honest as a defensive protection for maintaining existing individual and group interpersonal relationships.

By the time the child reaches adulthood, the patterns of communication have become well established. If relationships have fostered the expectation and acceptance of honesty in communication, the adult will send messages that are clear and direct. If, on the other hand, the child's communication pattern reflects a habitual use of lying, manipulating, and story telling techniques over and above what is considered normal or usual, then as an adult, masked or mixed messages are sent and game playing predominates. Lack of honesty in communication affects the transactions within the levels of relationships and tends to interfere with the ability to trust, feel secure, and be involved in dynamic relationships.

Openness refers to the individual's ability to communicate what he thinks and feels without fear of censure, ridicule, or retaliation. Openness deals with the characteristic way the individual receives and processes messages from others. Openness is observable and can be perceived in terms of degree. It is exemplified through receptivity to ideas, information, or people. It implies a willingness to share oneself. Openness is not to be equated or confused with total self-disclosure.

People have a right to privacy but may still engage in transactions that convey openness. For example, a person at work greets you with "Good morning, how are you?" Your response is, "Things are not so good today, but I'd rather not go into them right now." This example illustrates several points. First, it shows an honest declaration of where you are. Second, it is open in its realistic statement about self without detailing the particulars, as one might do with total self-disclosure. Third, lines of communication were maintained and an indication was given that at some future time you might be open for further sharing.

Openness is displayed in the child by direct and clear communication. Childlike openness is enhanced or inhibited by familial interactions and the way the primary group teaches the child to send messages—by positive example or by restricting openness through disciplinary action; rejection; failure to hear the messages; using verbal corrections; or subtle nonverbal innuendoes. Both the honesty and openness of the communication in early childhood are directly related to the degree to which trust amd security have been demonstrated from earliest interpersonal encounters.

Openness, like honesty, tends to decrease as communication complexity increases. The individual learns that openness leads to interpersonal risk and exposure of self. Feeling threatened, the individual communicates his thoughts and feelings more subtly in order to protect his present and future interpersonal associations. An individual's interpersonal relationships may appear satisfactory, but what does the individual do to himself in the process? Are the resultant relationships true? Are they significant? Meaningful? For some individuals, the answers to these questions are yes! For many others, the answers are no.

Generally, the natural components of communication—clarity, directness, honesty, and openness—contribute to and enhance an individual's relationship(s) with others. However, through the phases of growth and development and through the limitations imposed or perceived as imposed by society, an individual may sometimes sacrifice the naturalness of communication to preserve relationships. This is where the other components that influence interpersonal relationships come into play, that is, the perception of self in relation to the psychosocial and cultural factors influencing the developmental process. There is more to living than mere survival. During infancy, the mother-child relationship is markedly one-sided. Because the infant is totally dependent on others to meet his life-sustaining needs, he identifies with and conforms to the expectations of those most important to him. The attitudes, feelings, and behavior of individuals within the child's environment exert a strong influence on him and his relationship with others. Prevailing values of and attitudes toward such sociocultural factors as the concepts of morality, humanity, and sexuality; the norms for living, loving, learning, working, praying, and playing; the expectations regarding success and failure; and the discrepancies in social sanctions—all become part of the developing self.

As the child progresses from a dependent state toward a state of independence and finally interdependence, the self emerges as a separate identity. Exposure to and involvement with significant others aid him in the search for this self. As the individual moves toward adulthood, he struggles to identify, evaluate, retain, or reject those attitudes and values that contribute to a feeling of wholeness or oneness with self. The maturation process is gradual and allows the child to develop a realization of the "individual self" that becomes unique and different for each individual.

SUMMARY

Interpersonal relationships are an end as well as a means toward reaching maturity. As a means to an end, they enhance perception of self. They alter perception of self, and they contribute to the continuous modification of self, thereby producing a "dynamic self." As an end, interpersonal relationships are a combined demonstration of the individual's acquired ability and skill both to communicate and to formulate a set of values and attitudes.

SUGGESTED READINGS

Ackerman, N. W. *The Psychodynamics of Family Therapy*. New York: Basic Books, 1958.

Brammer, L. M., & Shostrom, E. E. *Therapeutic Psychology*. Englewood Cliffs, N.J.: Prentice-Hall, 1968.

Brandner, P. Women in Groups. *American Journal of Nursing*, Vol. 74, No. 9 (September, 1974), 1661–1664.

Burton, G. *Personal, Impersonal and Interpersonal Relations*. New York: Springer, 1964.

Downs, F. S. Technological Advances and the Nurse Family Relationship. *Nursing Digest*, Vol. 3, No. 3 (May/June, 1975), 23–24.

Heider, F. *The Psychology of Interpersonal Relations*. New York: Wiley, 1958.

Hubbard, P., Muhlenkamp, A. F., & Brown, N. The Relationship Between Social Support and Self-Care Practices. *Nursing Research*, Vol. 33, No. 5 (September/October, 1984), 266–269.

Johnson, D. W. *Reaching Out: Interpersonal Effectiveness and Self-Actualizations*. Englewood Cliffs, N.J.: Prentice-Hall, 1978.

Jourard, S. *The Transparent Self*. Princeton, N.J.: Van Nostrand Reinhold, 1971.

Klotkowski, D. Self Disclosure: Implications for Mental Health. *Perspectives in Psychiatric Care*, Vol. 18, No. 3 (May/June, 1980), 112–115.

Lair, J. *I Ain't Much, Baby—But I'm All I've Got*. Greenwich, Conn.: Fawcett Publications, 1974.

Lair, J. *I Ain't Well But I Sure Am Better*. Greenwich, Conn.: Fawcett Publications, 1975.

Powell, J. *Why Am I Afraid To Tell You Who I Am?* Niles, Ill.: Argus, 1969.

Sullivan, H. S. The Interpersonal Theory of Psychiatry. New York: W. W. Norton Co., 1953.

Yankelowicz, D. *New Rules in American Life: Searching for Self-Fulfillment in a World Turned Upside Down*. New York: Random House, 1981.

Zunin, L., & Zunin, N. *Contact: The First Four Minutes*. New York: Ballantine, 1972.

III

PSYCHOPATHOLOGY

A Differential Data Base for Professional Nursing Practice

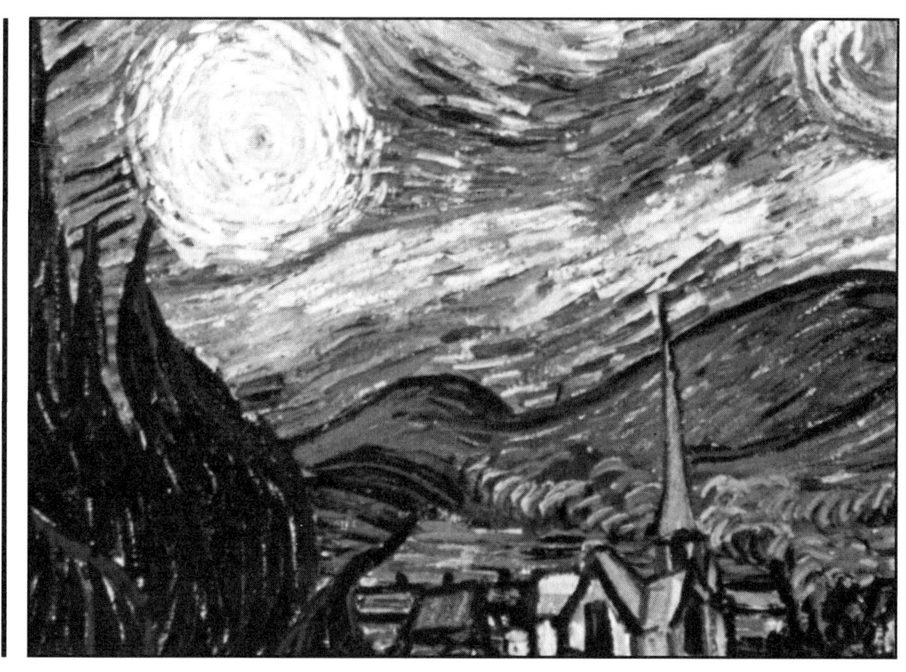

10

PSYCHOPATHOLOGY AND DIAGNOSTIC CRITERIA

A Frame of Reference

LEARNING OBJECTIVES

On completion of this chapter the reader should be able to:

1. Define **psychopathology**.
2. Identify and distinguish among the five axes used in the classification of mental disorders.
3. Discuss the implications that knowledge and understanding of diagnostic criteria have for nursing.

PSYCHOPATHOLOGY: AN OVERVIEW

What is psychopathology, and what are the criteria by which its presence is determined within a given individual? These two questions have puzzled mankind throughout recorded history. Man's effort to distinguish the normal from the abnormal, to develop criteria for differentiating between mental health and mental illness, as well as to distinguish between broad categories of mental disorders is well documented.

Psychopathology is a term used to designate the study of disease processes of the mind; it is the persistent, repetitive, recognizable, and exaggerated expression of distorted thought, disturbed feeling, and disruptive behavior. It is the study of emotional incongruence and psychological disequilibrium. Psychopathology encompasses the causes, clinical symptomatic manifestations, and dynamics affecting the mind and its functioning, which in turn influences the individual's total pattern of action and reaction within his daily life. Psychopathology is an outcome of an individual's inability to function according to and in concert with society's predetermined expectations of performance. In effect, it signifies the individual's failure, as judged by personal or social norms, to adapt, modify, or change behavior in response to the fluctuating internal and external needs or conditions of the psychosociocultural environment.

DIAGNOSTIC CRITERIA: CURRENT STATUS

The evolutionary process of designing and developing a system for classifying pathological manifestations of man's reactions to and involvement in life and living has been evidenced repeatedly. The medical profession's latest attempt to identify, organize, and differentiate between diagnostic categories culminated in the publication of the *Diagnostic and Statistical Manual of Mental Disorders* (DSM-III) in 1980. This movement toward a more effective means of categorization was influenced by a need to demonstrate the extent of current knowledge; provide consistency for intradisciplinary and interdisciplinary communication; furnish a reliable data base for ongoing research and funding; guide the planning of treatment regimes; and predict potential treatment outcomes.

In this latest edition of the *Diagnostic and Statistical Manual,* the American Psychiatric Association identifies a total of 16 major diagnostic classes and 187 specific diagnostic categories. This extensive and comprehensive method of classification indicates that the behavioral syndromes or patterns manifested are distinct, separate entities representing significant demarcations between classes and categories. Furthermore, such a system of organization and ordering connotes recognition of a multiplicity of clinically nonrelated entities that are physically, psychologically, and behaviorally undesirable and painful to the self, others, and society.

The DSM-III addresses and specifies criteria that guide the clinician in formulating a diagnosis. It employs a strongly descriptive approach in classifying psychological, behavioral, and physical phenomena. It uses a multiaxial format that recognizes the many variables that impinge on each designated condition. There are currently five axes, each of which addresses a different class of information. Each axis serves as a guide for collecting and assessing significant data. Axes I and II form the basis of classification for mental disorders. Specifically, **Axis I** details all the major diagnoses that have been identified as mental disorders, while **Axis II** specifies those diagnostic conditions that have specific reference to developmental and personality disorders. Each identified class and category include criteria that are described as essential features. Essential features are those multiple criteria whose presence must be evidenced if the specific diagnosis is to be made.

In addition, supplementary information is included in an attempt to insure the consistency and comprehensiveness of the descriptions. Pertinent information is supplied under each of the following headings: **associated features**, those signs and symptoms which may or may not be present; **age at onset**, the age of the individual when the disorder is first observed; **course**, the prognostic outcome of the disorder; **impairment**, degree and level of disability in social and occupational functioning; **complications**, those conditions or events that may occur as an outcome of the disorder; **predisposing factors**, those specific individual personality conditions or events that may tend to increase vulnerability, thereby placing the individual in a position of risk; **prevalence**, the epidemiological data regarding incidence; **sex ratio**, the frequency of occurrence in men and women; **familial pattern**, an indication of incidence within a particular family as opposed to incidence within the general population; and **differential diagnosis**, those diagnostic conditions that have similar clinical features and from which a distinction between them and the particular diagnosis needs to be made. The reader will find in the Appendix a listing of the American Psychiatric Associations' DSM-III Classification: "Axes I and II Categories and Codes."

Axis III allows for the inclusion of any existing physical disorder or condition that may have potential relevance for increasing comprehension of the primary diagnosis as well as influencing the treatment approach to be used with a specific patient. **Axis IV** addresses the severity of impairment with respect to the specific psychosocial or cultural stressors. It provides a system of coding by which the clinician is able to rank the effect identified stressors have on the development or intensification of the major disorder presented. Types of psychosocial stressors delineated as significant for judging severity of impact include marital status or condition; parenting; interpersonal relationships; occupational problems; living and financial conditions; developmental stages; physical health; traumatic events; or family difficulties. In other words, Axis IV takes into account any or all life events that may act as a predisposing or precipitating cause.

Axis V is a time-oriented axis. It attempts to identify the highest level of adaptive capability that a given individual was able to manifest during the year prior to recognition and diagnosis of the major mental disorder. Three areas for assessment included in this axis are the individual's interpersonal and social relationships with others, occupational functioning, and use of leisure time. The information obtained on this axis has a predictive and prognostic implication in that resumption of functioning following illness usually is similar to that displayed prior to onset of illness.

One significant item not addressed in the DSM-III is the theoretical framework for interpreting causation. In other words, no explanation is provided for the user with respect to the dynamics involved in the development and course of the disease process. According to the task force report, this omission was made as a deliberate choice, since the consensus of thinking was that each practitioner or potential user would be better able to utilize the DSM-III without becoming entangled in controversial side issues that arise out of diversity in theoretical bent and conceptual bias. Thus, this limitation is an attempt to promote unity among professionals by creating a contextual framework that is objective and universal, rather than subjective and personal.

RELEVANCE FOR NURSING PRACTICE

The increasing complexity of assessment criteria related to the establishment of differential demarcations between known and recognizable clinical entities makes it essential that the nurse have a fundamental grasp of current diagnostic nomenclature. Such knowledge enables the nurse to communicate effectively with other disciplines; participate collaboratively in patient care management; contribute to clinical research; and organize and use data in exercising problem-solving and judgmental processes in the designing of effective nursing interventions. Furthermore, since knowledge and use of a classification system presume a systematic and logical mechanism for ordering of data, and since ordering is indicative of rational action and rational action presupposes understanding, such kmowledge increases the nurse's total efficacy in the rendering of professional service on behalf of the patient. In addition, awareness of objective data divorced from subjective interpretation that stems from a particular theoretical orientation and conceptual framework allows the nurse to make maximum use of her creativity and uniqueness in clinical practice.

SUMMARY

We have supplied the reader with a brief, concise explanation of the current state of thinking regarding psychopathology, diagnostic criteria, nomenclature, and the specific features associated with the assessment process. The presentation of these fundamental concepts serves as an orientation to the ensuing discussion of specific, selected mental disorders contained in the following chapter. Such an orientation is intended to promote the understanding of conditions affecting the individual patient and to facilitate therapeutic effectiveness.

SUGGESTED READINGS

American Psychiatric Association. *The Diagnostic and Statistical Manual of Mental Disorders*, 3rd ed. Washington, D. C.: American Psychiatric Association, 1980.

Kaplan, H. I., Freidman, A. M., & Sadock, B. J. (Eds.) *Comprehensive Textbook of Psychiatry*, 3rd ed. 3 vols. Baltimore: Williams & Wilkins, 1980.

Williams, J. B. A., & Wilson, H. S. A Psychiatric Nursing Perspective on DSM-III. *Journal of Psychosocial Nursing and Mental Health Services*, Vol. 20, No. 4 (April, 1982), 14–20.

Woody, R. H. (Ed.) *Encyclopedia of Clinical Assessment*. 2 vols. San Francisco: Jossey-Bass, 1981.

11

PSYCHOPATHOLOGY

Differential Data Base, Dynamics, and Principles

LEARNING OBJECTIVES

On completion of this chapter the reader should be able to:

1. Identify, define, and describe the seven classifications of mental disorders presented in this chapter.
2. State the etiology for each of the seven psychopathological conditions presented.
3. Identify the characteristic symptomatology associated with each of the seven major classifications.
4. Discuss the dynamics associated with each of the seven major classifications.
5. Identify the broad concepts and principles for nursing care that are specifically related to each of the diagnostic classifications.

INTRODUCTION

This chapter presents an overview and synthesis of the seven most frequently encountered mental disorders: (1) organic, (2) substance use, (3) schizophrenic, (4) affective, (5) anxiety, (6) somatiform, and (7) personality. This chapter is not a comprehensive survey of mental disorders. The reader can refer to easily accessible resources in both books and journals for descriptive and comprehensive studies of mental disorders, the current nomenclature, and extensive treatment objectives. This chapter is designed to be of practical value for the reader and to serve as a basic reference for diagnostic criteria and application. There is no special adherence to any one particular theoretical school of thought. In essence, this chapter is a composite summation of data and diagnostic nomenclature regarding specific disease conditions, their distinguishing characteristics, etiology, dynamics, applicable nursing diagnoses, and the major concepts and principles underlying nursing care.

To orient the reader to the complexity of psychopathology and to provide an essential frame of reference, Table 11–1 outlines each of the seven psychiatric disorders selected for presentation. The reader will note that each of the broad classifications has certain dynamics or underlying causes in common, such as: some form of subjective discomfort and distress; exaggerated use of or excessive reliance on the automatic adaptive mechanisms; disturbed or interrupted interpersonal relationships; ineffective patterns of communication; inability to delay gratification; or an inability to meet and satisfy wants, needs, or desires in one or more areas of vital functioning. Nevertheless, each of the seven major disorders is diagnostically and therapeutically different. They differ in definition, types, idiosyncratic and associated characteristics, etiology, dynamics, age at onset, level of impairment, prognostic outcome, and related nursing diagnoses.

Table 11–1 provides an outlined, concise synthesis of commonly encountered and treated psychopathologic conditions. We have highlighted many fundamental theoretical and technical concepts in a condensed, readily comprehensible format intended to assist the reader to become better able to identify the major classes and categories of mental disorders and also to more easily identify the etiology, dynamics, and characteristics manifested by individuals suffering from these types of psychiatric conditions. In order to better assist with the integration of theory and practice, the last segment of the outline is devoted to identifying those nursing diagnoses that currently have been developed and approved by the North American Nursing Diagnosis Association (NANDA).

The nursing diagnoses detailed in Table 11–1 are not meant to be conclusive. The reader is reminded that legitimate nursing diagnoses can only be made when a complete assessment of a given client has been carried out. The placement of nursing diagnoses within the table is meant to illustrate a broad range of possibilities that might eventuate for a client with a particular medical psychiatric diagnosis. The reader is directed to Chapter 19 for a more in-depth discussion of nursing diagnosis as part of the nursing process and for a complete list of accepted diagnoses from NANDA.

In other chapters of this book the reader will find extensive and detailed descriptions of theory and practice principles of therapeutic interactive–interventions relating to stress and crisis, human feelings, communicative skills, and the therapeutic use of self and group process. Careful reading and review of these significant chapters will arm the reader with those essential skills necessary to effectively intervene and therapeutically advocate for those patients suffering the ravages of psychopathology and to plan for effective nursing care.

In the subsequent pages we have elaborated on seven major classes of psychopathology so that the reader may learn to identify the characteristic symptomatology associated with each of the disorders.

ORGANIC MENTAL DISORDERS

Cerebral dysfunction, a cognitive and emotional disturbance of neurophysiology or brain tissue functioning, produces and accounts for one of the most frequently diagnosed psychopathological conditions currently confronting and challenging man—organic mental disorder. **Organic mental disorder** is a broad term used to designate a complex variety of psychological and behavioral manifestations that have their genesis in altered physiological processes. Disruptions in organic functioning, whether due to the aging process, trauma or disease, substance use or abuse, or drug therapy, produce either temporary dysfunction or permanent tissue damage of the brain. Characteristically, the specific grouping and arrangement of clinical signs and symptoms differ widely and reflect variations based on the extent of tissue damage, site of damage, onset, and progression, along with the specific etiological factor, if known.

The primary symptoms associated with organic mental disorders consist of impairment of both recent and remote memory, with remote memory remaining fairly well intact for a longer period of time; marked deficiency in immediate recall; disorientation in the three spheres—time, place, and person; and gross impairment of intellectual functioning involving decreased comprehension, inability to problem solve or learn new facts, behaviors, or activities. All of these are found in any one of the diagnostic conditions, although the degree of severity is not necessarily the same for each.

Concomitantly, secondary symptoms that involve lability of affect, disorganized thought content, and aberrant behavior may be superimposed on the existing condition. The broad secondary symptom spectrum may include any combination of apathy, depression, or euphoria; marked anxiety and agitation; confabulation, fabrication, or paranoid ideation; withdrawal and regression; or hyperactivity or psychomotor retardation. The secondary symptoms observed in each individual case are considered to represent the individual's exaggerated response or reaction of his basic personality to his mental and physical disability. Therefore, the specific symptomatology apparently

TABLE 11–1. DESCRIPTIVE ANALYSIS OF MENTAL DISORDERS

	Organic Mental Disorders	Substance Use Disorders	Schizophrenic Disorders
Definition	A disorder in which the individual sustains psychological, physiological or behavioral dysfunction as a consequence of damaged brain tissue.	A disorder in which the individual demonstrates behavioral changes as a result of the regular ingestion of substances that produce central nervous system dysfunction.	Psychogenic reactions in which the individual experiences severe personality disorganization and disintegration along with marked distortions of reality testing and thought process for a minimum of 6 months.
Examples of categories	Primary degenerative dementia, senile onset. Primary degenerative dementia, presenile onset. Substance-induced disorders. Organic brain syndromes.	Alcohol abuse. Alcohol dependence. Barbiturate abuse. Opioid dependence. Amphetamine abuse. Tobacco dependence.	Disorganized. Catatonic. Paranoid. Residual. Undifferentiated.
Essential characteristics	Presence of at least one brain syndrome or demonstrable specific organic syndrome producing psychological or behavioral manifestations due to temporary or permanent brain dysfunction.	For a substance abuse diagnosis, the individual must demonstrate a pattern of pathological use and impaired social or occupational functioning of at least 1 month's duration. For a substance dependence diagnosis, the individual must evidence psychological dependence in either the form of tolerance or withdrawal.	The presence of a delusional system or hallucinatory experience; disruptions in thought processes; deterioration in usual pattern of functioning; onset prior to age 45; and duration of at least 6 months.

Affective Disorders	Anxiety Disorders	Somatiform Disorders	Personality Disorders
A psychogenic disorder in which the individual experiences marked personality disorganization and dysfunction as evidenced by severe disturbances in mood.	A psychological disability in which anxiety results from an individual's inability to cope with emotional conflicts or stressful environmental situations.	A maladaptive emotional reaction in which physical symptoms are expressed without accompanying demonstrable organic cause.	Entrenched, chronic, maladaptive characterologic patterns in which there is subjective distress or significant impairment in social or occupational functioning, or both.
Bipolar: mixed manic depressed Major depression: single episode recurrent Cyclothymic. Dysthymic.	Phobic disorders. Anxiety states. Post-traumatic stress disorder.	Somatization disorder. Conversion disorder. Psychogenic pain disorder. Hypochondriasis.	Paranoid. Antisocial. Borderline. Dependent. Compulsive. Passive-aggressive.
Prolonged disturbance of mood involving either elation or depression. *Manic episode*: elevated, expansive or irritable mood; hyperactivity; pressure of speech; flight of ideas; somnolence; distractibility; poor judgment. *Depressive episode:* loss of interest or pleasure; disturbances in appetite and sleep; weight loss; psychomotor agitation or retardation; decreased energy; feeling of worthlessness or guilt; indecisiveness; memory deficits; confusion; suicidal preoccupation.	Presence of anxiety.	Physical symptoms suggestive of a physical disorder with no confirming data demonstrating organic etiology. Positive indication that presenting symptoms are directly related to psychological factors.	Inflexible and maladaptive personality traits that represent the individual's habitual form of functioning and which produce significant social or occupational impairment or personal distress.

(*continued*)

TABLE 11–1. CONTINUED

	Organic Mental Disorders	Substance Use Disorders	Schizophrenic Disorders
Associated characteristics (selected)	Anxiety; depression; irritability; shame; confabulation; circumstantiality; ritualistic behavior, lability of mood; faulty impulse control; diminished psychomotor activity; apathy; incontinence; lethargy; cognitive dysfunction.	Disturbances in personality and mood; antisocial activity; involvement in countercultural life styles; suspiciousness or violence.	Pacing; rocking; apathy; immobility; poverty of speech; ritualistic behavior; depression; anxiety; anger; depersonalization; ideas of reference; illusions.
Etiology	Any condition or agent that produces central nervous system pathology and cerebral tissue impairment.	Habituation or addiction to the use of a chemical substance.	Multiple causation; most likely related to psychological, sociocultural, organic or hereditary factors.
Dynamics	Inteference with or destruction of cerebral tissue. Libidinal energy is released as a result of organic changes. Loss of ability to control libidinal drives. Interruption of learning and coping potential.	Sense of destruction or loss of internal world; therefore, restoration is sought to overcome emptiness. Fragmentation of self with a corresponding need to achieve a sense of organization and integration. Substitute for interpersonal relationships and control over environment. Escape from the stresses of reality	Loss of ego boundaries. Denial of reality. Severe regression. Security and identity are threatened. Interpersonal relationships are superficial. Failure or inability to trust self or others.

Affective Disorders	Anxiety Disorders	Somatiform Disorders	Personality Disorders
Manic episode: lability of mood (rapid shifts to anger or depression); delusions or hallucinations that are mood congruent; suicidal. *Depressive episode*: sadness; anxiety; fear; irritability; morbid preoccupations; excessive concern with physical health; panic attacks or phobias.	None for class; specific associated characteristics relevant for individual categories.	None for class; specific associated characteristics relevant for individual categories.	Disturbances of mood involving depression or anxiety; dissatisfied with impact behavior has on others or own inability to function effectively.
Traumatic stress; longstanding, unresolved conflict; poorly developed and integrated ego boundaries; unresolved diffuse anger and hostility. *Manic episode*: repeated failure in early life to measure up to parental expectations. *Depressive episode*: loss of significant others or objects.	Disruption in the developmental pattern or in interpersonal experiences; multiple, intrapsychic conflicts resulting from unresolved guilt, fear, prolonged stress, or crisis; conflict between what an individual believes society expects and the bipersonal self.	Preoccupation with self and bodily functioning; probably arises out of unresolved conflicts, however, no supporting epidemiological data to confirm or deny.	Faulty or arrested emotional development which interferes with adequate social control or superego formation; constitutional predisposition; deprivation of basic needs in early childhood; physical or emotional trauma, or both, in childhood or adolescence; conditioned response reinforced by sociocultural factors within the environment.
Manic episode: Unmet needs during infancy give rise to feelings of insecurity and dependency with resultant ambivalence. Confidence and self-assurance are defense against dependency. Represses hostility and guilt in effort to seek approval from others. Unrealistic expectations of self give rise to feelings of inferiority	Persistent overuse of repression to control emotionally charged thoughts, and feelings. The presence of socially unacceptable thoughts, feelings, wants, or desires that if actualized would cause loss of approval, acceptance, or love from others. Fear of censure, disapproval, or rejection threatens the self-concept.	Symptoms are used as a vehicle of expression for unmet dependency needs. Protection against low self-concept. The resultant symptomatology offers the individual an external means of expressing repressed material, thereby allowing both primary and secondary gains for the ego.	The individual operates from an egocentric viewpoint and remains narcissistic. Interpersonal relationships are not important unless they can be used to achieve specific need gratification. A concealed "taking" relationship predominates as opposed to a mutual "give-and-take" relationship. Avoidance of expectations, discomfort,

(*continued*)

TABLE 11–1. CONTINUED

	Organic Mental Disorders	Substance Use Disorders	Schizophrenic Disorders
Dynamics (*cont.*)		or responsibility. The person's pattern of living reflects an excessive use of denial and rationalization as primary methods of coping.	
Age at onset	Any age.	Alcohol—adolescence to 40s. Barbiturates—two patterns, 30 to 60 and teens or early 20s. All other substances—late teens to 20s.	Adolescence or early adulthood.
Impairment	Minimal to severe, may affect all levels of functioning; variations based on specific disease category.	Moderate to severe. Can be fatal.	May affect routine daily functioning, ranging from no effect to severe disability necessitating institutionalization.
Course	Variable—progressive episodic, static or resolving.	Progressive dependence; course varies with specific substance used.	Variable with periods of exacerbation and remission; depends on length of prodromal stage.

Affective Disorders	Anxiety Disorders	Somatiform Disorders	Personality Disorders
and inadequacy. Flight into reality. Attacks external environment. Uses rationalization and projection. *Depressive episode*: Real or imaginary loss perceived as rejection. Regressed hostility and hatred turned inward as a result of rigid superego. Penance in the form of guilt feelings for aggressive and hostile feelings. Denial of aggression produces helplessness and hopelessness.			stress-producing situations. Disproportionate projection and accusations toward persons, places, and objects in the environment. Blatant disregard for the norms and mores of society.
Manic episode: Before age 30. *Depressive episode*: Any age, including infancy.	Varies, depends on specific diagnostic category—range is from childhood to middle adult life.	Varies, depends on specific diagnostic categories—range is from childhood to old age.	Childhood or adolescence.
Manic episode: Considerable impairment in social and occupational functioning coupled with need for protection and supervision. *Depressive episode*: Impairment varies from mild to severe.	Mild to severe, depending on specific diagnostic category.	Marked impairment interfering with pursuit of usual daily living.	Marked impairment in social and occupational functioning.
Variable and episodic.	Ranges from brief, isolated episodes to persistent, chronic states.	Varies depending on specific disease category.	Data unavailable.

(*continued*)

TABLE 11–1. CONTINUED

	Organic Mental Disorders	Substance Use Disorders	Schizophrenic Disorders
Tentative nursing diagnosis:	Alteration in thought processes, related to:	Sensory/perceptual alteration, related to:	Social isolation, related to:
Etiology	Central nervous system dysfunction. Aging process. Neurotransmitter dysfunction. Chemical alteration.	Altered sensory reception, transmission, or intergration. Chemical alteration, CNS stimulants.	Life patterns. Alienation. Crises, maturational or situational. Severe psychological stress. Developmental stage fixation.
Defining characteristics	Inaccurate interpretation of environment. Cognitive dissonance. Memory deficit. Inability to follow directions. Confabulation. Disorientation to time, place, and person.	Altered abstraction. Altered conceptualization. Change in behavioral patterns. Restlessness. Irritability. Unpredictability. Change in problem-solving abilities. Reported change in sensory acuity.	Seclusiveness. Seeming lack of awareness of environment. Disregard for social customs relating to interactions. Reduced motor activity; sleeping during daytime. Poor eye contact. Expressions of feelings or rejection. Hallucinations. Failure to take responsibility for self-care.

Affective Disorders	Anxiety Disorders	Somatiform Disorders	Personality Disorders
Currently, no approved nursing diagnosis has been developed by the North American Nursing Diagnosis Association (NANDA) that might represent a primary nursing diagnosis for clients with this psychiatric disorder. It is recommended that the reader define an appropriate diagnostic entity and relay its usefulness in practice to the Clearinghouse of Nursing Diagnoses, St. Louis University School of Nursing, 3525 Caroline Street, St. Louis, Mo. 63104.	Anxiety related to: Threat to self-concept. Threat to personal security system. Unconscious conflict. Actual failure of adaptive coping skills. Unmet needs.	Self-concept—Disturbance in self-esteem related to: Repeated negative experiences. Attack on self-confidence, self-respect, self-worth, self-approval. Threat to daily routine. Inability to accept self.	Existing nursing diagnoses seem to be inapplicable. See note under "Affective Disorders."
	Greatly reduced range of perception. Selective inattention. Inability to concentrate. Purposeless activity. Sense of impending doom.	Fears, especially of failure. Low sense of self-worth. Minimization of own strengths and abilities. Failure to achieve goals.	

is related to the individual's premorbid personality, preexisting patterns or modes of adjustment, and socioeconomic, cultural, and environmental situation, as well as the extent of his individual and group interpersonal relationships. A well-integrated individual can withstand organic brain damage better than a person who has manifested a rigid, immature, or other mental, emotional, or psychological disability or inadequacy. Thus, the great variability of individual response to illness accounts for the diversity of secondary symptomatology.

The following two case studies detail the development and progression of the most commonly encountered organic disorders, alcohol withdrawal delirium and multi-infarct dementia.

Situation I

Mr. Edward Nolen, age 47, was admitted to a general hospital with a diagnosis of acute appendicitis. Within 48 hours following surgery, Mr. Nolen displayed increasing restlessness and agitation. He was found trying to wash his face and hands with the water from his ice pitcher, and when he saw the nurse he wanted to know if she could do something about the "room service in this hotel." He asked the nurse to order a "shot and a beer" for him and said that as soon as he finished getting dressed he would be glad to take her to dinner in the hotel dining room, that is, if she could assure him that the service in the dining room was better than the room service. When the nurse proceeded to explain that he was in the hospital, he became angry and verbally abusive. He picked up the phone and tried to place a call to the "head man in charge" to get this "interfering female" out of his room. Shortly afterwards, Mr. Nolen shouted for someone to come and get "these terrible creatures off his bed." In his agitation and in his attempt to get away, he pulled off his dressing, disconnected his I.V., and ruptured his incision.

Emergency intervention included immediate return to surgery for incision repair and planning for close, continuous observation and care of him postsurgery. His caloric intake was increased, Librium was ordered to alleviate and prevent further agitation, and a Vitamin B complex regime was instituted. Within 3 days after the second surgery Mr. Nolen was no longer disoriented, nor was there any evidence of hallucinations or delusions. When his sensorium cleared, the patient was distressed and apologetic about his behavior. Both he and his wife stated that although he was once a heavy drinker, he had joined Alcoholics Anonymous 5 years ago and had not had a drink since. They had been convinced that this episode could not happen again.

Situation II

Mrs. Dorothy Snelling is a 74-year-old white female who was admitted to the Greenbriar Nursing Home at the request of her daughter Nancy. In talking with the staff nurse, Nancy described her mother as a woman who had been very independent and who had taken great pride in her personal appearance. Over the past 4 years Nancy had noticed obvious changes. For example, Mrs. Snelling had trouble remembering where she put things such as her eyeglasses, pocketbook, and dentures and had on one occasion put the coffee pot in the refrigerator. She had been in the habit of walking the dog every afternoon and lately was having difficulty finding her way back home, so that Nancy would have to drive around the neighborhood looking for her. Gradually her behavior became more erratic and unpredictable. Six months ago Mrs. Snelling gave a valuable piece of jewelry to the boy next door because she believed he was her son John. John was killed in Korea. Over the next few months she became more irritable and demanding and would often accuse Nancy of trying to get rid of her. She lost interest in her appearance, was reluctant to bathe, and flatly refused to let Nancy wash and set her hair. Lately, the neighbors reported to Nancy that Mrs. Snelling spent much of her time standing inside the front door, yelling at them whenever they appeared outside. Last week Mrs. Snelling found her way to the corner drugstore where she purchased a package of Rit Dye and colored her own very white hair a bright red. Two days ago when Nancy came home she found the house filled with smoke. Mrs. Snelling was ironing and had placed the hot iron on the dining room chair when she finished and had forgotten to turn it off. Nancy found her sitting calmly in the kitchen reading the newspaper, completely oblivious of the hole in the chair or the smoke-filled dining room. This event finally convinced Nancy that her mother could no longer safely manage on her own.

The preliminary admitting diagnosis of multi-infarct dementia was made.

In Mr. Nolen's situation, the inflammation and subsequent surgical trauma combined to act as a psychophysiological stressor that precipitated the onset of his organic mental disorder. The reader should note that typically alcohol withdrawal delirium begins to manifest itself within the first 36 to 72 hours after the cessation of alcohol ingestion. However, as in the case of Mr. Nolen, it can also occur long after the alcohol is no longer present in the system.

Alcohol withdrawal delirium is an acute, reversible, organic mental disorder that if unrecognized and left untreated can result in death for the client. In fact, recent statistics reveal that a high mortality rate exists for this diagnostic condition. The 15-percent mortality rate has been attributed to suicide, accidents, and cardiac or renal failure. The nurse's observations and assessments are critical to early intervention.

In the case of Mrs. Snelling, the onset was insidious and progressive over time. The pathological process is not reversible, but early detection and treatment may very well retard its progression.

Most often initial treatment for an individual with an organic mental disorder takes place in a general hospital setting, since the presenting symptoms or basic etiological factors produce marked physiological change. In this setting, the initial focus of care is twofold. Whether one is dealing with a patient with alcohol withdrawal delirium, meningitis, arteriosclerotic heart disease, multiple sclerosis, or Parkinson's syndrome, the care is directed toward alleviating the physical symptomatology where the primary aim is maintenance of life support systems and return to physiological equilibrium. Concurrently, equal emphasis is given to sustaining the psychological coping mechanisms already in operation. Such emotional and psychological emphasis contributes to the preservation of the individual's psychological need system, safeguards personal integrity, provides emotional security, and curtails further personality disintegration.

Concepts and principles upon which nursing intervention is based include the following:

- Organic conditions produce mental dysfunction, alteration in mood, physical manifestations, and disrupted interpersonal relationships.
- Acute conditions require immediate interventive techniques to maintain life.
- Basic needs for survival take precedence.
- Progressive destruction of cerebral tissue produces an inability to adapt responsively to changing conditions or stress, leading to confusion and irritability.
- Chronic conditions require supportive care coupled with an attitudinal approach of hopefulness.
- Sensory and social deprivation increases regressive behavior.
- Loss or impairment of physical functioning contributes to increasing the level of fear, anxiety, and confusion within the person.
- As impairment increases in severity, ability to understand and care for self decreses proportionately.
- The need for close observation and protective supervision increases proportionately to a decrease in independent functioning.
- Any threat to self-esteem and self-respect can retard progress toward health.
- Feelings of self-esteem increase in direct proportion to the amount of respect the individual receives.
- Feelings of inadequacy, uselessness, and helplessness can be mitigated.
- Work and social activities serve to maintain self-esteem and enhance reality orientation.
- Gratification of the interpersonal needs for affection, recognition, and control promotes movement toward the maintenance of emotional equilibrium.

- Provision for personal satisfaction, comfort, and dignity are the basis for fostering self-worth.
- Change is disorganizing; regularity promotes a sense of continuity and belonging.
- Minimizing an individual's exposure to new people or new experiences will decrease the potential for adverse reactions.
- Alterations in mood, behavior, or level of consciousness may be indicators of change in the person's physical status.
- Consistency in the attitudes and behavior of health care personnel promotes security and provides reassurance.
- A severely impaired person is highly sensitive to attitudes conveyed through nonverbal behavior.
- Careful, well-planned, and structured routines will minimize progression of the disability and maximize opportunities for rehabilitation.

In Table 11–1, the reader will find a summary of pertinent information on organic mental disorders regarding characteristics, dynamics, onset, degree of impairment, and prognosis, along with tentative nursing diagnosis. Specific nursing interventions for clients experiencing distortions in thought can be found in Chapter 20.

SUBSTANCE USE DISORDERS

The use of chemical substances to alter or modify behavior is a practice that individuals have participated in throughout recorded history. The problem of substance use and abuse is a clinical entity that manifests itself in all cultures and age groups and at all educational and economic levels. This diagnostic category deals with the regular or continuous use of specific substances which, when introduced into the system, produce undesirable behavioral changes and affect central nervous system functioning. Behavioral changes that occur as a direct result of substance use or abuse include impaired social or occupational functioning, inability to limit the use of or to cease taking the substance, and the development of withdrawal symptoms after discontinuation of the substance.

Substance use is divided into two main classes—abuse and dependence. **Substance abuse** is defined according to three distinct criteria. First, abuse is characterized by a pattern of pathological use. This means that depending on the substance chosen, the individual engages in a repetitive regime despite intoxication, acknowledged harm to self, control efforts, and complications or urgency of need to maintain functioning. The second criterion identifies impairment in social or occupational functioning produced by repetitive use pattern; that is, disturbed interpersonal and family relationships, poor judgment and impulse control, inappropriate expression of aggression, and illegal or criminal activity, as well as a marked deterioration in physical and psychological functioning. The third criterion concerns itself with duration and identifies abuse as requiring the disturbance to be in existence for at least one month.

Substance dependence is more severe than substance abuse. A distinctive difference is that substance dependence requires a physiological dependent state on the substance used. This dependence is manifested by either tolerance or withdrawal. By **tolerance** is meant that the individual markedly increases the amount of the substance used in order to achieve the desired effect. **Withdrawal** is an abstinence syndrome that occurs subsequent to the abrupt cessation of the substance used.

Within the diagnostic classification of substance use there are five categories of substances that manifest both abuse and dependence: alcohol, barbiturates, opioids, amphetamines, and cannabis. Three categories of substances are associated only with abuse and include cocaine, phencyclidine (PCP), and hallucinogens. Only one substance is associated with dependence alone, and that substance is tobacco.

According to all documented evidence there exists no particular characteristic description that is universally applicable to the substance user. However, there are indications that those individuals who resort to substance use and abuse manifest to some degree an inability to tolerate and adjust to the stresses and strains of daily living. Their disequilibrium is such that they seek ways of blurring their current reality. Frequently there seems to be some indication that these individuals set for themselves expectations beyond their capacity to achieve that often results in a lifelong pattern of failure. Coupled with this failure pattern is a corresponding inability to cope with or accept success. Furthermore, substance users tend to demonstrate low self-esteem along with feelings of inadequacy as well as limited tolerance for frustration and an inability to exercise self-control. In addition, they demonstrate passivity, which may be used to mask aggressive tendencies. This hidden aggression is displayed in either clearly overt or more subtle actions indicative of resentment toward authority.

Concepts and principles upon which nursing care is based include but are not limited to the following:

- Substance use and abuse are prevalent in all strata of society.
- Any substance that gives pleasure or relieves discomfort may induce psychological dependence.
- Substance use disorders are treatable, and recovery is possible.
- The abuser finds his current reality intolerable.

- The need for dependence takes precedence over physical needs.
- The abuser exhibits low self-esteem and projects blame for felt inadequacies.
- Coexistence of an altered physiological state may place the client in a life-threatening situation.
- Fluid and electrolyte imbalances are common during withdrawal.
- The person who exhibits chemical dependence or abuse demonstrates an inability to make long-term commitments.
- Current meaningful interpersonal relationships are almost nonexistent.
- Substance use alienates significant others.
- The abuser is a master of manipulative tactics.
- Successful experiences are important to interrupt a lifelong pattern of failure and inadequacy.
- Stressors can be antecedent cues to drinking behavior.
- A social support network is necessary for rehabilitation.
- A structured supportive environment will facilitate the learning of alternative adaptive responses to stress.
- Environmental stimuli should be kept to a minimum because of low frustration tolerance.
- A demonstration of acceptance, concern, and understanding serve as a source of strength to the patient.
- Attitudinal change in the client is a necessary prerequisite to successful rehabilitation.
- Staff attitudes influence the rehabilitation process.
- Hopefulness can be maintained by formulating goals with levels of expectation commensurate with patients' presenting needs.
- Hopefulness can be communicated.
- Action-oriented behaviors are more likely to create hopefulness.
- Success breeds self-confidence; self-confidence enhances self-esteem.
- Recognition of assets by the client leads to increased self-worth.
- A substance abuser does not stop using mood-altering drugs until he discovers something better.
- Recovery involves taking control of one's life.
- Alternatives to drug abuse also serve as alternatives to other self-destructive or deviant behavior.

For additional information regarding etiology, dynamics, and onset for this broad classification of substance use disorders the reader is referred to Table 11–1. For additional data concerning addictive behavior and specific nursing interventions, the reader is referred to Chapter 22.

SCHIZOPHRENIC DISORDERS

Schizophrenia is a movement away from reality into an inner world of fantasy—a world that is at once bizarre, frightening, overwhelming, and yet, apparently infinitely more bearable than the "real world." The person with schizophrenia experiences such inner pain and conflict that his patterns of thinking, feeling, and acting become grossly distorted. Frequently, these exaggerated and disturbed manifestations are not only frightening to the individual but to those with whom he comes in contact. The individual with schizophrenia may be described as a person who is out of tune with the rest of society—someone who just doesn't make sense to others. The psychotic individual is one who overreacts, underreacts, or reacts uniquely and unexpectedly to the general demands of living.

Schizophrenia is a major mental disorder whose chief characteristic is gross deterioration in ego functioning. Severe personality disintegration and disorganization are manifested through disorientation in the cognitive and sensory spheres, withdrawal and isolation from the environment, and offensive or bizarre behavior that is often accompanied by pronounced regression. There are several diagnostic categories within the classification of schizophrenic disorders (see Table 11–1).

This mental disorder is probably the most prevalent of the psychotic disorders due to its early onset and chronic nature. Schizophrenia represents a group of reactions whose chief characteristics appear to be an inability to formulate reality relationships, disturbances in the boundaries of self-image, along with distortions in the affective and cognitive domains. The four primary symptoms connected with the schizophrenic disorders are ambivalence, autism, looseness of associations, and affective disturbances. The predominant behavior pattern exhibited is withdrawal. The predominant coping mechanism is regression.

The schizophrenic patient is unable to cope with the problems of living. His use of ego defenses is often ineffective and inappropriate, which results in intense and overwhelming anxiety. As the anxiety mounts, the patient isolates himself from others and displays a lack of concern for social demands in an attempt to ward off possible anticipated rejection from others, thus evidencing a widening social distance that progresses to the pathological state of loneliness. Characteristically, the schizophrenic's fantasy world is dominated by delusions of persecution, auditory hallucinations, and preoccupation with bodily functions.

Many theories have been postulated regarding the possible cause or causes of schizophrenia; however, a review of the current literature reveals that despite the number of studies that have been conducted, no single cause has as yet been identified. The most likely theory is that of multiple causation, taking into account such factors as the individual's vulnerability and sensitivity to stress; the type of personality the individual is or was prior to onset; the specific modes of adaptation the individual uses in the stress situation; the type of social, cultural, and economic background that influenced his development; his biophysiological and chemical makeup and familial hereditary factors.

The complexity of the symptom picture of schizophrenia has resulted in the identification of specific types. Included among these are the following.

Disorganized Type

This type of schizophrenic disorder demonstrates a severe disintegration of the personality. The background of the patient often reveals a history of numerous peculiar mannerisms, overscrupulousness about trivial matters, and preoccupation with religious or philosophical issues. The patient experiences disorganized thinking, a shallow and markedly inappropriate affect accompanied by excessive giggling, silliness, and severe regressive behavior. Hallucinations and delusions are common and are transient, unsystematized, and bizarre. Usually the patient will display obscene behavior and demonstrate a frank absence of any modesty or sense of shame. In addition, this individual is subject to impulsive, explosive outbursts of angry, hostile feelings and displays temper tantrums, which are generally in response to his fantasy life.

Catatonic Type

This clinical condition appears suddenly and is commonly observed to be of two subtypes—**catatonic excitement** and **catatonic stupor**. Typically, there may be alterations or swings between these two subtypes. Catatonic excitement is characterized by hyperactivity, that is, excessive and sometimes violent motor activity. Usual behavior includes marked agitation and impulsive and explosive acting out. Catatonic stupor is characterized by a loss of animation, mutism, negativism, and waxy flexibility. The patient is unable to function independently. He will remain motionless for long periods of time and seldom responds to verbal commands. However, while in this apparently detached state the individual does not lose awareness of his environment, even though he demonstrates no obvious external response.

Paranoid Type

The paranoid type generally becomes apparent in adult life. Characteristically, the patient's life pattern has been dominated by hostility, suspicion, and distrust. The patient's autistic manifestations are predominantly those of persecutory or grandiose delusions and auditory hallucinations of an accusatory or threatening nature. Much of the patient's ideation centers around sexual and religious content. In this type, regression is less pronounced, with a corresponding ability to sustain some semblance of personality organization and attention to the maintenance of physical appearance.

For further details to supplement this brief overview of the schizophrenic process, dynamics, and subclassification, the reader is referred to the suggested readings at the end of the chapter. In addition, Chapter 25 provides a complete account of a patient with a diagnosis of schizophrenia, paranoid type. This chapter describes the family constellation, and identifies developing symptomatology and precipitating stress factors that led to psychiatric hospitalization. Chapter 26 is a further elaboration and contains the completed nursing assessment and subsequent nursing intervention.

Undifferentiated Type

This category reflects a unique feature that is not found in the previously identified types. That is, in clinical situations an individual may be encountered who displays all of the essential characteristics of schizophrenia, yet does not display a majority of the essential features described under any of the above types. Furthermore, there may be, in fact, such a variety of essential and associated characteristics that clear-cut clinical differentiation is impossible. Thus, since differentiation is unclear, a specific subtype, **undifferentiated**, has been established.

Residual Type

The term **residual** is applied to schizophrenia when there is evidence to support the continued presence of diagnostic symptomatology after an individual has recovered from an acute episode. Its designation as residual indicates the chronic aspect of schizophrenia. Symptomatically, the individual manifests emotional blunting, eccentric behavior, and social withdrawal. Most often, this condition does not warrant continued institutionalization. Thus, the individual with residual schizophrenia often returns to his community to live and frequently resumes a role within the work force. However, his contribution, in terms of productivity and effectiveness of performance, is at a diminished level when compared to performance displayed prior to the original onset of illness.

Concepts and principles upon which nursing care is based include but are not limited to the following:

- Symptomatology is a maladaptive coping mechanism that is used as a defensive operation or protective device.
- Presenting symptomatology is evidence of unmet needs.

- Symptoms are a method of communication and can be understood through exploration and clarification with the client.
- The bizarre and often eccentric behaviors exhibited by the patient have symbolic meaning known only to him.
- The most frequent automatic coping mechanisms include rationalization, projection, depersonalization, and regression.
- Self-concept is not clearly defined.
- Validation of communication assists in defining the self-concept.
- The environment is perceived as hostile and threatening to self due to poorly developed or nonexistent ego boundaries.
- Loss of ego boundaries and identity produces feelings of depersonalization and movement away from reality.
- Fluctuations and variability between periods of rational and irrational behavior are characteristic of the schizophrenic process.
- Decreased reality testing is evidenced by presence of delusions and hallucinations.
- Misinterpretation of reality leads to increases in the level of anxiety, fear, and a sense of alienation.
- Individuals exhibit a limited capacity for intimacy.
- Tolerance for frustration is minimal.
- Rejection and resistance are maneuvers used to sabotage relationships.
- Resistance and distancing maneuvers are used to protect the self from hurt.
- Hypersensitivity and excessive symbolism interfere with the individual's capacity for socialization.
- Security operations should be supported until such time that the patient learns new ways of adapting.
- Physical and psychological needs merit equal attention.
- Care must be directed toward the building and the maintenance of healthy relationships based on trust.
- Consistency and persistence in approach are essential to the establishment of rapport, the building of trust, and promotion of interpersonal relationships.
- Clarification of communication is needed to decrease distortions in perceptual and cognitive functioning.
- Interpretation of communication is difficult because of the person's affective distortions.
- Genuine interest, honesty, warmth, and optimism are essential for establishing contact with psychotic persons.
- Reduction of environmental stimuli prevents sensory overload, thereby reducing threats to security and limiting regressive behavior.
- Reduction of anxiety and stress increases comfort and security.
- Purposeful activity promotes self-esteem and establishes contact with external reality.

- Activities and personal contacts should be directed to increasing self-esteem and feelings of adequacy.
- Effective nursing intervention requires that the nurse promote functioning by "doing with" rather than "for" the patient.

AFFECTIVE DISORDERS

Affective disorders is a broad classification that encompasses a number of diagnostic entities whose common and essential feature is a disturbance in **mood**. This mood disturbance is accompanied by distortions or exaggerations of cognitive, psychomotor, psychophysiological, and interpersonal functioning. The clinical conditions considered within this classification involve two major emotions, **depression** and **mania**. These emotions and the changes their presence produces within the individual are pervasive and sustained, thus influencing the total personality and performance of the individual.

The DSM-III has reorganized the classification system of affective disorders to include all conditions with an affective component, whether or not these conditions present distinctly neurotic or psychotic features. The new classification divides affective disorders into three separate categories: major affective disorders, other specific affective disorders, and atypical affective disorders. **Major affective disorders** indicate the presence of a full affective syndrome and are further subdivided into **bipolar disorder** and **major depression**. The second category, **other specific affective disorders**, stipulates that there exists only a partial affective syndrome that has been in existence for at least two years' duration. Under this category are classified the **cyclothymic disorder** and the **dysthymic disorder**. In the third category, **atypical affective disorders**, the diagnostic criteria indicate that the subdivisions of **atypical bipolar disorder** and **atypical depression** are residual categories to be employed when individuals having once been diagnosed as having had a major episode experience a recurrence whose features do not clearly meet the diagnostic criteria of the first two major categories.

Affective disorders usually manifest themselves between the ages of 20 and 35. Current theory supports the idea that genetic factors may be involved along with some biochemical or physiologic alterations. Analytic theory places emphasis on unmet oral needs, self-hatred, and loss of self-esteem. It is commonly accepted that the feelings of aggression and hostility are in response to threats to the security and self-esteem of the individual. The outward expression of aggression results in manic behavior, while the inward direction of aggression results in depressive behavior.

Unlike the schizophrenic, the individual with an affective disorder maintains a better integrated self-system, and his total functioning is less bizarre and distorted. To further clarify, compare, and contrast the significant differences between schizophrenia and the major affective disorders, the reader should refer to the outline in Table 11–2. It will be helpful in distinguishing the etiologic, symptomatologic, and dynamic differences in these two prevalent and frequently encountered disorders. The first two major categories—major affective disorders and other specific affective disorders—are briefly described in the following discussion.

Major Affective Disorders

Major affective disorders are distinguished by one or more episodes involving a severe and pronounced disturbance in mood. The disruption in mood is identified as being either manic or depressed. The major characteristic of a manic episode is an elevated, expansive, or irritable mood in connection with such symptoms as hyperactive behavior; purposeless activity; poor judgment; unrealistic expectations of self; distractibility; flight of ideas; wakefulness; and pressure of speech as evidenced by circumstantiality, rhyming, punning, and clang associations. The total picture involving cognitive, sensory, and psychomotor activity can be described as disorganized, flamboyant, enthusiastic, grandiose, dramatic, and oftentimes bizarre. The distinguishing feature of a depressive episode is a pervasive depressive mood that is associated with such symptoms as the following: disturbance in appetite and sleep patterns; a change in weight; psychomotor agitation or retardation; a marked decrease in energy level; a pronounced loss of interest or pleasure in self and activities; morbid preoccupation with death and dying; suicidal threats and attempts; cognitive disturbance in the form of inability to concentrate or follow directions; and the expression of feelings related to worthlessness and guilt. In major affective disorders, any given episode may be diagnosed as manic, depressed, or mixed depending on presenting symptomatology. If psychotic manifestations are also present in the symptom picture, these are also included in the diagnosis.

Typically, manic episodes appear to occur prior to the age of 30, while the depressive episode has been observed to occur in infancy and throughout the life span. Manic episodes present a clear and precise point of sudden onset followed by a rapid escalation of symptoms in a relatively short period of time. On the other hand, a major depressive episode may vary from sudden onset over a period of days to a more insidious onset occurring over a period of several months. When comparing durations of episodes, it appears that manic episodes are shorter and terminate more abruptly than major depressive episodes.

TABLE 11–2. GENERAL COMPARISON BETWEEN THE SCHIZOPHRENIC AND MAJOR AFFECTIVE DISORDERS

Elements for Comparison	Schizophrenia	Major Affective Disorders	
		Manic Episode	***Depressive Episode***
1. Prepsychotic personality	Introvertive. Aloof. Daydreaming. Shy and indifferent. Rejecting. Emotionally detached.	Extrovertive. Overtly aggressive. Manipulative. Confident and friendly. Sensitive. Pronounced feeling of well-being.	Unobtrusive. Passively aggressive. Rigid and fearful. Timid and retiring. Sensitive. Pronounced feeling of sadness and morbidity.
2. Causes	Multiple causes. Most likely related to psychological, sociocultural, organic and hereditary factors.	Traumatic stress. Long-standing unresolved conflict. Poorly developed and integrated ego boundaries. Unresolved diffuse anger and hostility. Repeated failure in early life to measure up to parental expectations.	(Same as Manic Episode) Loss of significant others or objects.
3. Dynamics	Withdrawal from reality. Preoccupation with fantasy. Fear of rejection. Regression to complete dependency. Loss of ego boundaries. Loss of personal identity. Inability to distinguish between objective reality and fantasy.	Unmet needs during infancy give rise to feelings of insecurity and dependency with resultant ambivalence. Confidence and self-assurance are defenses against dependency. Represses hostility and guilt in effort to seek approval from others. Unrealistic expectations of self give rise to feelings of inferiority and inadequacy. Flight into reality. Attacks external environment. Uses rationalization and projection.	Real or imaginary loss perceived as rejection. Repressed hostility and hatred turned inward as a result of rigid superego. Penance in the form of guilt feelings for aggressive and hostile feelings. Denial of aggression produces helplessness and hopelessness.

4. Symptoms			
a) Cognitive process	Associative looseness. Autistic or magical thinking. Concrete rather than abstract. Vague and neologistic. Illogical sequence of thought. Blocking. Depersonalization. Hallucinations and delusions. Perseverance. Incoherence. Religiosity.	Flight of ideas. Circumstantiality. Grandiose delusions. Distractibility. Rhyming. Punning. Clang association. Absence of self-criticism.	Poverty of ideas. Retardation of thought process. Self-accusatory and somatic delusions. Confusion and perplexity. Impairment of concentration and memory. Excessive preoccupation with a particularly personal meaningful life event. Suicidal preoccupation.
b) Multisensory integration	Inappropriate affect. Blunted or flattened affect. Inadequate, inconsistent, or exaggerated affect. Ambivalence. Indifference. Distrust. Shallowness. Anxiety. Loneliness. Apathy.	Euphoric, effusive, elated. Volatile and erratic. Aggressive, irritable and self-exaltive. Increasing intensity of pseudopositive feeling states. Omnipotence and omniscience.	Despondent, despairing. Gloomy, pessimistic. Unworthiness, guilt. Inadequacy, inferiority. Helplessness and hopelessness. Bitterness and anger. Fear, loneliness. Anxiety.
c) Psychomotor activity	Withdrawn. Negativistic. Ritualistic. Automatic. Impulsive. Regressive. Posturing.	Hyperactive. Boisterous, teasing, meddlesome. Arrogant and pompous. Sarcastic, insulting, and caustic. Irritable, abusive, or violent. Exhibitionistic, vulgar, and profane. Overtly seductive and obscene. Wakeful.	Underactive or agitated. Marked fatigue. Lack of appetite. Weight loss. Early morning wakefulness. Suicidal gestures. Lassitude. Bored. Crying.

Other Specific Affective Disorders

This clinical entity identifies chronic mood disturbance. Its identifying characteristic is the presence of long-standing illness of at least 2 years' duration with either continuous symptomatology or alternating periods of mild exacerbation and remission. Other specific affective disorders do not identify psychotic features as a part of the associated symptomatology.

This clinical entity is divided into two subtypes, **cyclothymic disorder** and **dysthymic disorder**. In cyclothymic disorder, the individual experiences a chronic mood disturbance of at least 2 years' duration. This condition may evidence symptoms associated with both the manic and depressive syndromes. However, their severity and duration are less pronounced and do not meet the criteria for a major episode. Furthermore, the depressive and hypomanic periods alternate with periods of normal mood. In dysthymic disorder, the chief characteristic is a chronic nonpsychotic disturbance of depressed mood or a loss of interest or pleasure in all or almost all activities and pastimes.

The following two case presentations serve to provide the reader with explicit examples of two classes of major affective disorders: the bipolar disorder, manic type and major depression, recurrent.

Situation III

Present Illness: Kathryn Howard is a 24-year-old, white, married woman who was admitted to a state hospital for the second time on a voluntary basis. She was first admitted to the state hospital in early February but was subsequently transferred to a small private hospital. After 1 week in that facility she was taken home by her husband and remained there until her present admission in early March. At this time, she was agitated, overtalkative, delusional, and the presence of hallucinations was suspected.

Past History: Kathryn was born in Chicago and has lived in Illinois all of her life except for the past 6 months, which were spent in Lancaster, Pennsylvania. She is the oldest of four. Kathryn finished high school and during her admission interview stated that she did not like school and had never made good grades except in English. Kathryn married at 18 and held a variety of jobs until her son was born about 3 years ago. Her husband, who is 27, is somewhat effeminate and immature. They had dated each other since Kathryn was in the ninth grade and neither had had any previous dating experience. Kathryn is Protestant and her husband, Joe, is Jewish, and for this reason both sets of parents have always disapproved of the marriage. Joe had been working as a disc jockey in Lancaster but lost his job because of his wife's behavior and at present is unemployed, receiving welfare. Now they live alternately with each set of parents. Kathryn's mother is 41; her father, 51, is a diabetic, has had recurrent skin cancer, and has just recently had surgery. One brother, age 23, has asthma, is retarded, lives at home and works in a laundry close by. Two other siblings, a sister, 13, and a brother, 4, are in good health and live with their parents.

Appearance and behavior: Kathryn is a well-developed, adequately nourished woman who looks and acts like a 15-year old. She is oriented in all three spheres. Her speech is rapid, constant, and irrelevant, and she speaks with a "little-girl voice." She demonstrates a flight of ideas, delusions, and a labile mood that alternates between euphoria and slight depression. She talks of getting pregnant from men who slipped into her hospital bed and raped her. She says, "My husband is a fag. My mother didn't give me the right attention and it has to come out some way. I think I might be a man. I have a large Adam's apple. I am writing a book. People send me messages. I can predict for the President of the United States. The President is a communist. I have supernatural powers. I am helping all these girls. God talks to me. I know nobody believes me."

Kathryn's memory is intact, she displays no insight, and her judgment is impaired. She is hyperactive, spends a great deal of time pacing, shouting orders, and advising others, and sleeps about 4 hours per night.

Situation IV

Present Illness: George Garner is a 44-year-old, black, married male who was admitted to an acute care setting. On admission he was in a state of psychomotor retardation, depressed, and responded only to direct questions in a whispering monotone.

Past History: George was born in Birmingham, Alabama. His family moved to the Cleveland area when he was 3 years old. He is the third of nine siblings. His two older brothers and a younger sister were killed in an automobile accident 15 years ago. The remaining three brothers and two sisters are married and well. His parents are both dead.

George graduated from college, earned a teaching certificate, and is currently a high school principal. He met his wife, Mildred, while in college, and they were married shortly after their graduation. They have no children.

He was promoted to his present position just 2 months ago. For a month prior to admission, he had shown an increasing inability to perform his duties. His lack of initiative and depressed emotional state was noticed by his wife, family, students, and colleagues.

His history revealed one other psychiatric hospitalization when he was 30 years old, just 1 month after his automobile accident. His wife reports that he had had periodic "fits of depression" where he would cry, wring his hands, and refuse to eat, but "they didn't last long." She says that his usual behavior is quiet, and retiring and he is never very happy. His wife further related that after the death of each of his parents he became very morose and frequently expressed the thought that he should die. Mildred stated that she thought this episode was like all the rest and that it would go away after awhile, but she really became concerned when she found him standing motionless in the middle of the bathroom holding a straight razor in his hand. He would not respond to her or tell her what he was doing. It was at this point that she called his brother, and together they brought him to the hospital.

Appearance and behavior: George is a tall, thin, almost emaciated man who looks and acts like an "old man." In the hospital, he refuses to eat, sleeps an average of 4 hours a night, and replies in barely audible monosyllables when questioned. He usually stands or sits with head bowed, eyes downcast, has a dejected facial expression, and will not join in activities with other patients or personnel. He is oriented to reality. However, he expresses a self-accusatory delusional system in which he blames himself for the deaths of his brothers and sister in an auto accident in which he was the driver.

These case histories, although markedly different in terms of social history and presenting symptoms, have a common denominator that is displayed through affective and behavioral patterns that represent an exaggerated aggressive response to living. In Situation III, Kathryn's response is externalized onto the environment, resulting in loud, hyperactive, and overtly aggressive dominating behavior. In Situation IV, George's aggression is turned inward on himself, resulting in rejection of the worthwhile self, overwhelming guilt, and self-punishment.

Concepts and principles upon which nursing care is based include but are not limited to the following:

Survival for the client depends on the meeting of his basic needs.

MANIC EPISODE

- Exaggerated responses to stimuli necessitate a physical and emotional environment that is nonstimulating.
- Mania is manifested by an acceleration of thought processes.
- Neutrality and objectivity in light of hyperactive behavior enable the nurse to provide consistency in the application of external controls.
- Hyperactivity leads to exhaustion.
- Respect of interpersonal space prevents acting-out behavior.
- Stability of environment and firm limit setting promote identification of realistic ego boundaries and act as external controls.
- Maintenance of interpersonal and environmental distance allows the patient freedom of movement.
- The verbal expression of hostile feelings acts as a safety valve and should not be discouraged.
- Extreme hostility may be directed toward others through acts of violence.
- Physical violence is preceded by cues of impending uncontrollable behavior.
- Redirection of behavior discharges excess energy.

- Argumentation and contradiction exacerbate existing symptomatology.

DEPRESSIVE EPISODE

- The potential for suicide is always present.
- Close observation is necessary for the clients' safety and protection.
- Decreased potential for danger can be achieved through monitoring the environment.
- Negative attitudes, comments, or the nonverbal communication of others are readily incorporated into self-depreciatory ideation.
- Feelings of hopelessness and helplessness interfere with socialization.
- A subtle, pleasant, interested approach will reinforce a sense of dignity and worth.
- Worthwhile, useful menial tasks enable the individual to rid himself of guilt and allow him to feel a sense of accomplishment.
- Planned scheduled activities are needed to increase social contracts, distract preoccupation with self, and lessen the feeling of hopelessness and helplessness.
- Legitimate praise decreases self-depreciatory behavior.
- Feelings of guilt and lack of self-esteem prevent movement toward wellness.
- Decision-making progresses in complexity based on client readiness.
- Nursing care should focus on lessening the client's feelings of guilt and increasing self-esteem.
- Safety and protective measures are necessary to guard against self-destructive behavior.

ANXIETY DISORDERS

Anxiety disorders demonstrate a broad range of responses to overwhelming anxiety. The predominant behavioral pattern within this clinical syndrome is that of **ritualism**. The clinical symptoms seen within this diagnostic classification are viewed as ineffective substitutes for satisfactory need gratification. They are generally of a symbolic nature, reflecting the underlying conflict, and usually interfere with the maintenance of interpersonal relationships. The underlying conflict can be traced to disturbances within childhood developmental experiences, particularly those in which primal cravings and vital stimuli were not met or were thwarted and resulted in the imposition of rigid restrictions. In adult life the outcome is conflict, which produces tension and the need for defensive and security operations. Thus, the patient is responding to internal or external stress. His response permits him to avoid the initial stressful situation while allowing him to obtain gratification for his previously unmet dependency needs. The following excerpt from a case history illustrates a rather classical picture of a generalized anxiety disorder.

Situation V

Mr. Starre is a 42-year-old, Caucasian, married man who works as a foreman in a steel mill. He is the father of three children, two boys and a girl, ages 17, 15, and 12 respectively. In the past 2 years, he has experienced progressive feelings of acute uneasiness. Originally, he displayed periodic restlessness and evidenced some minor disturbances in his sleep pattern. Gradually, he began to complain of indigestion, palpitations, loss of appetite, constipation, cold sweats, insomnia, and impotence. In addition, he became more irritable, short-tempered, and demanding, and imposed more and more rigid restrictions, not only on his two sons but also on the men he supervised at work. His sick days began to outnumber his work days. He sought frequent medical assistance but stated that he didn't feel any better despite the variety of medications he was taking. Mr. Starre had been admitted to various hospitals for complete physical examinations and diagnostic evaluation. He refused to believe that all the test results were negative and maintained that he was a "sick man." On his last admission he became very angry when the physician suggested that a psychiatric consult should be considered. He demanded that he be discharged so that he could "find himself a doctor who really knows what he is doing."

Mr. Starre's behavior represents a deep-seated and long-term problem. The anxiety displayed has intensified over time so that his total functioning as an individual—as a father, husband, and foreman—has been severely disrupted. He manifests excessive use of rationalization and denial. If left untreated, more severe ego dysfunction can be anticipated which, in turn, can lead to a complete alienation of his family, friends, and co-workers.

Most authorities believe that anxiety disorders are less severe and disabling than other psychiatric disorders; nevertheless, they can and do produce marked interference with effective and efficient functioning. Table 11–3 outlines in greater detail the chief clinical entities within this broad diagnostic classification and highlights the dynamics, the defensive operations, and the specific symptomatology displayed along with the general concepts and principles for nursing care.

There are important points for the nurse to remember while caring for the anxious patient. First, realize that the individual is experiencing real discomfort and distress. Second, the overwhelming anxiety and corresponding fears that are felt by the patient are as significant as any physical pain or condition. Third, symptoms are *consciously* unwanted and viewed by the individual as undesirable; they produce irritation and create distress, are felt to be strange and to produce discontent in daily living. Fourth, the clinical picture is not always definitive and more than one condition or type may exist simultaneously. And fifth, the specific symptoms associated with this diagnostic category are not limited; diagnosis may be an organic mental disorder, substance use disorder, or schizophrenic disorder. For more detailed information on the concept of anxiety, we refer the reader to Chapters 7 and 21.

Concepts and principles upon which nursing care is based include but are not limited to the following:

- Anxiety is psychic pain that arises from conflict between the id and the ego.
- Anxiety is manifested through biophysical, psychosocial, and cognitive modes of response.
- Anxiety can be transmitted interpersonally.
- Anxiety interferes with cognitive functioning, with a resultant loss of objectivity.
- Acknowledgment of somatic concerns reduces the level of anxiety.
- As the level of anxiety increases, there is a corresponding increase in the expenditure of energy with less effective adaptation, requiring more assistance from the care provider.
- Early recognition of mounting anxiety can prevent an acute episode.
- Defensive operations are used to protect the ego and maintain integrity.
- The presence of anxiety signals a need for adaptation.
- Intervention is imperative before anxiety mounts and becomes uncontrollable.
- Ventilation of feelings reduces the level of anxiety.
- Ability to verbalize discomfort brings temporary relief from mounting anxiety.
- Automatic coping devices afford limited relief from psychic pain.
- Rituals release tension and temporarily reduce the level of anxiety.
- Interruption of ritualistic behavior increases the patient's anxiety and guilt.
- Physical complaints require investigation.
- Reinforcement of positive coping behaviors enhances self-esteem.

TABLE 11–3. AN OVERVIEW OF ANXIETY DISORDERS

Condition	Definition	Dynamics	Symptom Picture	Concepts and Principles for Nursing Care
Phobic disorders	A reaction of intense, recurrent, unreasonable fear attached to a specific object, activity, or situation.	Incomplete repression with **displacement** of anxiety onto an external focus which the individual can then avoid. Particular phobias assume a **symbolic** significance with respect to underlying emotional conflicts or unacceptable desires.	Intense, prolonged, irrational, and disabling fear. Avoidance of the phobic stimulus. Recognition of the response as disproportionate to the stimulus.	Phobias are **real** to the individual. Avoidance patterns are necessary to survival. The nurse assumes initiative in seeking out the patient and provides opportunities for the verbal expression of feelings. Control of phobic responses can be effected by application of learning theory in the form of behavior modification through desensitization, shaping, and conditioning.
Anxiety states	A reaction in response to no apparent or insufficient environmental stimulus of at least one month's duration.	Unresolved emotional conflict evokes overwhelming anxiety. Specific symptomatology provides an external means for expressing repressed material. Resolution of conflict is avoided through symbolic expression, that is, symptoms.	Free-floating anxiety of an acute or chronic nature. Variations in level of intensity. Symptom picture includes psychological manifestations (depression, guilt, confusion, and agitation) and physical manifestations (tachycardia, palpitations, paresthesias).	Since anxiety is transmittable interpersonally and since the client is highly responsive to suggestion and stimuli, the nurse must recognize, understand, and deal with her own level of anxiety. Specific behavior of the patient connotes unmet

			Maintenance of symptomatology is sustained through primary and secondary gains.	needs. Conscious awareness of anxiety is the first step in the interruption of repetitive behavioral patterns. Readiness and motivation to change behavior are essential for controlling anxiety and resolving underlying conflicts. Support is conveyed through an attitude of self-worth and hopefulness.
Post-traumatic stress disorder	A reaction to traumatic life events to which the individual is unable to adapt or adjust.	A stressor impacts to the extent that disequilibrium is produced. Coping mechanisms are inadequate to facilitate resolution. Residual associations remain; general resistance resources continue to be inadequate resulting in persistent disequilibrium.	Reexperiencing of the traumatic event causing withdrawal, isolation, and restricted emotional responses. Cognitive and autonomic disturbances.	Assessment includes detailed examination of precipitating stress factor and the patient's corresponding reaction. Somatic therapies are utilized to decrease anxiety, interrupt preoccupation, and restore socialization. Interventions are directed toward the reduction and prevention of chronic disability. Physical, social, or occupational rehabilitation is an essential component of the treatment process. Maintenance of personal integrity is a key attitudinal component of care.

- Increased motor activity is often a sign of impending crisis.
- Direct confrontation regarding client responses increases client's awareness to threatening stimuli.
- A warm, concerned human environment enhances the patient's security and reduces the level of anxiety.
- Assisting the client to recognize strengths and weaknesses contributes to a realistic self-assessment.
- Readiness, timing, and spacing of observational information prevents the client from being overwhelmed.
- Distraction from preoccupation with egocentric thoughts is possible through redirection.
- Continuous, consistent, and positive reassurance decreases agitation.
- Knowledge and understanding of "normal activity" will provide the nurse with the data base to assess the level of patient dysfunction.
- Acceptance by the nurse of the patient's avoidance pattern contributes to the patient's sense of security.
- Substitutions for avoidance behavior should be introduced when the client evidences a readiness for change.

SOMATIFORM DISORDERS

This classification of disorders is distinguished by the predominance of physical symptomatology identified by the patient as producing distress, discomfort, and pain. Although the patient clearly describes the symptoms, there is no corroborating evidence of organic disturbance or dysfunction. On the other hand, there may be presumptive evidence that associates the presenting symptomatology with psychogenic factors. The symptoms are real for the client, not under volitional control, and involve primarily the autonomic as well as the sensory or motor nervous systems. In this disease classification, physical symptoms are representative of unconscious conflict. The specific symptomatology expressed by the individual connotes symbolic communication of the underlying distress. The symptoms serve a twofold purpose. First, they are a means of expressing unacceptable emotions of fear, anger, sadness, or inadequacy. Second, they are a means of meeting needs for attention, approval, dependency, and security.

Specific conditions identified within this broad classification include **somatization disorder, conversion disorder, psychogenic pain disorder, hypochondriasis**, and **atypical somatiform disorder**. The first four major categories are briefly described in the following discussion.

Somatization Disorder

The predominant clinical features of this category are the presence of recurrent and multiple physical symptoms that predispose the individual to seek out medical attention for relief. The symptom picture is vague and is presented in an exaggerated manner. Symptoms usually involve complaints associated with organ systems, such as gastrointestinal, in the form of abdominal pain; cardiopulmonary, evidenced by dizziness; or reproductive, as indicated by painful menstruation. Corresponding affective disturbances may be seen in the form of heightened levels of anxiety and depression. Physical findings are not significant. The first manifestations of this condition appear in early adulthood, and evidence seems to indicate that it is more common in females than in males.

Conversion Disorder

Conversion disorder is a reaction in which the individual unconsciously transforms his underlying conflict into specific kinds of motor or sensory dysfunction suggestive of the presence of a physical condition. Again, there is no supporting documentation indicating the involvement of a pathophysiological mechanism. Environmental conditions surrounding the individual point to the existence of conflict or unmet needs and can be identified as a causative factor in precipitating or intensifying the symptom picture. In addition, the presence of the symptomatology earns for the individual a secondary gain that accounts for the relative lack of concern in the face of the potential severity and nature of the impairment.

By definition, a **secondary gain** is the attached value or gratification that the individual experiences as a result of the way in which the sociocultural environment reacts to the person's illness. A secondary gain is not an integral part of the presenting symptoms per se, but is viewed unconsciously by the individual as a benefit derived from the presence of illness. For those individuals diagnosed as having a conversion disorder, one such gain might be avoidance of some action or participation in some activity which is deemed either unacceptable or undesirable. Another secondary gain might be that the individual is able to obtain support from significant others within his environment. which otherwise might not be forthcoming. Specific physical manifestations of this condition include such symptoms as blindness, paralysis, deafness, aphonia, laryngitis, or convulsions.

Psychogenic Pain Disorder

The most salient feature evident in this condition is the presence of severe and prolonged pain for which no specific cause can be established. However, in some cases of **psychogenic pain** there is minimal evidence of pathological change, although physical findings cannot account for the patient's description of its intensity and degree of incapacitation. The psychological factors influencing the course of the condition are identical to those that operate in the conversion disorders. Initial onset is frequently seen in adolescence, although the condition may erupt at any stage in the life span. Severe psychosocial stressors which the individual has limited resources to combat are seen as predisposing factors in the development of this condition. Impairment varies with the intensity and duration of the episode and may range from mild social and occupational dysfunction to total immobilization.

Hypochondriasis

The symptom picture for hypochondriasis features a distortion in interpretation of existing physical signs or sensations that lead the individual to an unrealistic belief that their presence is indicative of a serious debilitating disease process. Thorough physical examination does not support such a conclusion, although a physical disorder may be present. The underlying dynamics of this condition seem to be related to a narcissistic view of self in which the individual substitutes an image of himself as being physically ill in order to avoid dealing with the self as a less than worthwhile human being. This condition is found to be equally distributed among men and women and occurs most frequently during adolescence. Social and occupational functioning may remain relatively intact, provided the individual's preoccupation with self and bodily functioning is limited. However, in some cases, individuals can and do adopt sick role behavior, resulting in the establishment of an invalid life style that precludes participation in normal daily activities.

Concepts and principles upon which nursing care is based include but are not limited to the following:

- Mind and body work in concert as an integrated whole.
- Physical symptoms are not under volitional control.
- The symptoms and corresponding impairment cannot be changed as a result of intellectual reasoning.
- Symptoms have a symbolic value to the client reflective of primary and secondary gains.
- Secondary gains serve as a reward and reinforcement of the disorder with its associated symptoms.
- Presenting symptoms usually involve the voluntary and sensory systems.
- The physical symptoms serve to lessen any consciously felt anxiety in a socially acceptable way.

- The perception of symptoms is real for the patient; therefore, the need for relief is also real.
- Environmental stressors intensify symptomatology.
- Observation is critical in order to obtain a realistic data base for ruling out the presence of physiological cause.
- The ability to distinguish and describe subjective feeling states enhances the client's self-awareness and autonomous functioning.
- Strategies for adaptation against anticipated anxiety or frustration can be learned.
- Symptom reduction can be achieved through the deliberate use of relaxation techniques.
- A calm, warm, supportive approach conveys understanding and acceptance.
- It is necessary for the nurse to understand the patient's feelings and behavior and not pass judgment on his actions.
- Labeling of the patient interferes with the initiation of a therapeutic approach.
- Autonomy can be achieved through self-regulation and self-management.
- Socialization can be enhanced through the implementation of activities to generate a feeling of self-satisfaction.
- Intervention is directed toward caring for the whole person and not focused on specific symptomatology.
- Reduction of anxiety promotes restoration of psychological equilibrium.
- Attention is directed from preoccupation with self and symptomatology toward purposeful activities that are designed to promote interest and success.
- Nursing care is based on the acknowledgment of the attitudes of personal integrity, personal worth, and open-mindedness.

PERSONALITY DISORDERS

The **personality disorders** can best be described as a disorganized way of living. They are probably the most challenging and the least understood of the psychiatric disorders. Unlike many of the other diagnostic classifications, the personality disorders originate from a cathexis of lifelong experiences resulting in basic disturbances in the individual's ability to interact appropriately with society within the context of societal norms. Since the personality disorders demonstrate a repetitive pattern of behavior that manifests specific deficits within the personality structure, the individual experiences problems in living, rather than specific symptoms as with other psychiatric disorders.

The type of maladjusted behavior evidenced indicates that the observable pathology is outwardly directed toward and against others. Because of its lifelong, deeply ingrained, and persistent nature, causation is attributed to faulty or arrested emotional development during the first three years of life where there has been apparent interference with the development of adequate social control or superego formation. Therefore, during early childhood experiences the individual has most likely been deprived of satisfactory gratification of the basic needs of love, security, trust, and responsibility.

The characteristic symptom pattern associated with personality disorders incorporates one or more of the following:

- Poor or marginal interpersonal relationships.
- Severely limited ability to feel or experience emotions (patient is often described as "cold" or "unfeeling").
- Easily distractible.
- Poor self-motivation.
- Marked lack of persistence except in areas of self-gratification.
- Limited stress tolerance.
- Impulsivity.
- Verbally or physically explosive, especially when crossed.
- Poor discriminative and reflective judgment.
- Fails to profit from experience.
- Lacks foresight.
- Distorted or absent moral code or value system.
- Behavior is generally manipulative, self-defeating, or destructive.

With each succeeding revision of the nomenclature there has been marked reorganization and realignment of the specific diagnostic categories included in this section. Personality disorders include a myriad of conditions covering a wide array of personality, character, and behavioral maladjustments in living. We refer the reader to the suggested reading material at the end of the chapter for more detailed information on the specific conditions that were identified in Table 11–1.

The case history of Paul Miller is a typical example of two of the clinical conditions seen in this broad diagnostic category. His diagnoses are passive-aggressive personality disorder and antisocial personality disorder.

Situation VI

Paul Miller is a 19-year-old, black male, who was admitted to a state hospital after having severely beaten both of his parents while under the influence of alcohol. His parents reported that "he was always a problem" and was continuously in and out of trouble at school. At the age of 14,

Paul was with his friend in a stolen car when they were stopped by the police who, according to the patient, later "beat them" and brought them to a juvenile detention home. Subsequently, Paul was placed on probation for 2½ years. Since that time Paul developed an animosity toward the police and believes that the police are "doing wrong and not doing justice to the people." The patient has had several confrontations with the police, but he refused to elaborate on the specific incidents. However, in talking with the nurses on the ward, he did relate portions of some of these experiences. He admits to having robbed the homes of some elderly people across town. He stated that in his conscience he does not feel that there is anything wrong with this. "After all, I didn't steal from our neighbors." He further commented, "This is a dog-eat-dog world. I was brought up on the streets." He admitted that he started to drink at the age of 16. Since that time he has had many episodes of excessive drinking and when he came home he was, according to his parents, violent, hostile, and unmanageable. One year ago, he related that he struck his father for the first time and later he also struck his mother. His mother stated that she is "scared of him." A few months ago, Paul left his parent's home and went to live in an apartment with a friend. He worked sporadically at various kinds of odd jobs but never for very long. Paul describes himself as "a good worker, who deserves more than what I get paid" and "a good friend with people I get along with."

His parents voiced concern about their son's behavior, stating that they had tried different ways to reach him in an effort to prevent his drinking habit but were not successful. They thought they had the solution when he came home last week, drunk and threatening. They called the police. But by the time the police had arrived, Paul had severely beaten both his parents. He was taken to the city jail and later transferred to the hospital. His parents were treated at a nearby hospital emergency room and released. They have hopes that perhaps this hospitalization will help him to find a morally and socially acceptable way of life.

In the hospital, the patient made new friends and became more interested in politics. He made several statements about the conditions in the United States, and his room is full of political literature, most of it leftist, for example, *Quotations from Chairman Mao Tse-tung*, *Report to the Ninth National Congress of the Communist Party of China*, and *Mass Line*, a newspaper of the American Communist Workers Movement. He stated that he is trying to find a life on his own, that he is not yet a Communist but is learning and trying to understand what is going on.

He wrote a letter to his parents in which he tried to convince them of his new political views and tried to explain what these things mean to him. He wrote, "The nation is run by the government and the government is run by the rich. All of the masses of the working people are the backbone of the country. In a matter of years, not many, there will be a revolution and there will be a great change in government and all Fascist courts, police, judges, and other unrealistic forces trained in using the great masses of the people then will no longer be."

In the same letter, he describes some of his experiences at the hospital: "When I inquired the purpose of the pills which they had given to me, they would say they were "to keep me calm and from being nervous and upset.' Since, they have said, 'Don't you sleep much better since you have taken the pills in the daytime?'—although I have taken none all of this time, but two."

During various therapy sessions Paul's mood changed from time to time. Sometimes he was very cooperative and friendly, talking freely, logically, and coherently about his personal problems and his personal life history. When his drinking habits were discussed, he repeatedly stated he felt he was old enough and adult enough to take the responsibility of this and said he was able to stop himself from becoming drunk but he also said he has pleasure from being drunk and wants to do it again. He describes himself as "a lumpen proletarian who belongs to the proletariat but prefers an easy way of life if possible with luxury, pleasure, etc." He says he "likes to have everything the best." If he has to choose, he wants to have "the best car, the best home, the best suit, the best shoes, and everything the best. I want to enjoy a family and have at least one boy and a daughter, but no more than four children." He says that he does not like a normal way of education and does not like to work in a factory—he prefers to be "the man who delivers and carries things on the truck." He further characterizes himself as having "a hot temper and one who acts easily and quickly." He demonstrated this aspect of his personality in several of the sessions by jumping up, waving his arms, and talking in a loud voice when the topics focused on issues or subjects he disliked.

He enjoys going to occupational and recreational therapy and spends much of his time talking politics with other patients, especially those younger than himself. Periodically, he insists that he has to be released as soon as possible. He is becoming slightly more critical of his drinking habits and states he is sorry for hitting his parents. He believes he is ready to go home, return to his family, and try to start a new life.

On initial encounter, those individuals who manifest personality disorders give the impression of being intelligent, charming, pleasant, friendly, and nonchalant people. However, closer scrutiny of the behavior and verbal comments such as those made by Paul Miller in this case presentation indicate that the facade is often misleading.

In planning intervention for patients with personality disorders the nurse will find the following concepts and principles helpful:

- Stressful life situations tend to increase aberrant behavior.
- Symptoms are used to mask feelings of inadequacy, worthlessness, and fear.
- Impulsive acting-out, including suicide and homicide, often emerge in response to frustration.
- Manipulative and aggressive behavior are used by the client to avoid meaningful relationships.
- Limit setting and consistent structuring of the environment enhance opportunities for learning socially acceptable responses.

- Limits are set according to the client's ability to accept responsibility for self.
- A direct, honest approach reinforces positive behavior.
- Consistency in staff responses promotes realistic self-awareness.
- Entrapment can occur when unrealistic goals are set and promises are made that cannot be kept.
- Compliance with the therapeutic regime is achieved through collaboration and sharing with the client.
- Confrontation rather than interpretation of behavior facilitates the internalization of alternative adaptive strategies.
- The nurse-patient relationship must incorporate learning experiences directed toward maturation.
- Intervention must be guided by the consistent use of rational authority that permits freedom and experimentation within specified limits.
- The nursing responsibility requires provision for experimentation coupled with assistance toward realistic self-evaluation by the patient.
- The nurse must recognize that the patient will frequently attempt to place responsibility for the satisfaction of his needs on others.
- Inability to recognize or control personal feelings toward the patient will impede the therapeutic process.

The nurse should keep in mind that those individuals afflicted with personality disorders seldom see themselves as needing help. They view themselves as being in step and consider the rest of the world in contention with them. They tend to be consummate actors attempting to fool others and in the process, end up fooling themselves instead. They play at life and living, many times never fully realizing what it is that they are missing. Their plight is sad, for they miss one of life's most unique experiences—loving and being loved.

SUMMARY

This chapter is a concise synthesis of predominant psychopathology. It provides essential, relevant, factual information. It serves as a basis for distinguishing and differentiating among pathological phenomena. It is a fundamental frame of reference designed to promote the nurse's understanding of psychopathology operational within individual patients. From this base the nurse should be able to participate intelligently with other members of the interdisciplinary team.

As an essential care provider the nurse is apt to find that patients do not always conform to the textbook picture. People are unique and defy classification, categorization, and labeling. In fact, patients usually manifest a crisscrossing of symptomatology. Thus, the textbook serves only as a frame of reference, since it is with the individual patient, his concerns, needs, and problems, that the nurse must deal. Knowledge of the pathological process is important only insofar as it contributes to furthering the nurse's assessment or appraisal of the individual patient's need system.

The focus of nursing is always on the patient and not on his illness. It is not the diagnostic label that receives treatment, intervention and recognition, but rather the individual who is suffering, cries out in his loneliness, lives with overwhelming anxiety, cannot differentiate the real from the unreal, or experiences self-defeating helplessness and hopelessness. The nurse's primary task is to assist those in distress to establish pathways that lead to healthier, happier, and more successful adjustments in living.

SUGGESTED READINGS

Aaronson, L. S. Alienation and Paranoia. *Perspectives in Psychiatric Care*, Vol. 15, No. 1 (1977).

American Psychiatric Association. Task Force on Nomenclature and Statistics. *Diagnostic and Statistical Manual of Mental Disorders*. 3rd ed. Washington, D.C.: American Psychiatric Association, 1980.

American Psychiatric Association. *Quick Reference to the Diagnostic Criteria from DSM-III*. Washington, D.C.: American Psychiatric Association, 1980.

Arietti, S. Roots of Depression: The Power of the Dominant Other. *Psychology Today*, Vol. 12, No. 11 (April, 1979), 54–55, 57–58, 92–93.

Arnold, H. M. Four A's: A Guide to One-to-One Relationships. *American Journal of Nursing*, Vol. 76, No. 6 (June, 1976), 941–943.

Back, S. *Narcissistic States and the Therapeutic Process*. New York: Jason Aronson, 1985.

Berger, F. Alcoholism Rehabilitation: A Supportive Approach. *Hospital and Community Psychiatry*, Vol. 34, No. 11 (November, 1983), 1040–1043.

Blumm, J. When You Face the Alcoholic Patient. *Nursing '81*, Vol. 11, No. 2 (February, 1981), 71–73.

Boyd, C., & Mast, D. Addicted Women and Their Relationships With Men. *Journal of Psychosocial Nursing and Mental Health Services*, Vol. 21, No. 2 (February, 1983), 10–13.

Campbell, R. J. The Language of Psychiatry. *Hospital and Community Psychiatry*, Vol. 32, No. 12 (December, 1981), 849–852.

Cicaux, A. Anorexia Nervosa: A View from the Mirror. *American Journal of Nursing*, Vol. 80, No. 8 (August, 1980), 1468–1470.

Claggett, M. S. Anorexia Nervosa: A Behavioral Approach. *American Journal of Nursing*, Vol. 80, No. 8 (August, 1980), 1471–1472.

Cohen, S. *The Substance Abuse Problems*. New York: The Haworth Press, 1981.

Coyrell, W., & Tsuang, M. T. DSM-III Schizophreniform Disorder: Comparisons with Schizophrenia and Affective Disorder. *Archives of General Psychiatry*, Vol. 39, No. 1 (January, 1982), 66–69.

Davis, J. M., & Moas, J. W. *The Affective Disorders.* Washington, D.C.: American Psychiatric Press, Inc., 1983.

Dean, P. R. The Neurotic Process: An Overview and Its Application to Nursing. *Journal of Psychiatric Nursing and Mental Health Services,* Vol. 17, No. 12 (December, 1979), 35–37.

Dixson, D. L. Manic Depression: An Overview. *Journal of Psychiatric Nursing and Mental Health Services,* Vol. 19, No. 5 (May, 1981), 28–31.

Drake, R. E., et al. Suicide Among Schizophrenics: A Review. *Comprehensive Psychiatry,* Vol. 26 (January/February, 1985), 90–100.

DSM-III Case Book: A Learning Companion to the Diagnostic and Statistical Manual of Mental Disorders, 3rd ed. Washington, D.C.: American Psychiatric Association, 1981.

DSM-III Training Guide to the Use of the American Psychiatric Association's Diagnostic and Statistical Manual of Mental Disorders, 3rd ed. Larchmont, New York: Brunner/Mazel, 1981.

Estes, N. J., & Heinemann, M. E. *Alcoholism: Development, Consequences, and Interventions,* 2nd ed. St. Louis: C. V. Mosby, 1982.

Faberow, N. Suicide Prevention in the Hospital. *Hospital and Community Psychiatry,* Vol. 32, No. 2 (February, 1981), 100–102.

Ford, C. V. *The Somatizing Disorders: Illness as a Way of Life.* New York: Elsevier Biomedical, 1983.

Fox, H. A. The DSM-III Concept of Schizophrenia. *British Journal of Psychiatry,* Vol. 138 (January, 1981), 60–63.

Frances, A., & Strauss, J. S. DSM-III Case Studies. *Hospital and Community Psychiatry,* Vol. 32, No. 6 (June, 1981), 385–386.

Furey, J. A. For Some, The War Rages On. *American Journal of Nursing,* Vol. 82, No. 11 (November, 1982), 1695–1696.

Gallop, R. The Patient is Splitting. *Journal of Psychosocial Nursing and Mental Health Services,* Vol. 23, No. 4 (April, 1985), 6–10.

Goodwin, D. W. The Genetics of Alcoholism. *Hospital and Community Psychiatry,* Vol. 34, No. 11 (November, 1983), 1031–1034.

Gordon, V. C., & Ledray, L. E. Depression in Women. *Journal of Psychosocial Nursing and Mental Health Services,* Vol. 23, No. 1 (January, 1985), 26–34.

Griest, J. H. (Ed.). *Treatment of Mental Disorders.* Fair Lawn, N.J.: Oxford University Press, 1982.

Grinspoon, L. (Ed.). Attention Deficit Disorder. *The Harvard Medical School Mental Health Letter,* Vol. 2, No. 3 (September, 1985), 1–4.

Grinspoon, L. (Ed.). Multiple Personality. *The Harvard Medical School Mental Health Letter,* Vol. 1, No. 10 (April, 1985), 1–4.

Grinspoon, L. (Ed.). Senile Dementia—Part I. *The Harvard Medical School Mental Health Letter,* Vol. 1, No. 11 (May, 1985), 1–3.

Grossniklaus, D. McC. Nursing Interventions in Anorexia Nervosa. *Perspectives in Psychiatric Care,* Vol. 18, No. 1 (January/February, 1980), 11–16.

Hagerty, B. K. Obsessive-Compulsive Behavior: An Overview of Four Psychological Frameworks. *Journal of Psychiatric Nursing and Mental Health Services,* Vol. 19, No. 1 (January, 1981), 37–39.

Halikas, J. A. Psychotropic Medication Used in the Treatment of Alcoholism. *Hospital and Community Psychiatry,* Vol. 34, No. 11 (November, 1983), 1035–1039.

Hicky, B. The Borderline Experience: Subjective Impressions. *Journal of Psychosocial Nursing*, Vol. 23, No. 4 (April, 1985), 24–29.

Huppenbauer, S. L. A Portrait of the Problem. *American Journal of Nursing*, Vol. 82, No. 11 (November, 1982), 1699–1703.

Hylands, J. The Wernicke-Korsakoff Syndrome. *Nursing '79*, Vol. 9, No. 7 (July, 1979), 26–29.

Jacobson, A. Melancholy in the 20th Century: Causes and Prevention. *Journal of Psychiatric Nursing and Mental Health Services*, Vol. 18, No. 7 (July, 1980), 11–21.

Johnson, B. S. *Psychiatric-Mental Health Nursing Adaptation and Growth*. Philadelphia: Lippincott, 1986.

Kahn, E. Psychotherapy With Chronic Schizophrenics. *Journal of Psychosocial Nursing and Mental Health Services*, Vol. 22, No. 7 (July, 1984), 20–25.

Kaplan, H. I., & Sadlock, B. J. *Modern Synopsis of Comprehensive Textbook of Psychiatry/III*, 3rd ed. Baltimore: Williams & Wilkins, 1981.

Keller, M. B., et al. Long-Term Outcome of Episodes of Major Depression: Clinical and Public Health Significance. *Journal of the American Medical Association*, Vol. 252 (August 10, 1984), 788–792.

Kendler, K. S., Gruenberg, A. M., & Tsuang, M. T. Subtype Stability in Schizophrenia. *American Journal of Psychiatry*, Vol. 142, No. 7 (July, 1985), 827–832.

Kerfoot, K. M., & Buckwalter, K. C. Post-partum Affective Disorders: The Manias and Depression of Childbirth. *Nursing Forum*, Vol. 20, No. 3 (1981), 297–317.

Kerr, N. J. Pathological Narcissism. *Perspectives in Psychiatric Care*, Vol. 18, No. 1 (January/February, 1980), 28–36.

Kiely, M. A. Alzheimer's Disease: Making The Most of The Time That's Left. *R.N.* (March, 1985), 34–41.

Kjervik, D. K. Dual Personality: Assessment and Reintegration. *Journal of Psychiatric Nursing and Mental Health Services*, Vol. 17, No. 7 (July, 1979), 28–32.

Knapp, T. J., & Peterson, L. W. Behavior Analysis for Nursing and Somatic Disorders. *Nursing Research*, Vol. 26, No. 4 (July/August, 1977), 281–287.

Kroner, K. Are You Prepared for Your Ulcerative Colitis Patient? *Nursing '80*, Vol. 10, No. 4 (April, 1980), 43–45.

Kunkel, J., & Wiley, J. K. Acute Head Injury: What To Do When . . . and Why. *Nursing '79*, Vol. 9, No. 3 (March, 1979), 22–23.

Mark, B. Hospital Treatment of Borderline Patients: Toward a Better Understanding of Problematic Issues. *Journal of Psychiatric Nursing and Mental Health Services*, Vol. 18, No. 8 (August, 1980), 25–31.

McEnany, G., & Tucker, B. E. Contracting for Care. *Journal of Psychosocial Nursing and Mental Health Services*, Vol. 23, No. 4 (April, 1985), 11–18.

McFarland, G. K., & Wasli, E. L. *Nursing Diagnoses and Process in Psychiatric Mental Health Nursing*. Philadelphia: Lippincott, 1986.

Millon, T. *Disorders of Personality: DSM-III: Axis II*. New York: Wiley, 1981.

Modley, D. M. Paranoid States. *Journal of Psychiatric Nursing and Mental Health Services*, Vol. 16, No. 5 (May, 1978), 35–37.

Moore, J. A., & Coulman, M. U. Anorexia Nervosa: The Patient, Her Family and Key Family Therapy Interventions. *Journal of Psychiatric Nursing and Mental Health Services*, Vol. 19, No. 5 (May, 1981), 9–14.

Morey, L. C., & Blashfield, R. K. A Symptom Analysis of the DSM-III Definition of Schizophrenia. *Schizophrenia Bulletin*, Vol. 7, No. 2 (February, 1981), 258–268.

Naegle, M. A. The Nurse and the Alcoholic: Redefining an Historically Ambivalent Relationship. *Journal of Psychosocial Nursing and Mental Health Services*, Vol. 21, No. 6 (June, 1983), 17–24.

Norman, E. M. The Victims Who Survived. *American Journal of Nursing*, Vol. 82, No. 11 (November, 1982), 1696–1698.

O'Brien, P., Caldwell, C., & Transeau, G. Destroyers: Written Treatment Contracts Can Help Cure Self Destructive Behaviors of the Borderline Patient. *Journal of Psychosocial Nursing*, Vol. 23, No. 4 (April, 1985), 19–23.

Offer, D., Marohn, R. E., & Ostrov, E. *The Psychological World of the Juvenile Delinquent*. New York: Basic Books, 1979.

Post, R. M., & Uhde, T. W. Treatment of Mood Disorders with Antiepileptic Medications: Clinical and Theoretical Implications. *Epilepsia*, Vol. 24, Suppl. 2 (1983), 597–S106.

Rickelman, B. Brain Bio-Amines and Schizophrenia: A Summary of Research Findings and Implications for Nursing. *Journal of Psychiatric Nursing and Mental Health Services*, Vol. 17, No. 9 (September, 1979), 28–33.

Schmagin, B. G., & Pearlmutter, D. R. The Pursuit of Unhappiness: The Secondary Gains of Depression. *Perspectives in Psychiatric Care*, Vol. 15, No. 2 (1977), 63–65.

Schopler, E., & Dalldor, J. F. Autism: Definition, Diagnosis, and Management. *Hospital Practice*, Vol. 15, No. 6 (June, 1980), 64–69.

Schuckit, M. A. Alcoholism and Other Psychiatric Disorders. *Hospital and Community Psychiatry*, Vol. 34, No. 11 (November, 1983), 1022–1027.

Silverstein, M. L., et al. Changes in Diagnosis from DSM-II to the Research Diagnostic Criteria and DSM-III. *American Journal of Psychiatry*, Vol. 139, No. 3 (March, 1982), 366–368.

Skodol, A. E., Spitzer, R. L., & Williams, J. B. Teaching and Learning DSM-III. *American Journal of Psychiatry*, Vol. 138, No. 12 (December, 1981), 1581–1586.

Smith, J. W. Diagnosing Alcoholism. *Hospital and Community Psychiatry*, Vol. 34, No. 11 (November, 1983), 1017–1021.

Spitzer, R. L. An In-Depth Look at DSM-III. *Hospital and Community Psychiatry*, Vol. 31, No. 1 (January, 1980), 25–32.

Tousley, M. M. The Paranoid Fortress of David J. *Journal of Psychosocial Nursing and Mental Health Services*, Vol. 22, No. 2 (February, 1984), 8–16.

Twerski, A. J. Early Intervention in Alcoholism: Confrontational Techniques. *Hospital and Community Psychiatry*, Vol. 34, No. 11 (November, 1983), 1027–1030.

Van Der Kolk, B. A. (Ed.). *Post-Traumatic Stress Disorder: Psychological and Biological Sequelae*. Washington, D.C.: American Psychiatric Press, Inc., 1984.

Vourakis, C., & Bennett, G. G. Angel Dust—Not Heaven Sent. *American Journal of Nursing*, Vol. 79, No. 4 (April, 1979), 649–653.

Webb, L. J., et al. Accuracy of DSM-III Following a Training Program. *American Journal of Psychiatry*, Vol. 138, No. 3 (March, 1981), 376–378.

Whitney, F. W. How To Work with a Crook. *American Journal of Nursing*, Vol. 81, No. 1 (January, 1981), 86–91.

Woodward, C. A. Wernicke-Korsakoff Syndrome: A Case Approach. *Journal of Psychiatric Nursing and Mental Health Services*, Vol. 16, No. 4 (April, 1978), 38–41.

IV

THE PROFESSIONAL

The Development of Care and Concern

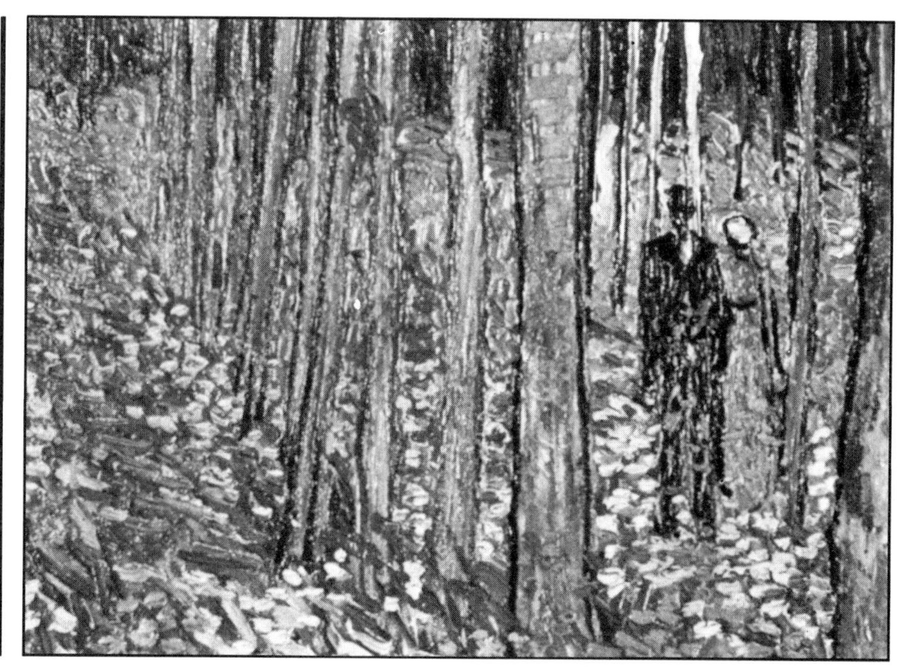

12

THE THERAPEUTIC SELF

LEARNING OBJECTIVES

On completion of this chapter the reader should be able to:

1. Develop an understanding of the concept **therapeutic self.**
2. Increase self-awareness through systematic examination of the personal and professional self.
3. Foster growth and development of the therapeutic self.
4. Define the term **attitude** as used throughout this book.
5. Identify the six positive attitudes essential in the delivery of nursing care.
6. Discuss the use of these attitudes in the delivery of client care.

The concept of the therapeutic self plays a major role in the development of a positive attitudinal approach to client care. In this chapter, we will discuss this concept and the meaning of the therapeutic self. In addition, we will identify and elaborate on those positive attitudes we feel are a necessary foundation in the nurse's practice and will promote her appropriate and meaningful intervention with each patient.

THE SELF AS A PERSON AND AS A PROFESSIONAL

Reading the phrase **the therapeutic self**, the nurse asks, "What does it mean?" and "How do I achieve it?" Inherent in this phrase is the idea that I, the nurse, make a difference. Immediately, within the mind there should be an image that I can do something to bring about or effect change. In other words, I am a *change agent*. What I do, what I say, what I think, and what I feel make me unique, and my uniqueness is the key to caring. If change is to occur, it is up to me to bring it about.

The kind of change I bring about must be positive, that is, I must enable the patient to move toward an optimal health care goal. To achieve this positive change, I must look at myself and examine my assets and liabilities, first as a person, and second, as a professional. First I must examine my characteristics and traits—my total personality.. To accomplish this, I must consider the following questions:

- What value system do I hold?
- What is my level of irritability?
- What mood changes do I experience? And when?
- Do I have an easygoing attitude toward myself and others?
- Do I have a sense of humor?
- Am I able to laugh at myself?
- What are my habits or patterns relating to my appearance, speech, and posture?
- What are my reactions to similar or different situations?
- Do I underestimate or overestimate my abilities?
- Can I make decisions?
- Can I accept my shortcomings?
- Do I like and respect myself?
- How do I relate with others?
- How do I see myself in relationship to authority figures, peers, loved ones, and strangers?
- Am I patient, or do I complain excessively?
- Am I considerate of others, or do I take them for granted?
- Do I acknowledge and respect the differences I find in other people?
- How do I function within my entire living experience?
- Do I exercise my ability to meet my own basic needs in a variety of situations?
- Do I deal with problems as they arise?
- How open am I to new experiences and new ideas?
- Do I make use of my own creative and natural talents?
- Am I practical, sensitive, impulsive, idealistic, quiet, reserved, outgoing, effervescent?

Your responses to these questions indicate the kind of individual you are and how you function in your daily living. After reviewing these questions, it should become apparent that a qualified practitioner must know herself—her reactions, capabilities, and limitations.

Armed with this assessment of the personal self, you will be able to proceed to discover the extended and expanded dimensions of the professional self. Without the knowledge gained from an honest appraisal of the personal self, the therapeutic self can be, and is, in jeopardy of being ineffective as a change agent.

Next I must examine the occupational, working segment of my total personality—my professional self. Some questions I must consider:

- What is my basic level of knowledge and preparation?
- To what extent do I implement my previous learning?
- Do I hold myself responsible for my performance?
- What were my reasons for choosing nursing as a career?
- What degree of satisfaction do I receive from the work I do?
- To what extent do I adhere to my professional code of ethics?
- What influences do I exert over the lives of others and to what degree?
- Do I push people around? Do I allow myself to be pushed around?
- Can I say no?
- Can I set realistic goals for myself and with my patients?
- What fears do I have?
- What hopes do I express?
- What kind of judgments am I called upon to make?
- What amount of giving is required of me?
- What degree of personal investment must I make and direct toward the pursuit of increased knowledge?

To complete the examination of the professional self, the nurse also needs to consider the ongoing assessment of daily functioning as a practitioner; the type of relationship established and maintained with nurse colleagues and other professionals; the degree of commitment to the nursing profession; the level of involvement with the professional organization; and the level of knowledge about and involvement with the nurse's community and its resources. This personal examination serves as a basis for establishing the nurse's identity and acts as a point of departure for further growth and development of the therapeutic self. In essence, the process outlined above enables the nurse to identify who and what the self is, where the self is, how the self functions, and why the self functions as it does.

In addition to the nurse's awareness and knowledge concerning self, there is another dimension to the concept of the therapeutic self. It is the idea of **being yourself**. To be yourself implies recognition of personal strengths and weaknesses and the ability to work with and use them to the best advantage in therapeutic patient care. How does the nurse use an acknowledged strength or weakness constructively?

By being genuine, honest, open, and flexible. In being herself, the nurse *shares* feelings as opposed to trying to mask or cover them. This sharing is a very meaningful part of honest and open communication. In the process of sharing, the nurse feels free to feel sadness, happiness, loneliness, gladness—free to be as a person. A tear, a hand on the shoulder in comfort, a smile or a joke shared with a patient can convey, as no other means, the reality of the nurse as a person and as a professional. This humanness is the essence of professionalism.

However, being yourself does not give the nurse license to forget, deny or abuse basic principles, or to act impulsively without thought for the consequences, or to relate *every* personal experience with the patient. Being yourself means being your professional self, that is, bringing to the therapeutic situation all the knowledge, skill, and judgment that can assist, support, and encourage the patient to move toward health. *The therapeutic self is that personal awareness, knowledge, and understanding which when put into operation results in a positive experience for the patient, his family, and his community.*

POSITIVE ATTITUDES

The operational or internalized concept of the therapeutic self permits the nurse to develop those positive attitudes that will enable her to provide the best possible nursing care. In many nursing texts where the student is instructed to develop positive attitudes for patient care, we find such terms as friendliness, matter-of-factness, permissiveness, and reassurance. These terms represent the type of approach the nurse is to use; that is, they indicate what the nurse does as opposed to the attitudes the nurse holds. By **attitude** we mean the opinion or view the nurse has toward nursing, people, hospitalization, caring, colleagues, health and illness, and life and death. Some of the necessary attitudes the nurse must cultivate in approaching patients are the attitudes of **personal worth, integrity, open-mindedness, advocacy, hopefulness,** and **involvement**.

Personal Worth

An attitude of **personal worth** is the viewpoint the nurse holds about self and others. Implicit in this attitude is the acknowledgment that each individual is uniquely different and as such is uniquely valuable. The attitude of personal worth acknowledges and accepts differences in such things as cultural and ethnic origin, but values the difference. This attitude exists within the context of mutual respect and dignity. It operates within the self-system of the individual and recognizes the autonomous rights of others. An attitude of personal worth promotes a positive self-concept and enhances self-esteem. It is a reflection of universal love.

The basis for this attitude is the extent of the nurse's awareness and understanding of such things as cultural differences and social influences affecting people, respect for humanity, and patience in dealing with human frailty. For example, the nurse displays an attitude of personal worth when she anticipates and acknowledges religious eating habits and adapts hospital service to meet the needs of the individual, when she provides privacy and comfort for a patient undergoing a physical examination, or when she explains completely to the patient, more than once if necessary, any procedures he must undergo. The nurse's approach should demonstrate a conviction that the dignity, individuality, and equality of people must be protected at all costs. Within this kind of framework, then, the nurse does not approach a patient in a rigid, stereotyped fashion.

Two sets of nursing actions in which the nurse is encountering a newly admitted patient for the first time are used to illustrate this attitude of personal worth. The patient is Mr. Santhat Nivatzongs, a 56-year-old male Caucasian, who was admitted to the hospital with a diagnosis of paranoid schizophrenia. Miss Walker, a staff nurse, is assigned as his primary therapist. He enters the unit accompanied by Miss Jones, a nursing assistant from admitting who is a friend of Miss Walker. They are on the same hospital bowling team. As they approach the nursing station, Miss Walker observes that Mr. Nivatzongs' eyes dart from side to side and that he glances furtively into open doorways as they pass. He also walks quite close to the right-hand side of the corridor, almost brushing the wall. Miss Walker notes that as they come to a halt before her and she reaches across Mr. Nivatzongs to take the chart from the nursing assistant, Mr. Nivatzongs quickly backs away as if he were afraid of physical contact. Miss Walker's initial assessment is that her new patient is distrustful, fearful, and insecure.

Situation I

Taking the chart from the nursing assistant, Miss Walker said, "Hi ya 'Jonesy'! How goes it?" Then, glancing at the chart and toward the patient, Miss Walker spoke again saying, "Mr. ah, ah, Mr. SAN . . . THAT NIVA . . . NIVA. Well, I can't pronounce it, so I guess I'll just call you 'Mr. San Niva'—OK by you?" Without waiting for a reply, Miss Walker turned to the nursing assistant and began discussing their team's chances in the upcoming league playoffs. Mr. Nivatzongs remained standing quietly on the sidelines.

Situation II

As Mr. Nivatzongs approached the nursing station, Miss Walker moved forward, smiled, and greeted both people by name, saying, "Good morning, Miss Jones, Mr. Nivatzongs. I am Miss Walker, a staff nurse on this unit." Turning directly toward the patient, she asked, "Have I pronounced your name correctly? Please help me if I haven't." Miss Walker established eye contact and waited expectantly. Mr. Nivatzongs shook his head saying, "No, no, you did OK." "Thank you, Mr. Nivatzongs. Let's go into one of the conference rooms where we can sit down. I can tell you about our unit and answer any questions you might have. But before we do, I want to speak with Miss Jones for a few moments. Do you mind?" During this brief exchange, Miss Walker kept her entire attention focused on Mr. Nivatzongs and waited for his replies. Receiving an affirmative nod of his head, Miss Walker directed her attention toward the nursing assistant saying, "Thank you, Miss Jones, for showing Mr. Nivatzongs to our unit. I'll see you at lunch, and perhaps we can plan some ways to improve our scores." Turning again to Mr. Nivatzongs, she said, "Let's step across the hall to the conference room."

In the first situation Miss Walker's behavior was grossly unprofessional and disregarded the personal worth of all participants—the patient's, the nursing assistant's, as well as her own. The nurse treated the patient as a nonentity, ignoring his display of distrust and possible fear. In addition, Miss Walker's casual familiarity and personal comments to the nursing assistant detracted from both her own and Miss Jones' status as members of the health team and as potential therapeutic agents.

The attitude of personal worth was clearly manifest in the second illustration. In it, Miss Walker respectfully acknowledged each person. She recognized the patient's wariness of his new surroundings and stated a plan of action that had potentiality for reducing mistrust and fear. Her approach was warm, yet not effusive; her comments direct and to the point. Her recognition of his individual identity regarding the pronunciation of his name conveyed dignity, respect, and equality.

Personal Integrity

When we say that the nurse must demonstrate an attitude of personal integrity, we mean that the nurse maintains an honesty toward herself in her dealings with herself and with others. An old but still viable cliché that conveys our meaning quite clearly is: "To thine own self be true." Demonstration of this attitude makes visible the code of ethics under which the nurse operates and which in all conscience cannot be violated. Integrity of the self implies that the nurse is just, fair, honest, dependable, and conscientious and willing and able to acknowledge commitment to the profession, to patients, and to self. Personal integrity demands that the nurse accepts challenge and is committed to a willingness to take risks.

Personal integrity acts as a catalyst to promote the advancement of the profession, prevent stagnation, and move the professional self toward its highest potential. It operates from an altruistic base and demands of the self, acceptance of responsibility, and accountability for actions. Personal integrity does not permit compromise of issues involving quality and standards of care. Personal integrity reflects pride in self and pride in the profession; it replaces the "I cannot" with "I can" and provides the nurse with a power base to effect change.

The attitude of personal integrity is illustrated in the following situation.

Situation III

Miss Steele is a recent graduate who has been assigned to a surgical unit of a large privately endowed metropolitan hospital. She has been on the unit for about 4 weeks and has just been scheduled to share with Mrs. Robinson, another staff nurse, a functional medication assignment for the next 2 week period. The unit is divided into two wings. Each nurse takes responsibility for preparing and administering the routine medications for each wing. Between them they agree to alternate administering PRN requests for medication as they are received. Over the next 2 to 3 days, Miss Steele becomes aware of a pattern in patient requests and the patients' responses to the medications she has administered. For example, if she responded to a request for pain medication from a patient who had previously been given medication by Mrs. Robinson, the time interval between requests was much shorter. In addition, some patients made the observation that the previous medication did not seem to reduce the pain and would ask if there was a difference and could they have what she, Miss Steele, gave them rather than the other kind. At lunch on the third day, she broached the topic to another staff nurse on the same unit in an effort to validate her observations. The other nurse responded that she had not noticed anything like what Miss Steele described and that she, Miss Steele, was new to nursing. This nurse also stated that Mrs. Robinson had been nursing for years with no possible hint of any unprofessional or unethical behavior. "After all," said the other nurse, "all you have is a suspicion without any 'real facts.' Let it alone: you could cause a lot of trouble for yourself and for Mrs. Robinson."

Miss Steele thought long and hard about the situation and the possible outcome. If she reported her observations and they were not correct, she could damage not only her own professional reputation, but that of Mrs. Robinson. Other nurses and members of the health team might label her a "troublemaker" or a "goody-two-shoes" who thought she knew it all—a tenuous position for a new graduate. Certainly, if Mrs. Robinson came to hear about her suspicions, she would be hurt, angry, and could possibly bring a suit for defamation of character. Yet, on the other hand, if her observations were correct, what then? Patient welfare was placed in jeopardy.

Miss Steele came to a decision. She felt she had a duty to herself, her patients, and her profession. She decided to place herself in a position of risk in order to remain true to her commitment and developed a plan of action. Quietly, over the remaining days of her medication assignment, without calling undue attention to herself, she began to gather data. Miss Steele made a careful log of each patient on the unit, noting the drug ordered; time and frequency of administration; by whom; and any observable effects or comments made by each patient. When she had gathered her data, which substantiated her initial assessment, Miss Steele approached Mrs. Robinson.

Personal integrity involves a commitment to standards and ideals. It reflects an adherence to ethics in practice. It is characterized by such traits as dependability, trustworthiness, and investment of self.

Open-Mindedness

Open-mindedness is an attitude conveying the idea that a willingness to change is present within the nurse. It stems from the sincere desire on the part of the nurse to learn from others and to make use of the knowledge thus gained. Open-mindedness demands flexibility and receptiveness to modify or change existing belief systems. It signifies that the nurse is ready to adapt. It allows her an opportunity to exercise judgment based on objective data as opposed to judgment based on preconceived beliefs, biases, or prejudices. It is conveyed through acceptance, respect, and understanding.

Open-mindedness is an attitude permitting the nurse to really hear what is being said despite the fact that she may hold a contrary opinion. Open-mindedness is accepting the right of others to hold values and make decisions that may differ from one's own. To develop an attitude of open-mindedness the nurse should continuously ask herself *why, how, what,* and *under what circumstances?*

To illustrate this attitude of open-mindedness, the following situation is presented.

Situation IV

Mr. John Edwards, R.N., was entering the termination phase of his relationship with Mrs. Armstrong, a 38-year-old female who has been hospitalized with a diagnosis of major depression, single episode. They had been discussing her discharge. Mrs. Armstrong, who prior to her marriage was a head buyer in a large department store, was expressing a desire to see if she could resume similar employment when she returned home. She has four small children, ages 2, 3, 5, and 7. Mr. Edwards, who himself has a wife and three children, believes very strongly that women with small children should not work outside the home. His wife concurs, and they have a very good relationship. Now, as he discussed this idea with Mrs. Armstrong, he found himself becoming uncomfortable and cut her off in mid-sentence on more than one occasion during the session. Nonverbally, he frowned several times, moved forward in his seat so that he was practically looming over Mrs. Armstrong, and, as the session ended, he stood up over her stating that they will have to go into it more thoroughly next time. Mrs. Armstrong kept her eyes downcast and whispered timid agreement.

During report, he elaborated on Mrs. Armstrong's progress and made some rather cutting remarks about her wish to work outside the home. After his report, there was a slight pause and one of his colleagues interjected, "Mr. Edwards, did you hear what you just said?" Mr. Edwards looked at the speaker inquiringly. "It sounds as if you are kind of hung up on the idea of women with small children not working. I know you and your wife, Joan, feel about the same on this issue, but perhaps Mrs. Armstrong and her husband look at the idea differently." Mr. Edwards shrugged his shoulders, muttered, "Maybe," and continued reporting on the other patients he was seeing on a one-to-one basis. The subject was dropped.

On his way home that afternoon, Mr. Edwards mulled over the day's events, thinking about his session with Mrs. Armstrong and the remarks made by one of the nurses during report. Perhaps his responses to Mrs. Armstrong had been colored by his own beliefs; perhaps they did have different values. What is right for one person is not necessarily right for another. As he pulled into his driveway, he resolved to approach Mrs. Armstrong the next day and share these thoughts with her. And even though he still felt strongly about his point of view, he freely acknowledged that everyone did not think and feel as he did. His obligation was to his patient and her need was to work out a satisfactory situation for herself and her family, not one that would fit in with his.

Thus, open-mindedness is an essential attitude if free and effective communication is to exist between patient and nurse. The whole concept of a therapeutic relationship is risked if the bias of the therapist is permitted to cloud professional judgment.

Advocacy

Advocacy as an attitude for the nurse is a relatively new and challenging idea in professional nursing practice. Advocacy is an attitude of support that safeguards the rights and integrity of the patient. It demands that the nurse expand the health concept of doing unto a person for his own good to include standing up for the good of the patient. When a nurse takes the attitude of advocacy, she supports the patient in those decisions he feels are right and necessary for the maintenance of his personal integrity. Assumption of this attitude demands that the nurse act by providing the patient with necessary information to reach an informed decision and act by ensuring that the decisions made can be carried out according to the patient's wishes. These two actions cannot be separated, that is, you cannot perform one without the other. In its most simplistic form, the attitude of advocacy is the expression of genuine loving and caring for others. It is based on the premise that each of us shares in conjunction with others, a commonality of needs, rights, and basic humanness. Advocacy is operational within the individual's physical, social, and emotional support systems.

Advocacy is a matter of fighting for the good of the patient. We believe that it is never undertaken when the outcome may be harmful to the patient's total welfare. When the situation may be harmful either physically or emotionally, as when a patient who has made a suicidal gesture wants to leave the hospital or terminate therapy against professional judgment, the nurse cannot advocate such a decision. For us, such a situation would require that the nurse seek support from nurse colleagues as well as professionals from other disciplines to sustain therapeutic intervention.

We recognize, however, that our belief is predicated on our own philosophy, value system, and ethical orientation. Further, we recognize that advocacy in such a situation as we describe may very well fall into the realm of actions considered as an ethical dilemma. We acknowledge that some nurses, as well as other health care professionals, might question the nurse's right to prevent suicide. The judgments and decisions involved in this and similar situations require careful, thoughtful deliberation.

Situation V

Mrs. Small, a 43-year-old divorced, Caucasian female, was admitted to the psychiatric unit of a hospital following a 6 month period of increasing depression and inability to function adequately as a legal secretary and as a mother of two teenage children. She refused to go to work, prepare meals, or do household chores. She spent her days in bed and complained of crying for no apparent reason. Her family physician suggested that Mrs. Small seek psychiatric consultation. As a result, she was hospitalized for psychiatric treatment.

After 8 days of hospitalization, Mrs. Small stated that she was "feeling better" and had received "much needed rest." She thought she was ready to return to her job and her children, who were being cared for by her mother. Mrs. Pryor, a staff nurse, encouraged Mrs. Small to remain in the hospital for further treatment and therapeutic intervention that might then be followed through on an outpatient basis. Mrs. Small insisted on being discharged and was verbally abusive of other patients and the psychiatrist. She repeatedly declared herself "not crazy," became agitated, and frequently burst into tears.

Mrs. Pryor had observed and charted Mrs. Small's loss of sleep, restlessness during the day, poor appetite, and consequent weight loss. Mrs. Small remained in bed most of the day and refused to participate in any therapeutic or recreational activities on the ward. Nonetheless, Mrs. Small insisted on her discharge and demanded release as "her right" since she had been hospitalized voluntarily. Mrs. Pryor increased her con-

> tacts with Mrs. Small and allowed the patient to ventilate and share her feelings. At the same time Mrs. Pryor informed and consulted with the psychiatrist, the psychologist, the clinical social worker, and the other nurses about these developments. Mrs. Pryor felt that Mrs. Small was still depressed and was possibly a suicidal risk so that she could not advocate and support Mrs. Small's request for a discharge from the hospital. Mrs. Pryor shared with the treatment team that she respected the right of the patient to make decisions but was concerned for Mrs. Small's physical and emotional well-being if she were to leave the hospital. The treatment team agreed with Mrs. Pryor, and together they formulated a plan of intervention to assist Mrs. Small to work through her crisis. The psychiatrist reevaluated Mrs. Small's medication and intensified his supervision of psychotropic intervention. The psychologist agreed to contact the legal firm that employed Mrs. Small in order to assess her functioning on the job and to plan for whatever testing might be necessary for her vocational rehabilitation. The clinical social worker agreed to contact Mrs. Small's mother and request support for continued hospitalization and reassurance about the children's well-being. The family was encouraged to visit. Mrs. Pryor was to assume the role as primary therapist with Mrs. Small and would see her on a daily basis.
>
> Mrs. Small reluctantly agreed to remain in the hospital for a maximum of 3 more weeks. During one of the therapy sessions with Mrs. Pryor, Mrs. Small admitted that she was feeling anxious, overwhelmed, and discouraged since she felt she was not improving rapidly enough and was, in fact, contemplating going home to commit suicide.
>
> During the next 3 weeks Mrs. Small showed a marked improvement in her affect, appearance, appetite, and sleep pattern. She began to converse with the staff and other patients, and she participated in group discussions and recreational activities. She stated she enjoyed the visits from her parents and children and had telephoned her employers to discuss her future with them. Mrs. Small was subsequently discharged from the hospital. Mrs. Pryor arranged for her to continue therapy on an out-patient basis at the neighborhood mental health clinic. Mrs. Small returned to her job and with assistance enrolled in art school two evenings a week.

This actual case history serves an an example of effective advocacy and demonstrates the intervention of the nurse on behalf of the patient. Note that Mrs. Pryor acknowledges the patient's insistence on discharge, but is able to maintain objectivity in view of the patient's demands, negativism, and verbal abuse.

To further illustrate the attitude of advocacy, let us look at a situation in which the nurse is caring for a patient who has difficulty in his home situation in addition to the medical problems for which he is seeking care. The nurse has identified aspects of the problem that lie beyond the realm of a nurse's capabilities and expertise. The nursing action at this point would require a recommendation to the patient that a social agency could be of assistance. Previously, nurses were told that they stop there and leave the rest up to the patient. However, a patient advocate would provide him with a list of names and telephone numbers and might even phone for him. What if the nurse finds that after the recommendation is made, the patient vehemently opposes it? The nurse's attitude of advocacy demands supporting him in his decision to reject the services of the agency and, at the same time, exploring with the patient possible alternatives which might be more acceptable.

Hopefulness

Another attitude that is essential for the nurse to cultivate in approaching patients is that of hopefulness. Hopefulness is looking at a situation from the bright side. By no means do we propose a Pollyanna attitude. What we do advocate is that the nurse feel within herself an optimism, a recognition that professional attitudes, knowledge, and skills do make a difference, that even in the most hopeless situations, the nurse can use this knowledge and skill to be of support and bring peace and comfort to the patient and assist the patient to find meaning in his illness. Hopefulness is an attitude that nurtures the individual. It has both a renewing effect and an enduring function. Hopefulness is a commitment to life, to growth, and to a belief in the future; it is a commitment to actively seek out those new experiences that can promote and maintain an optimal level of functioning. Hopefulness is based on the premise that solutions exist and change is possible. Hopefulness is essential to man's biological and psychological existence and well-being. Without hopefulness, the individual is at risk and vulnerable to despair. Hopefulness is generated in an environment that is conducive to freedom of choice, where honesty is valued, where realistic goals are identified, and in which the individual can exercise control over self and his environment. This attitude can only be experienced where there exists between the care giver and the care receiver a sharing, caring, and nurturing relationship.

Hopefulness is conveyed through touch, "bright shining eyes," a "light step," a warm smile, and a kind, interested word. These and other such actions on the part of the nurse convey to the patient that here is a human being who knows what life and death are all about and whose care and attention demonstrate concern. The message of hope is subtly transmitted through commitment to caring.

Situation VI

Mr. Stephen Yankey, 36, is the owner of a large marina. His business expanded from a small repair shop to a large concern serving the needs of boaters in a wide geographic area. As his business expanded, he became less and less confident about his ability to succeed and make a go of it.

> Two years ago he was hospitalized for an acute anxiety reaction. At that time he was able to pull himself together, marshalling his inner resources so that he remained in the hospital less than 3 weeks.
>
> He is again being hospitalized for a recurrence of severe anxiety, which is producing an almost complete disintegration of total functioning. His wife reports that during the past 6 months he has become increasingly more anxious and less able to handle his business concerns. He was exercising increasingly poor judgment and was unable to make or stick to decisions.
>
> To his nurse, Miss Webster, he freely verbalizes his feelings of utter helplessness. He approaches her many times throughout each day asking the same questions and making the same statements. "Will I get better? When will I get better? I'll never be the same again, will I? What am I going to do? I can't stand being like this. I can't think, I can't concentrate, Miss Webster. Tell me what I should do." Miss Webster listens thoughtfully and patiently to his repetitious verbalizations and responds clearly and concisely with honest, factual information. In addition, Miss Webster attempts to keep environmental stresses at a minimum while offering continuous support and reassurance. She encourages him to discuss and explore with her stress-provoking issues and what actions, if any, provide relief from his overwhelming feelings. Together they explore and work to develop coping devices to deal with stress.

In this situation, the nurse's attitude conveyed hopefulness, that is, the expectation that he could return to successful functioning. She willingly acknowledged with Mr. Yankey his need of external support and provided that support.

Involvement

The last of the attitudes we would like to call attention to is that of involvement. Involvement demands a personal and professional responsibility of the highest order. The attitude of involvement means that the nurse places priority first on the practice of nursing and last on the self. This does not mean that the nurse is not concerned about her economic welfare, working conditions, and other personal conditions that might affect the nurse's total well-being. It does mean that in the day-to-day operation of professional activities, the nurse functions to the best of her ability regardless of the personal circumstances in which she finds herself. It also means that if the circumstances are such that they may result in poor practice, lack of safety for the patient, or disregard for professional ethics, the nurse is obliged to use whatever means available to rectify the circumstances.

In the example under "Personal Integrity," the attitude of involvement is clearly demonstrated in the luncheon conversation that takes place between Miss Steele and the other nurse from her unit. In this conversation, Miss Steele is seeking collegial collaboration. She presents an attitude of involvement by sharing and attempting to validate her concerns. The other nurse demonstrates just as clearly her noninvolvement when she says, "Let it alone, you could cause a lot of trouble for yourself. . . ." This admonition to Miss Steele conveys the idea that one does not make waves. However, professional responsibility necessitates occasional wave making to safeguard patient welfare and to protect professional integrity. Involvement is necessary.

SUMMARY

In this chapter we have presented our concept of the therapeutic self and the attitudes essential for development of a mental health approach to patient care. It is our firm belief that these concepts are the most viable tools needed by a nurse in any fundamental area of practice or level of patient care responsibility. It is up to the nurse to recognize and cultivate the unique, individual, personal, and professional potentialities of self.

SUGGESTED READINGS

Adelson, P. Y. The Back Ward Dilemma. *American Journal of Nursing*, Vol. 80, No. 3 (March, 1980), 422–425.

Bindschadler, H. P. Dare To Be You. *American Journal of Nursing*, Vol. 76, No. 10 (October, 1976), 1632–1633.

Brill, N. I. *Working with People: The Helping Process*. Philadelphia: Lippincott, 1978.

Carson, V. Meeting the Spiritual Needs of Hospitalized Psychiatric Patients. *Perspectives in Psychiatric Care*, Vol. 18, No. 1 (January/February, 1980), 17–20.

Clark, C. C. Inner Dialogue: A Self-Healing Approach for Nurses and Clients. *American Journal of Nursing*, Vol. 81, No. 6 (June, 1981), 1191–1193.

Davis, E. D., & Pattison, E. M. The Psychiatric Nurses' Role Identity. *American Journal of Nursing*, Vol. 79, No. 2 (February, 1979), 298–299.

Deubrec, M., & Vogelpahl, R. When Hope Dies—So Might the Patient. *American Journal of Nursing*, Vol. 80, No. 11 (November, 1980), 2046–2050.

Doll, A. The Things Patients Say about Their Nurses. *Nursing '79*, Vol. 9, No. 5 (May 1979), 113–114, 116–118, 120.

Fay, P. Sounding Board: In Support of Patient Advocacy as a Nursing Role. *Nursing Outlook*, Vol. 26, No. 4 (April, 1978), 252–253.

Frankl, V. E. *Man's Search for Meaning*. New York: Washington Square Press, 1969.

Geiger, R., et al. The Value of Life. *Nursing '79*, Vol. 9, No. 5 (July, 1979), 30–37.

Hartel, D. E. Stress Management and the Nurse. *Advances in Nursing Science*, Vol. 1, No. 4 (July, 1979), 91–100.

Herbener, G. F. Recognizing Personal Coping Styles to Get Along Better With People. *Nursing Life*, Vol. 4, No. 1 (January/February, 1984), 28–32.

King, E. S., R. N. Should We Get Emotionally Involved? Hell Yes! *R.N. Magazine*, Vol. 40 (June, 1977), 48–53.

Kramer, M., & Schmalenberg, C. *Path to Biculturalism*. Wakefield, Mass.: Contemporary Publishing, 1977.

Kramer, M., & Schmalenberg, C. The Nurse's Responsibility to the Consumer. *American Journal of Nursing*, Vol. 78, No. 3 (March, 1978), 440–442.

Kurtzman, C., Block, D. E., & Freud, Y. S. Nursing and Medical Students' Attitudes Toward the Rights of Hospitalized Patients. *Journal of Nursing Education*, Vol. 24, No. 6 (June, 1985), 237–241.

Limandry, B. J., & Boyle, D. W. Instilling Hope. *American Journal of Nursing*, Vol. 78, No. 1 (January, 1978), 78–80.

Logan, C. Praise: The Powerhouse of Self-Esteem. *Nursing Management*, Vol. 16, No. 6 (June, 1985), 35–36, 38.

Maloney, E. *Interpersonal Relations*. Dubuque, Iowa: Wm. C. Brown, 1966.

Manfredi, C., & Pickett, M. "The Take Time Series": A Program on Coping With Stress. *Nursing Forum*, Vol. 20, No. 3 (1981), 322–328.

McGee, R. F. Hope: A Factor Influencing Crisis Resolution. *Advances in Nursing Science*, Vol. 6, No. 4 (July, 1984), 34–44.

Mott, S. R. Personality Correlates of a Psychiatric Nurse. *Journal of Psychiatric and Mental Health Services*, Vol. 14, No. 2 (February, 1976), 19–23.

Mullins, A. C., & Barstow, R. E. Care for the Caretakers. *American Journal of Nursing*, Vol. 79, No. 8 (August, 1979), 1425–1427.

Newman, M., & Berkowitz, B. *How To Take Charge of Your Own Life*. New York: Harcourt, Brace, Jovanovich, 1977.

Partridge, K. B. Nursing Values in a Changing Society. *Nursing Outlook*, Vol. 26, No. 6 (June, 1978), 356–360.

Peplau, H. E. An Open Letter to a New Graduate. *Nursing Digest* (March-April, 1975), 36–37.

Peplau, H. E. The Psychiatric Nurse Accountable? To Whom? For What? *Perspectives in Psychiatric Care*, Vol. 18, No. 3 (May/June, 1980), 128–134.

Pilette, P. C. Overcoming The Tyranny of Our Professional Role. *Nursing Management*, Vol. 14, No. 3 (March, 1983), 57–60.

Reich, S., & Geller, A. The Self-Image of Nurses Employed in a Psychiatric Hospital. *Perspectives in Psychiatric Care*, Vol. 15, No. 3 (July/September, 1977), 126–128.

Robb, S. S., Peterson, M., & Nagy, J. W., Jr. Advocacy for the Aged. *American Journal of Nursing*, Vol. 79, No. 10 (October, 1979), 1736–1738.

Rogers, C. R. *On Becoming a Person*. Boston: Houghton Mifflin, 1961.

Ryan, J. B. Scrutinizing Mental Health and Me. *Journal of Psychiatric Nursing and Mental Health Services*, Vol. 16, No. 11 (November, 1978), 32–35.

Schneider, J. S. Hopelessness and Helplessness. *Journal of Psychiatric Nursing and Mental Health Services*, Vol. 18, No. 3 (March, 1980), 12–21.

Schoenhofer, S. O. Support as Legitimate Nursing Action. *Nursing Outlook*, Vol. 32, No. 4 (July/August, 1984), 218–219.

Seeger, P. Self-Awareness and Nursing. *Journal of Psychiatric Nursing and Mental Health Services*, Vol. 15. No. 8 (August, 1977), 24–26.

Shikora-Wachter, N. Scapegoating Among Professionals. *American Journal of Nursing*, Vol. 77, No. 3 (March 1977), 406–409

Simms, L. M., & Lindberg, J. B. *The Nurse Person*. New York: Harper & Row, 1978.

Simon, S. *I am Loveable and Capable: A Modern Allegory on the Classical Put-Down*. Niles, Ill.: Argus Communications, 1978.

Sinkier, G. H. Identity and Role. *Nursing Outlook*, Vol. 18, No. 10 (October, 1970), 22–24.

Smith, L. L. "To Be, or Not To Be . . ." *Journal of Psychiatric Nursing and Mental Health Services*, Vol. 15, No. 10 (October, 1977), 37–39.

Smoyak, S. A. The Confrontation Process. *American Journal of Nursing*, Vol. 74, No. 9 (September, 1974), 1632–1635.

Stacklum, M. M. New Student in Psychology. *American Journal of Nursing*, Vol. 81, No. 4 (April, 1981), 762.

Ujhely, G. B. Am I My Brother's Keeper? *Perspectives in Psychiatric Care*, Vol. 17, No. 5 (September/October, 1979), 204–210.

Zander, K. The Nurse As a Professional: Gaining the Respect We Deserve. *Nursing Life*, Vol. 5, No. 1 (January/February, 1985), 42–47.

Zimmerman, B. N. Human Questions Versus Human Hurry. *American Journal of Nursing*, Vol. 80, No. 4 (April, 1980), 719.

13

THE THERAPEUTIC USE OF SELF

LEARNING OBJECTIVES

On completion of this chapter the reader should be able to:

1. Define the **nurse–patient relationship**.
2. State the purpose and importance of the nurse–patient relationship.
3. Identify the basic concepts that are prerequisites for the successful achievement of the therapeutic goal.
4. Define and distinguish among **love**, **empathy**, **sympathy**, **understanding**, and **acceptance** as used within the nurse–patient relationship.

BASIC CONCEPTS IDENTIFIED

In nursing, interpersonal relationships take on added significance primarily because the nurse uses the interpersonal process as the major tool to assist the patient in maintaining or restoring an optimal level of health and in the prevention of illness. Every encounter the nurse has with a patient, no matter how brief or for whatever purpose, should be used to either establish or maintain a therapeutic relationship. The **nurse–patient relationship** is a **therapeutic alliance**. It is a transactional encounter. It is a goal-oriented, educative event that occurs between the patient and the nurse. The specific purpose of the relationship is to foster gradual changes through a series of events designed to help the patient deal with current reality, problems, needs, and crises and to encourage a process of resolution.

The implementation of and engagement in a nurse–patient relationship involves certain specific basic concepts. These basic concepts are love, empathy, sympathy, understanding, and acceptance. The nurse's use of these basic concepts permits the establishment of **rapport** between herself and her patients. They are prerequisites to achieving therapeutic goals. These essential elements that the nurse must bring with her to the relationship are acquired through her professional education and her personal growth. To what degree is the nurse expected to use these elements in the relationship? This depends on two factors: (1) the actual identified needs of the patient, and (2) the ability of the nurse to help the patient meet his needs.

BASIC CONCEPTS DEFINED

Love

Love is a demonstration of care and concern toward another human being. **To care** is: to commit one's self; to invest one's time, effort, and knowledge; to utilize specific skills born out of a willingness to help; a desire to share one's therapeutic self with another in problem solving; and to be willing to become involved during stress and discomfort. To care means that the nurse approaches the patient with assurance. **Assurance** is a quality that connotes the confidence that the nurse has in her professional ability to engage in therapeutic helpfulness. **To be concerned** is: to demonstrate respect for the individual as a unique human being; to acknowledge his intrinsic worth; and through one's behavior convey interest, compassion, warmth, and comfort to the patient. When the nurse expresses care and concern, the patient experiences a sense of self-worth, belonging, security, and hope. Thereby the seeds of trust are sown. Unless the nurse achieves this level of interaction with the patient, movement toward the goals of a therapeutic relationship cannot be accomplished.

Nursing actions that convey this concept of love to the patient range from the very simple, as in the extension of common courtesies, to the very complex, as in the skillful application of a body of knowledge to practice. Some examples of simple activities include a smile and nod of the head in greeting; addressing or referring to a person by name; apologizing when appropriate; supplying correct and necessary information; and responding truthfully to questions. More complex activities include attending to individual likes and dislikes; taking time to explain and to repeat explanations if need be; listening to a story told for the tenth time; providing an extra pillow or blanket;

opening or closing a window; and being gentle or firm as appropriate. Nursing actions demonstrating an even greater degree of complexity might be seeking the patient's collaboration in establishing mutually desired goals; keeping promises; insuring privacy; setting realistic expectations for patient behavior; and repeatedly approaching the patient despite continuous rejection. The nurse can find many other ways to express love as she engages in the daily routine of the ward and treatment regimes. When done with love, the routines become therapeutic.

Empathy

Empathy is the capacity to comprehend another's experiences without actually having encountered the same or similar condition(s) within the context of your own life. As a component of the nurse–patient relationship, empathy is the ability on the part of the nurse to feel "with" and "for" the patient. When expressed within the relationship, it enables the nurse to sense, to share in, and to accept the patient's emotional point of view.

Empathy occurs when the nurse is able to set aside her own values, opinions, and judgments and "see" the situation as it appears to the patient. Its use enables the patient to feel that he is understood. Thus, the use of empathy in practice enables the nurse to support the patient and assist him in finding meaning in each of his experiences.

The following case incident illustrates the concept of empathy in nursing practice.

> On a medical unit in Centerville General Hospital, the night nursing staff reported that Mr. Wilson was up at frequent intervals during the night and would often roam the corridors looking about with a scrutinizing eye. When approached by the night staff and told to return to his room, he would grumble and say, "Just leave me alone. I'm OK," or when offered a sleeping pill he would say, "Never take the stuff." The day staff complained of him as a "problem patient" because he spent the day sleeping. One night Miss Norton, a relief nurse, found Mr. Wilson wandering the hospital corridor and instead of reporting him, she took the patient into the nursing station to talk to him. During this conversation, Mr. Wilson revealed that, although retired, he had been a night watchman for 30 years and had spent daylight hours sleeping. He also stated that he had never broken this pattern and, even now, did much of his household work at night.

Miss Norton's use of empathy with this patient allowed her to understand the patient's behavior and to identify his feelings as opposed to applying personal views, values, opinions, and judgments that would have resulted in the patient continuing to be labeled as a "problem." A prerequisite for the effective use of empathy is that the nurse have a fairly clear understanding of herself and how she operates. The nurse with empathy exudes an aura of continued concern, interest, tolerance, patience, and nonjudgmental support.

Sympathy

Sympathy refers to a momentary feeling and the resultant action triggered by a specific situation. A display of sympathy on the part of the nurse is a recognition of the discomfort, pain, or distress experienced by the patient. This recognition evokes an immediate response in the nurse to alleviate the condition. The application of sympathy to patient care is appropriate and needed. The nurse must exercise judgment in the application of sympathy and take precautions to prevent sympathy from turning into pity. Pity is inappropriate because it reduces nursing care to an ineffective level by decreasing the patient's self-worth, rendering the nurse equally helpless with the patient through overidentification, and lastly, having a dehumanizing effect because the patient wants help rather than wanting to inflict suffering on another.

Sympathy is regarded by the behavioral sciences as an element that can lead to detrimental outcomes of the therapeutic process through the loss of objectivity and countertransference, that is, the therapist's assumption of pseudopower and pseudocharacteristics as projected by the patient. Nevertheless, the nursing profession views sympathy as a therapeutic concept.

The concept of sympathy is depicted in the following case incident.

> It was 1:36 A.M. and Mr. Willie Davis was dying. His wife was at his bedside. At 2:05 A.M. he expired. Throughout the vigil, Miss Parker, R.N., had moved silently in and out of the hushed hospital room. Miss Parker had known and cared for Mr. Davis over a period of several months. After his death, Miss Parker led the weeping wife from the room and escorted her to a nearby lounge. As they reached the lounge, Miss Parker enfolded Mrs. Davis in her arms, hugged her, and shared in her tears. A silent message of comfort was conveyed from Miss Parker and recieved by Mrs. Davis.

This vignette illustrates a nursing action designed or intended to alleviate, even if only for a brief moment, the pain of loss of the grieving widow. It was a spontaneous gesture—an expression of sympathy.

Understanding

Understanding is both an intellectual function as well as a feeling state. As an intellectual function, understanding is a cultivated ability in which an individual demonstrates an awareness of the many subtle differences that influence a person and the development of his thoughts, feelings, and actions. The affective or feeling state of understanding is the ability of the nurse to accept and show appreciation for another's thoughts, feelings, and actions. Understanding is demonstrated when the nurse views the patient as an individual and recognizes his uniqueness by selecting those specific nursing actions that best meet his needs.

The degree of understanding the nurse can achieve depends on her ability to love, to empathize, and to sympathize with her patients. The nurse conveys understanding by listening attentively to her patient, learning about his uniqueness (cultural, religious, social, familial), maintaining a nonjudgmental position, extending warmth and kindness, seeking clarification of his communications, and seeking validation for her interpretations. The nurse must exert a continuous, conscious effort to engage in those behaviors that promote understanding.

Acceptance

Acceptance is receptivity without judgment. It is positive recognition and respect for a person. Acceptance is an unconditional state of neutrality that acknowledges a person's right to be different. Acceptance is awareness of an individual's pleasant and unpleasant ideas, emotions, or behavior without censure or retaliation.

Acceptance is cognizance that the verbal and nonverbal communications expressed in any specific living experience are the outcome of an individual's total development and are, most likely, the best coping methods he is able to demonstrate at that point. Acceptance is applied to the person, but not necessarily to the behaviors demonstrated and does not imply agreement, approval, or tolerance for the behaviors.

An intellectual acknowledgment of acceptance is not enough. It must be accompanied by the emotional state of acceptance as demonstrated through an attitudinal change. Attitudes that are most needed and that serve as a foundation for the development of acceptance are those of open-mindedness, personal worth, and personal integrity.

The nurse demonstrates acceptance by supporting and encouraging the individual's efforts to satisfy his needs. Acceptance makes explicit the use of a basic principle in health care, that is, to begin where the patient is and to make use of his potential capabilities to achieve an optimum level of wellness.

SUMMARY

The basic concepts of love, empathy, sympathy, understanding, and acceptance that the nurse nurtures and demonstrates toward her patient enable her to engage in a therapeutic interpersonal relationship either on an individual or group basis. These concepts are more than elements of personality; they are, in fact, a necessary part of nursing activity.

SUGGESTED READINGS

Barbieri, W. K. No Pity. *American Journal of Nursing*, Vol. 76, No. 9 (September, 1976), 1482.

Bernardo, M. L. Developing the Professional Nursing Relationship. *Nursing Forum*, Vol. 21, No. 1 (1984), 12–14.

Carkhuff, R. *Helping and Human Relationships: A Primer for Lay and Professional Helpers*, Vols. I and II. New York: Holt, Rinehart and Winston, 1969.

D'Addio, D. Reach Out and Touch. *American Journal of Nursing*, Vol. 79, No. 6 (June, 1979), 1081.

del Campo, E., & Hartigan, J. Psychiatric Nursing Therapy: Philosophy and Methods. *Journal of Psychiatric Nursing and Mental Health Services*, Vol. 16, No. 8 (August, 1978), 34–37.

Dickinson, Sister C. The Search for Spiritual Meaning. *American Journal of Nursing*, Vol. 75, No. 10 (October, 1975), 1789–1793.

Dormer, A. B. The Miracle of Caring. *Journal of Psychiatric Nursing and Mental Health Services*, Vol. 18, No. 8 (August, 1980), 21–24.

Ehmann, V. E. Empathy: Its Origin, Characteristics and Process. *Prospectives in Psychiatric Care*, Vol. 9, No. 2 (March–April, 1971). 72–80.

Fromm, E. *The Art of Loving*. New York: Harper & Row, 1956.

Gardner, K. G. Supportive Nursing: A Critical Review of the Literature. *Journal of Psychiatric Nursing and Mental Health Services*, Vol. 17, No. 10 (October, 1979), 10–15.

Hardin, S. B., & Halaris, A. L. Nonverbal Communication of Patients and High and Low Empathy Nurses. *Journal of Psychosocial Nursing and Mental Health Services*, Vol. 21, No. 1 (January, 1983), 14–20.

Hein, E., & Leavitt, M. Providing Emotional Support to Patients. *Nursing '77*, Vol. 7, No. 5 (May, 1977), 38–41.

Johnson, M. A. *Developing the Art of Understanding*. New York: Springer Publishing Co., 1967.

Kalisch, B. J. What is Empathy? *American Journal of Nursing*, Vol. 73, No. 9 (September, 1973), 1548–1552.

Leininger, M. Caring: A Central Focus of Nursing and Health Care Services. *Nursing and Health Care*, Vol. 1, No. 3 (October, 1980), 135–143.

MacDonald, M. R. How Do Men and Women Students Rate in Empathy. *American Journal of Nursing*, Vol. 77, No. 6 (June, 1977), 998.

Older, J. Four Taboos That May Limit the Success of Psychotherapy. *Psychiatry*, Vol. 40, No. 3 (August, 1977), 197–204.

Peitchinins, J. A. Therapeutic Effectiveness of Counseling by Nursing Personnel: Review of the Literature. *Nursing Research*, Vol. 21, No. 2 (March/April, 1972), 138–148.

Pilette, P. C. Overcoming the Tyranny of Our Professional Role. *Nursing Management*, Vol. 14, No. 3 (March, 1983), 57–60.

Pluckhan, M. L. *Human Communication—The Matrix of Nursing*. New York: McGraw-Hill Book Co., 1978.

Shanken, W. J., & Shanken, P. How To Be A Helping Person. *Journal of Psychiatric Nursing and Mental Health Services*, Vol. 14, No. 2 (February, 1978), 24–28.

Wilkiemeyer, D. S. Affection: Key to Care for the Elderly. *American Journal of Nursing*, Vol. 72, No. 12 (December, 1972), 2166–2168.

V

THE PROFESSIONAL IN PRACTICE

Skill Development

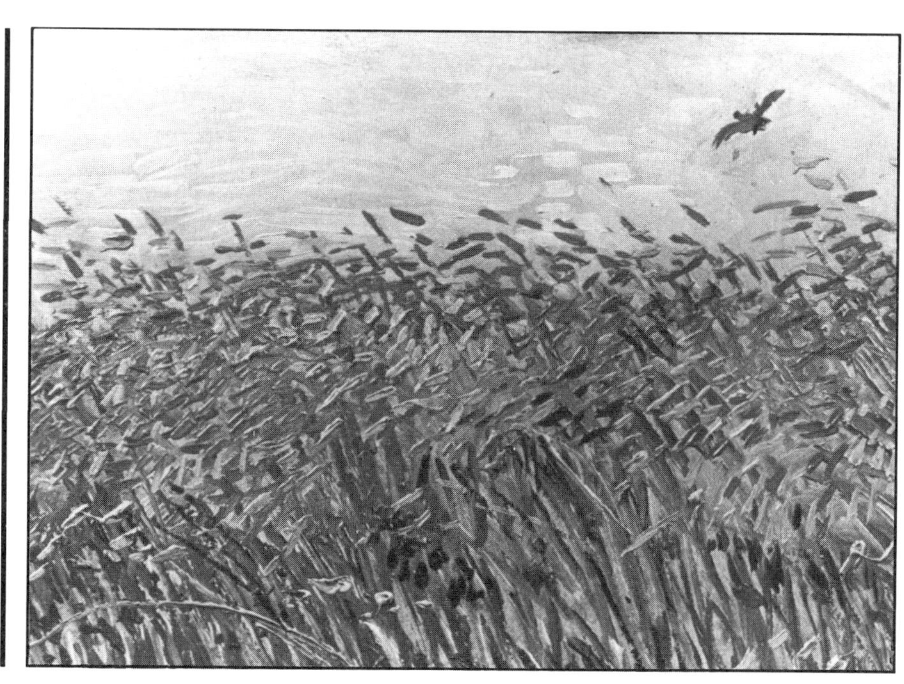

14

COMMUNICATION

Method—Process—Practice

LEARNING OBJECTIVES

On completion of this chapter the reader should be able to:

1. Define the term **communication.**
2. Distinguish between **social** and **therapeutic communication.**
3. Identify and describe the operational definition of the communication process.
4. Identify the barriers to effective communication.
5. List the three major categories into which effective communication practices may be divided.
6. Identify the specific nursing behavior associated with each of the communication categories.
7. Discuss the way in which the therapeutic techniques of communication can be used.

The concepts and practices of communication play a significant role in the social interactional process among people. As a therapeutic tool, communication becomes an even more significant adjunct within the therapeutic–interactional process. In this chapter, we will synthesize and clarify those aspects that are fundamental to the nurse's understanding of just what communication is and, most importantly, how both the nurse and the patient can benefit from its successful application. We present this material with the hope that the nurse can come to a better understanding of the importance communication plays in the development of the therapeutic self.

COMMUNICATION DEFINED

Communication is a frequently used term in today's society. Everybody's "communicating," but just what are they doing? What exactly is communication? We know that **communication** is a *process*, a logical, step-by-step progression of operations directed toward specific expected outcomes. As such, communication is the means we use to relate and share our thoughts, feelings, attitudes, needs, desires, pains, turmoils, and crises with others. The process of communication uses words and expressions that can be interpreted or heard differently. Communication takes place between people and can be either verbal or nonverbal.

We know that communication is instrumental in achieving satisfaction and aids in the solution of problems. We also know that communication can be a source of distress or discomfort. But what else is it?

Communication is:

- A dynamic social process involving an exchange of ideas between two or more people.
- A behavior used to express feelings.
- A system of operations that includes language, gestures, or symbols to convey intended meaning.
- A method by which information is transmitted, received, and understood.
- A mutual transactional process used to facilitate a relationship with others.
- An essential element in the establishment of the nurse–patient relationship.

THERAPEUTIC COMMUNICATION

Therapeutic communication differs from the usual social communicative process in that the messages that are sent and received are designed to deal with presenting problems and dissatisfactions from stressful living situations; to help the patient learn to use or increase coping abilities; and to develop or fortify ego strengths. The thrust of this form of communication is to create a space for the patient to engage in learning experiences—a physical and emotional space free of the encumbrances that result from the pressure of "aloneness and helplessness" the patient often feels when confronting a problem or crisis. The nurse initiates a focusing on the identified needs and goals of the patient. These are a given priority throughout the therapeutic process and, because of its dynamic nature, the process requires continuous reevaluation, which can result in revision of priorities or goals and in assisting the patient to reorder his needs and desires. Another unique characteristic of the therapeutic communication process is that as the process continues and evolves, the patient assumes a more active verbal and nonverbal communicative role.

PRINCIPLES FOR EFFECTIVE COMMUNICATION

We have identified at least four basic criteria the nurse can use to determine whether or not effective communication is achieved between herself and her patient.

First, the nurse recognizes that verbal and body language mean different things to different people. Too many times, people take for granted that the words they choose to use to express themselves are understood exactly as intended. This is not so. It is well known that a majority of problems people encounter center on misunderstanding and misinterpretation of communications. For communication to be clear and direct, the words must be mutually understood by sender and receiver. Therefore, it is important for the nurse to choose those words that have the most universal understanding and application. The nurse must consider and ask herself, "Does this word or phrase apply to this particular situation and have meaning for this person? Could misunderstanding be avoided by a more careful selection of terms?" For example, if someone said to us, "Look out," our immediate response would be to look for an environmental threat. We would most likely not go to the window and "look out."

The nurse must periodically validate and clarify with the patient to determine if the messages are received and are understood. The nurse can do this simply by asking him if he understands, or she can request that the patient tell her, in his own words, the essence of the message. The nurse must also observe nonverbal responses, such as a change in the tone of voice, which might be indicative of misunderstanding. The nurse's responsibility then takes the form of encouraging the patient to express his concern, voice his doubts, and question what he does not understand.

Second, the nurse recognizes the presence patterns in the transmission and reception of messages. While words have specific meanings, the way in which these words are put together, in transmission and in reception, also has meaning. Identification of patterns is essential if communication between the nurse and her patient is to be clear and explicit.

An individual learns through the developmental process a particular mode of expression. He communicates discomfort, distress, anxiety, hostility, and other feelings through a particular communication pattern he has set up with others. Reliance on this pattern becomes habitual. Such patterns of behavior often interfere with the open-minded sending and receiving of messages. Therefore, the nurse should know to observe for such patterns as the kind and amount of emphasis placed on particular words; the repetitive use of words or phrases; changes in tonal quality and pitch when specific subjects are discussed; or body movements indicating an approach toward or retreat from the sender.

If the nurse identifies the presence of patterns both within herself and within the patient, she is in a better position to achieve the specific purpose of the communication. For example, an individual who consciously or unconsciously wishes to avoid revealing information about self will either tend to place himself in a side-to-side communication position as opposed to selecting a face-to-face seating arrangement, or he will not engage in direct eye contact with the nurse. The nurse's awareness and recognition of this pattern of behavior allow her an opportunity to validate the impressions received. It also provides the nurse with an opportunity to focus on an area that might have a great deal of significant meaning for the patient.

Third, the nurse recognizes the importance personal experiences play in the interpretation of communication. An individual's perception of what is communicated is colored by his present and past experiences as well as his future expectations. For example, after the death of a family member a period of grieving occurs in which the surviving member(s) feel(s) a sense of loss and sadness. However, suppose the deceased family member was a domineering, self-centered, caustic, intimidating, and manipulative individual. In this situation, the survivor(s) may not view the death as a loss but may instead experience a sense of freedom and relief. If so, it would be erroneous for the nurse to assume that the survivor is mourning and "putting up a good front." In other words, the nurse cannot assume that generalities apply to a particular set of circumstances. The nurse must know the patient as a person and understand him within his own frame of reference before valid interpretations can be made.

Awareness of personal experiences and their effect on communication also applies to the nurse. In her position as receiver and sender of messages, the nurse's perspective is also framed within a personal context. If, for example, the nurse had a parent who was an alcoholic and from whom she had been alienated, interacting with a client who was discussing his drinking problem might influence responses indicative of a negative bias. Thus, self-awareness on the part of the nurse is important in order to reduce the potential for misinterpretation.

Fourth, the nurse recognizes the degree to which her patient can abstract and conceptualize as part of the communication process. The ability to abstract and conceptualize demands a high level of intellectual functioning. Individuals are endowed with variations of this ability. Environmental situations, psychological causes, or physiological changes are also responsible for variations. Effective communication requires that the individual internalize the message. The resultant appropriate response to the message demonstrates this internalization through discrimination and exercise of judgment in filtering out the pertinent from the unnecessary.

The nurse who engages in a therapeutic relationship must be aware of the possible levels of abstraction and conceptualization so that she can set realistic expectations. Often the patient can only think concretely; that is, his ability to abstract is almost nonexistent. This is true of patients diagnosed as being mentally retarded, having an organic brain syndrome, or having sustained early sociocultural, emotional deprivation. In psychotic patients we often find that internalization of transactions related to the environment is extreme, and consequently, they lose contact with or avoid reality and often develop a delusional or hallucinatory system to deliberately minimize their multisensory input.

It is appropriate for the nurse to identify and negotiate goals that are limited in scope and can be achieved by the individual. Adequate recognition on the part of the nurse prevents communication from becoming a frustrating process as opposed to a therapeutic process. In the mental health field one of the most frequent errors of psychotherapeutic intervention is that many professionals tend to analyze every word, action, or body movement. This technique may be detrimental to the patient because it can lead to the professional misinterpreting the messages communicated or losing the objective ability to understand and work through relevant data with the patient. It is of vital importance to the successful outcome of the therapeutic communicative engagement that the nurse learn to see and assess what messages are significant, to what degree, and what to accept at face value.

To evaluate the effectiveness of communication, the nurse must consciously and thoughtfully apply each of the above principles. If any one of the principles is omitted in the assessment process, the nurse is left with an incomplete picture of the patient's understanding of what is being communicated. This incomplete picture may incorrectly and negatively influence the nurse's interpretation of the patient's needs. It may also produce barriers to communication that may tend to decrease or retard the establishment of trust and rapport. This decrease could result in prolonging the patient's need for therapy.

THE COMMUNICATION PROCESS: OPERATIONAL DEFINITION

Communication is a complex art that requires learning and mastery. Therapeutic communication is based on the application of a set of principles. The principles are used as guidelines in the development of the structure and form involved in the communicative process. The process itself depends on the application of therapeutic techniques, which are used to facilitate the movement of the participants toward the identified goal. No one is born with the knowledge and ability to be therapeutic. Acquisition of principles and skills is not automatic. Therapeutic communication is hard work and demands that the nurse be actively involved. How? It requires that the nurse demonstrate sensitivity toward others and a willingness to give of self. This sensitivity and willingness to share self occur as the nurse comes to an awareness of who she is as a person, where she is at any moment, how she arrived there, the set of values she holds, the knowledge of what she is able to achieve, and the degree to which she can extend herself.

The communication process is composed of a series of six operations in which the nurse assumes an active, dynamic role. Meaningful communication cannot occur unless these operations are put into practice in each nurse–patient interaction.

Be There

To be there, the nurse must be fully conscious and aware of the purpose of the interaction. It requires that the nurse's full attention be focused on the individual(s) with whom she is interacting. Accessibility and availability do not fulfill the requirements of being there. **Being there** implies interest, expectancy, readiness, and attentiveness. These qualities can be demonstrated by such nursing behaviors as ignoring or eliminating distractions, looking directly at the patient as opposed to gazing about the room, remaining quietly composed as opposed to fidgeting in the chair, sitting erect and slightly forward as opposed to leaning back and away from the patient, and giving verbal encouragement for the patient to begin the interaction.

Observe

Standing about, looking around, and sitting in a nurse's station are patterns of behavior engaged in by many nurses under the guise of observation; however, this is not therapeutic observation. **Observation** is deliberate, planned, and systematized. To observe is to see the total patient. It is a data-gathering process that requires accuracy and objectivity in seeing the individual as a person who is separate and distinct from others as he functions within the context of his reality and environment.

Observation is the process of obtaining objective and subjective data. In objective data gathering the nurse makes use of her multisensory inputs—information gained through the five basic senses together with the information gained through specific nursing techniques or procedures, such as taking the patient's vital signs in an attempt to assess his physical and emotional functioning. In subjective data gathering the nurse employs the therapeutic communicative techniques to elicit from the patient his perceptions of himself and his functioning. Within the context of the nurse–patient interaction, to observe is to be cognizant of responses and to look for cues and patterns with regard to the patient's feelings, thoughts, and behavior.

Listen

Listening is the art of paying attention to the speaker. Many nurses hear and do not listen, that is, they hear only what they want to hear. To listen demands a great deal of effort and concentration. It also requires sensitivity to words, tonal qualities, silences, hidden messages with significant content, generalizations, and unrecognized feelings. To listen the nurse must actively seek to reduce environmental and personal distractions.

Listening, like observation, requires objectivity and accuracy. There are four major types of listening processes: defensive, selective, deliberate, and empathic. The nurse's understanding of each of these forms of listening is important because it helps her develop better use of the therapeutic self, aids and ameliorates the communicative process, and facilitates the establishment of rapport with the patient.

Defensive listening is the process of hearing by either filtering the messages so as to hear only that which is perceived or to place personal and negative values on the message. This type of listening inhibits spontaneity and rapport. A patient often is prepared "to hear the worst" or to be "accused" by the nurse, resulting in misinterpretation or confusion. The sources of defensive listening are often guilt, shame, fear, and feelings of inadequacy or worthlessness. The sources of this type of listening are the same for all, nurse or patient. When a nurse engages in defensive listening, she prevents the real message from being heard and distorts its meaning. We devoted Chapter 12 to the development of the therapeutic self because an honest assessment of the self greatly minimizes defensive listening and allows the nurse to understand and explore defensive listening with the patient.

Selective listening is an inherent practice attributed to human nature. We all like to hear what we want to hear, even though it may not have been said by the other person. We also have the habit of hearing only part of what is being said or communicated. Selective listening is detrimental to the interactive–interventive process because it severely limits message reception. In selective listening, the nurse is more often responding to her own needs rather than to the needs of the patient. This type of listening occurs when an individual allows herself to operate out of personal experience, preconceived ideas, stereotyping, prejudice, or false assumptions. Whatever the cause, distortion and distancing are the outcomes.

Listen

When I ask you to listen to me
and you start giving advice
you have not done what I asked.

When I ask you to listen to me
and you begin to tell me why I shouldn't feel that way,
you are trampling on my feelings.

When I ask you to listen to me
and you feel you have to do something to solve my problem,
you have failed me, strange as that may seem.

Listen! All I asked, was that you listen,
not talk or do—just hear me.
Advice is cheap: 10 cents will get you both Dear Abby and
Billy Graham in the same newspaper.
And I can do for myself; I'm not helpless.
Maybe discouraged and faltering, but not helpless.

When you do something for me that I can and need to do
for myself, you contribute to my fear and weakness.

But, when you accept as a simple fact that I do feel what I feel,
no matter how irrational, then I can quit trying to convince
you and can get about the business of understanding what's
behind this irrational feeling.
And when that's clear, the answers are obvious and I
don't need advice.

Irrational feelings make sense when we understand what's
behind them.

Perhaps that's why prayer works, sometimes, for some people
because God is mute, and he doesn't give advice or
try to fix things. "They" just listen and let you
work it out for yourself.

So, please listen and just hear me. And, if you want to
talk, wait a minute for your turn; and I'll listen to you.

Anonymous

Deliberate listening is essential for therapeutic effectiveness. It is a process in which the nurse commits herself intentionally and with forethought to the interpersonal experience. Receptivity and openness are key components to deliberate listening. One often hears the expression, "I heard every word he said!" to emphasize that the listener got the message clearly, distinctly, and without error. Another example is that of the listener replying, "I understand." Both of these statements illustrate the deliberate attentiveness of the listener and demonstrate the absence of defensive and selective hearing. They represent a type of hearing that excludes placing personal value judgments upon what is being said. **Attentiveness** is the essence of deliberate listening. In therapy, deliberate listening is vital. If the patient knows he is being heard and understood, he is at ease, his anxiety decreases, and he willingly volunteers more information about himself and his emotions. On the other hand, the patient must also learn deliberate listening. To assist in developing this type of listening, the nurse must, especially when discussing very significant data, be sure to validate that the patient has understood. If not, the question or statement should be clarified until the message is received and understood.

Empathic listening is the core of therapeutic intervention. Empathic listening may be defined as a conscious, voluntary listening process through which the nurse establishes contact with the client's internal frame of reference. In this process, the nurse actively and with forethought relinquishes her own ideas, beliefs, values, and perceptions and immerses herself through incorporation into the client's world. A simple way to describe this complex process is that the nurse tries to see the world through the eyes of the client. This type of listening demands that the nurse be perceptive, sensitive, and alert to client cues, that is, that the nurse exhibits a heightened awareness to the subtle nuances of social and cultural differences within the client. Empathic listening requires a constant flow of feedback of both feeling and content that is conveyed with warmth, caring, and congruity. Inferences and judgments are drawn, but only after careful clarification and validation have taken place. In essence, empathic listening demands that the nurse recognize the client's feelings and communicate that recognition back to the client. Furthermore, the nurse must be cognizant that in empathic listening, she places herself in a position of risk of being changed by the experience. Therefore, in empathic listening, the nurse willingly commits self to an opportunity for growth.

Respond

It is not uncommon to find a nurse responding to a patient with hackneyed phrases. This occurs because of "non-thereness," inadequate observation, and inattentive listening. The resultant communication is ineffective, inaccurate, and misrepresentative. **To respond** is to indicate to the sender, either verbally or nonverbally, that the message is received but is not necessarily understood. It is an opportunity to talk and to share. A response may take many forms and serve many purposes. It may be used to supply information in answer to a question; express mutual understanding derived from an empathetic experience; provide a greeting in acknowledgment or recognition; ask for clarification of issues and viewpoints; or provide feedback in the promotion of understanding. In responding, the nurse assumes the responsibility of helping the patient clarify the meaning and intent of his verbal and nonverbal expressions. The response of the nurse is not an impulsive reaction. It is the thoughtful and selective application of knowledge to the particular situation at a given moment. If the response is acceptable, the communication process continues uninterrupted and leads to goal fulfillment. If the response is unacceptable, communication may break down.

Interpret

Accurate and valid interpretation requires time, effort, and patience. The nurse can alienate and isolate a patient by making a too-rapid interpretation. **To interpret** is to derive meaning from that which is being communicated. The explicit and implicit meanings that are conveyed to the sender are not always clear; therefore, interpretation depends on the nurse's application of her knowledge of individual lifestyles as well as her understanding and acceptance of differences. The degree to which the nurse is able to consider various possible interpretations depends to a large extent on her ability to feel comfortable with her own words and with the language or modes of expression used by the patient, as well as a sound theoretical foundation. Interpretation requires that the nurse display honesty and sincerity in the search for meaning, since any artificiality in the nurse's approach is almost always immediately detected and viewed as a negative response by the patient. Inaccurate interpretation is a disservice to the patient because it may contribute to the acceptance of erroneous information as fact or may cause the patient to set up resistance to the interactive–interventive process.

Validate

The last and most complex operation in the communication process is validation. Once the nurse selects the most significant of all possible interpretations of the communicated message, she is in a position to present these to the patient for verification. **To validate** is to corroborate or substantiate the interpretations that have been made within the context of the nurse–patient interaction. It is an ongoing process. In most situations, interpretations need immediate validation, as in the case of feelings that may be implied but not directly expressed, or when the nurse suspects a different usage for a particular word or phrase. In other instances, presentation of interpretations to the patient for validation depends on the readiness of the patient to accept and use the validated material in a constructive manner. Because readiness is a critical factor affecting change and goal achievement, timing is of utmost importance in the execution of the validation process.

Not only does the nurse validate her interpretations with the patient, she also seeks to validate them with colleagues or supervisors. The purpose of this aspect of validation is twofold. First, it enables the nurse to maintain her objectivity. Second, it provides a means by which the nurse can follow through on the critical analysis and evaluation of the interaction process in light of her performance and in view of the stated therapeutic goals. It is through the active pursuit for validation that the nurse can realistically assess and perfect her skills in communication, thereby permitting her to grow, experience personal and professional satisfaction, and increase her therapeutic effectiveness.

The communication process is a step-by-step dynamic procedure used in both social and therapeutic communication. The responsibility for initiating and maintaining therapeutic communication rests with the nurse. With her also remains the obligation to follow each step of the process, regardless of the patient's initial ability to participate. In the application of the process the nurse must exercise judgment and move only as the patient is able to move. If the communication process were followed and practiced in normal day-to-day living, there would be little need for the establishment of therapeutic communication.

COMMUNICATION BARRIERS

As human beings we never cease to communicate; however, that which we communicate is not always clearly understood. A variety of internal and external factors influence the manner in which the message is sent, received, and comprehended. If the communicator is unaware of these factors and their influence on the communicative process, he is unable to deal with them. The net result is a breakdown in the communication process. For clarity and understanding, we identify four major barriers to communication. Encompassed in these is a majority of the most common internal and external factors influencing communication.

Inaccurate Perception of Self and Others

As with every other facet of living, knowledge of self is a prerequisite for communication. A person's attitudes, beliefs, and values shape the transmission, reception, and understanding of conscious and unconscious messages. A breakdown occurs when an individual assumes that his attitudes, beliefs, and values are shared by another. And even if there are similarities, because of individual differences, they will not be identical. Variations should be expected and given consideration. For example, two middle-class mothers, Mother A and Mother B, each with a family of four, verbalize to each other about the necessity to practice economy in a world of rising costs. Both talk of clipping coupons and taking advantage of "good buys." From their conversation, you would initially gather that both women shop in the same manner. In talking further with Mother A, you find that she shops at one store and points out savings in terms of gasoline, time, and energy. While in talking with Mother B, you find that she does her weekly shopping at several stores and points out savings in terms of a wider selection, redemption stamps, and self-satisfaction about "getting bargains." Economy is a shared value, and each woman takes for granted that the other shops in the same way. However, the manner in which they practice economy and the beliefs they hold regarding attainment are markedly different. A question that might well be asked at this point is: Why didn't they go into more detail with each other? The answer is that, because each valued economy and shared similar practices, each "assumed" that the other carried out all shopping habits in a like manner and therefore didn't explore further.

Another example to illustrate what happens when there is inaccurate perception of self and others in the therapeutic situation is one that involves misinterpretation of role.

> As part of the student's clinical experience in a psychiatric setting, a nursing student had been assigned to a patient, Mr. X. The patient was informed that a nursing student would be talking with him. When the student approached Mr. X, she introduced herself and stated the reason for her daily contacts with him. Mr. X indicated that he understood, and they proceeded to discuss his reasons for being hospitalized. Subsequently, the student accompanied Mr. X to his activities in order to complete the observation and assessment of his functioning. Mr. X began to shift his perception of the student from the professional role to one of a "friendly visitor." His perception became even further distorted as he viewed the student nurse as a "girlfriend." The student became upset and consulted her instructor.

This distortion occurred because the nursing student failed to establish and repeatedly clarify her role with Mr. X in this learning experience. Thus, she placed herself and the therapeutic alliance in jeopardy by assuming that Mr. X would continue to remember her role after being provided with only one explanation.

Little or no understanding of one's own attitudes, values, and beliefs produces communication breakdown through the expression of inconsistencies. These inconsistencies in words and behavior lead to sending mixed messages, which, in turn, result in confusion and misunderstanding by the receiver. They also detract from the credibility of the sender. We use clichés to describe an individual who demonstrates this type of communication breakdown: "She talks out of both sides of her mouth;" "You never know where you stand with her—you're damned if you do, and damned if you don't;" or "Actions speak louder than words." These inconsistencies may also be responsible for engendering within the receiver feelings of irritation, impatience, anger, and perhaps even disgust or distrust. Effective communication cannot survive where such negative feelings exist.

Lack of self-knowledge or knowledge of another with regard to attitudes, beliefs, or values provides a medium for the development of bias and prejudice. The natural response displayed by an individual confronted with the possible existence of a bias or prejudice is to deny its presence. Refusal to acknowledge the possibility of bias or prejudice defeats communication in that it produces a closed circuit. The individual is unable either to send or receive accurate messages surrounding a particular person, situation, or set of circumstances.

Inaccurate perception of self or another may be produced by other internal and external factors such as one's concern for status and prestige. Status and prestige are equated by some with power—power of position, expertise, competence, or force. Breakdown in communication occurs as a result of the misinterpretation or misuse of power. Take for example, the individual who is preoccupied with creating an impression of importance, superior knowledge, competence, or wealth. This individual may dwell on his social standing, educational background, credentials, or success in the stock market. This type of communication, because of excessive egocentricity, turns people off and thereby negates any avenue for positive communication.

Due to ethnic and cultural background, an individual has a built-in value system. Yet he may not clearly understand that he operates under the imposed traditions and values of that system. Those with whom the individual attempts to communicate also operate under the influence of an inherent ethnic and cultural social system. Operation without recognition of and consideration for self or another leads to the formation of barriers in communication. Such things as the specific language used by a group may not be clearly understood or may be understood in a different context than intended. Pronunciation, accent, or word connotations may interfere with the communication process.

The two illustrations that follow graphically portray the difficulties associated with linguistics and the nurse's need to be alert to such potential situations.

> Mrs. Ruiz, a native of Puerto Rico, was admitted to the hospital for observation following complaints of severe abdominal pain. A nursing

student was assigned to assist with Mrs. Ruiz's admission to the medical floor of a large metropolitan hospital. The student delivered the prepackaged bedside equipment. As she put each item in place, she named each for Mrs. Ruiz—bath basin, kidney basin, water pitcher, soap dish, and so forth. Later, when the student returned to the room, she found Mrs. Ruiz trying to void in the kidney basin. Upon questioning, Mrs. Ruiz stated that since she had been told it was a kidney basin, she used it to relieve her kidneys.

Many times communication is closed down because the sounds are "funny" or confused with other words. Here is an actual incident:

Tommy, age 5, was being oriented to the pediatric unit following his admission for a tonsillectomy. During the process of acquainting him with his new environment, the nurse pointed out several areas, including the linen chute. Tommy's eyes got very big, and he turned to look at her in amazement. As they proceeded to walk, Tommy reached toward the nurse and tugged at her uniform. When the nurse looked at him, he asked, "How do you shoot linen in there?"

Failure to Focus on Message or Sender

Barriers to communication found in this category result from the listener's inability to zero in on the concerns and messages the sender wishes to convey. Sometimes, in an effort to establish a commonality in the communication bond, speakers frequently change topics to an extent that neither party is able to derive meaning from the messages. The outcome is a sender and receiver who both experience an increased level of frustration and who move away from, instead of toward, establishing rapport.

Feelings of inadequacy, real or imagined, prevent an individual from achieving desired communication. This inability produces within the individual anger or hostility, which he directs toward the self or projects onto another. Various kinds of "cut-off" behaviors result from these feelings.

One type of cut-off behavior is the expression of **impatience**. Impatient behavior is evidenced by continuous verbal interruptions—when the listener says he understands or already knows, even before the speaker is finished talking—or by such nonverbal behavior as turning away from the communicator, responding to distractions in the environment, or using facial expressions that convey boredom or lack of interest in the message. Through these behaviors, the receiver is telling the sender to "hurry along and get it over with." When this happens there is a failure to pick up on the key words or cues that are indicative of the sender's main concern. Further progression toward goal attainment is then blocked.

Prying is another manifestation of cut-off behavior. Prying is an attempt to uncover material irrelevant to the sender's main message, which he is not ready to reveal. It may be asking for details—gory or sexual—that have no relation to the problem or process but merely gratify the curiosity of the receiver. Prying is destructive and dehumanizing because the individual seeking therapeutic intervention is made to feel that he cannot retain the right to withold nonpertinent information. It demonstrates disrespect, lack of interest, and unconcern for the individual. A patient is sensitive to this unprofessional behavior and frequently expresses negative feelings about the receiver to others. The only purpose that prying serves is to satisfy one's need for power, control, or gratification of one's own needs. Often the information gleaned from prying is used by the nurse as subject material for gossip among other professionals, which is inappropriate and destructive to any relationship.

Failure to focus on the sender or the message is the outcome of inattentive listening. It is another form of communication block. **Inattentive listening** is selective hearing, that is, hearing what one wants to hear when it is convenient to hear it. Inattentive listening is one of the most prevalent pitfalls occurring in ordinary, everyday communication. Just consider the following excerpt of a conversation between husband and wife. When the wife reminds her husband that the basement needs to be cleaned on Saturday, he acknowledges the message with a nod of his head, apparently indicating that he heard what was said. On Saturday, as he prepares to leave for a golf game with his buddies, his wife asks him about the cleaning project. His response to her is, "Why didn't you remind me sooner?" The wife replies, "But I did! On Thursday!" Sound familiar? Or, how about children who are engrossed in a television program before supper and have not heard Mother say, "It's time to set the table!" But if she had said instead, "There's a bag of potato chips on the shelf. Help yourselves!" there would have been a stampede to get to the shelf first. It is clear from these examples that inattentive listening occurs when the priorities of the participants are not the same.

Control is often an issue in communication and is the result of feelings of inadequacy. It is a maneuver used to divert the communicative process away from emotionally charged or self-revealing data. Control is manifested in several ways; for example, the speaker can monopolize the conversation, forcing the listener into a silent, passive role. This domineering sender has time for only his views, his opinions, and his belief systems and therefore rarely pays attention to the receiver. Another method of control is via incessant, trivial, and superfluous details that mask relevant messages. With this method the recipient is so deluged with issues and details that he cannot acknowledge, understand, or interrupt the rapid flow of communication. A third way in which control is manifested is through the use of minimal verbal activity. In this instance the messages are short and often vague, providing the receiver with little understanding of either the message or its purpose. A fourth means of control used in the communication process is through the use of hackneyed words or phrases. The deployment of stock phrases keeps the level of communication on a superficial, uninvolved basis and conveys to the receiver a lack of genuine interest. How often have you met a friend or acquaintance who says to you, "Good morning! How are you?" and continues on his way. He has accomplished a socially acceptable greeting but has not waited for your reply. Are you left with the impression that he is interested about what you think and feel?

The nurse must realize that not only patients try to exert these kinds of control. The therapeutic professional can also make interventive errors by exercising the same methods of control; the dynamics, however, differ in scope. The professional can control the therapeutic communicative process by remaining superficial, talking too much about generalities, or by focusing on secondary (background) data in order to avoid emotionally charged data. This error is a subconscious effort to mask a fear of therapeutic failure in effectively and successfully handling data with the patient.

Inaccurate Interpretations of Message

Communicators must always remain conscious of the fact that perception is highly individualistic and that therefore it is relatively easy to fall into the communication traps of making generalizations and assumptions and of overidentifying. In these traps, the original intent is lost, and the receiver is left with the feeling that the message or the sender is not important enough to be heard and responded to appropriately.

To generalize is to form an illogical, exaggerated premise based on insufficient factual information. Generalization is the process by which a set of circumstances that are applicable in a majority of settings are applied indiscriminately to every set of circumstances without consideration for the "specific" differences that apply to an individual person's life experiences. To illustrate, here is an example of an actual incident.

> Miss Kane, a black student nurse, was assigned to give a patient, Mrs. Jones, a back rub. Mrs. Jones was an Appalachian who had recently moved to a large industrial city with her husband and three children. Her speech was still thick with the accent of her native area. Miss Kane observed that Mrs. Jones became rigid when she began the back rub; she interpreted this as a sign of Mrs. Jones' racial prejudice.

In relating the incident to her classmates, Miss Kane stated that Mrs. Jones told her that she had never had a stranger bathe her or rub her back. Miss Kane had completely overlooked these comments as possibly significant causes for Mrs. Jones' tension.

An **assumption** is defined as attributing meaning to a message based on one's own frame of reference. Suppose a person says to you, "I'm going to take a rest." This comment can be interpreted in many ways. While to rest generally means to sit or to lie in a motionless position, we all know individuals who rest by pursuing an active hobby, exercising, taking a shower, paying a visit to the beauty shop, or going for a drive in the country. To avoid the assumption trap and to interpret accurately, you must seek clarification of the communicated message. You must discover what "rest" means to that person. Neither the necessity for accurate interpretation nor the acknowledgment of a person's uniqueness of individual perception can be emphasized strongly enough. Just think about the popular gift books, ceramics, or song entitled "Happiness is . . .," and you realize the many meanings the term implies! But remember—it has a particular significance for each individual person in a particular setting at a particular point in time.

Overidentification occurs when an individual hears what is being said and immediately interprets the message according to his own value systems or frames of reference. It occurs because what is being said may be similar to the listener's own experience. Accordingly, the listener either agrees, disagrees, approves, disapproves, or in some other way makes a value judgment about the message or the sender. In other words, the listener "jumps to conclusions" and regards the conclusion he reaches as valid.

Making assumptions and overgeneralizations leads the receiver of the communicated message into responding with specific communication tactics. Some of the more common tactics are: stating his personal opinions as fact, giving a "pep talk," providing advice, offering "pat answers" for problems, or offering false reassurance. In each of the preceding, self-worth, self-expression, uniqueness, individuality, concern, empathy, and acceptance are all denied, and thoughtful consideration of the meaning and intent of the communicated message is bypassed. Objectivity and rationality are lost. The respondent does not hear with understanding; therefore, the communication exchange is terminated.

Failure to Maintain Personal Integrity

Communication is often abruptly terminated because the participants fail to be honest with themselves and with the person with whom they are communicating. Integrity is symonymous with honor. Personal integrity is based on the amount of respect one has for self, which in turn influences the respect one is able to demonstrate toward another. Breaking promises, withholding information, giving misinformation, or providing a too-detailed description or explanation are communication tactics that demonstrate a lack of personal integrity. Honesty within the communication process is suspect when promises are made and not kept. Giving one's verbal word is just as binding as signing one's name to a written contract. One should neither make a promise one does not intend to keep nor withhold information to which another is legitimately entitled. A person has a right to know those facts that concern him and his particular situation or might influence him to act in a particular way. It is not unusual to hear words like, "I'm not going to tell him, for his own good," or "What he doesn't know won't hurt him." These are false premises and are usually employed when the speaker is afraid to be "real" or is afraid that he will be called upon to accept responsibility for another's action or reaction. A person has a right to self-determination, that is, to decide for himself what is or what is not "good" for him.

Misinformation is often transmitted because the speaker lacks knowledge and attempts to save face by supplying any answer. What the speaker fails to realize is that giving misinformation is far more damaging to his projected image than an honest, open, "I don't know." Self-respect can be enhanced by such an admission; misinformation can only tarnish it.

In conclusion, communication barriers lead to dead ends. They cause misunderstanding, apprehension, anxiety, and confusion for both sender and receiver. They are pitfalls that must be avoided at all costs. Learning to communicate is like learning to walk. First, you must be able to crawl, then to stand and hang on, and finally, to take your own independent steps. In those first steps, you feel you are walking on eggs. Becoming skillful in the art of communication, like learning to walk, requires patience, practice, perseverance, and determination.

EFFECTIVE THERAPEUTIC COMMUNICATION PRACTICES

Therapeutic communication, unlike social communication, is a goal-oriented, planned, purposeful pursuit. It is neither left to chance nor undertaken without thoughtful consideration and preparation. Before the nurse begins to implement the therapeutic nurse–patient relationship in an effective manner, she must become aware of specific communication practices and develop skill in the execution of these practices. We have devised three major categories into which communication practices may be divided. They are as follows:

I. Practices geared to establishing a climate for communication
   1. Select a setting that insures privacy and confidentiality.
   2. Schedule and use the same setting for subsequent sessions.
   3. Select a time that is mutually agreeable.
   4. Assess and modify the environment to promote physical and psychological comfort.
   5. Eliminate possible environmental and personal distractions.
   6. Provide for appropriate seating.
   7. Modify interpersonal spacing according to patient's and nurse's needs.
   8. Explain time limits.
   9. Modify length of interaction according to patient's tolerance for close, interpersonal contact and ability to concentrate.
   10. Start and end session on time.
   11. Contract with the patient for the method of recording the communication.
   12. Assume a body posture that conveys interest, attention, and respect.
   13. Maintain an unbiased or friendly facial expression and attitude.
   14. Speak with a clear, well-modulated tone of voice.
   15. Maintain eye contact.

II. Practices geared to developing approaches to facilitate communication
   1. State the goals of the interaction.
   2. Allow and encourage the patient to assume the initiative in the interaction process.
   3. Encourage and support a free exchange of ideas, thoughts, and feelings.
   4. Permit the patient to move at his own pace.
   5. Guide the interaction from the simple to the complex.
   6. Direct the focus of the communication on reality, on the patient, and on his needs in the here and now.
   7. Focus on problem areas.
   8. Send messages in a form the patient can understand.
   9. Send messages using language that has meaning for both nurse and patient.
   10. Send messages according to the patient's rate of ability to receive.
   11. Identify themes and recurring behaviors.
   12. Modify practice and technique according to the need of the patient.

III. Practices geared to implementing a verbal exchange that focuses on specific identifiable skills
1. Use indirect questions or comments to facilitate interaction.
2. Use direct questions only when specific information is needed.
3. Give short, clear, and direct responses.
4. Encourage the patient to elaborate.
5. Reflect feelings or ideas.
6. Note changes in subject matter.
7. Identify and explore discrepancies between verbal and nonverbal behavior.
8. Introduce new thoughts and ideas when the patient indicates readiness to hear, discuss, or accept.
9. Wait during periods of silence.
10. Use feedback to determine understanding of transmitted messages.
11. Identify with the patient specific concerns regarding himself and his relationship with others.
12. Summarize dialogue between participants.
13. Explore each of the identified concerns through description and clarification.
14. Compare and validate perceptions.
15. Extract, from content, data for interpretation.
16. Formulate with the patient possible alternatives or solutions.
17. Support the patient in his attempt to test out the solutions.
18. Evaluate with the patient results of testing.
19. Identify strengths and weakness of the communication process within the interactive–interventive event.
20. Assess the level of involvement of the participants in the interaction.
21. Evaluate the level of nurse–patient participation using as standards the principles for effective communication found on pages 268–271 and the stated goals of the interaction.
22. Write objectives for nursing care based on the interpretation of the evaluation.
23. Revise goals for subsequent interactions based on interpretations of evaluation.
24. Identify objectives for improving nurse effectiveness.
25. Keep an accurate record of the interaction.

THERAPEUTIC TECHNIQUES OF COMMUNICATION

Effective communication functioning within the nurse–patient relationship depends on an understanding of others and the process of communication. It also depends on the ability of the nurse to employ certain identified techniques of communication. These techniques are tools by which the nurse carries out communication practices. The tools are important only in the sense that they facilitate the communication process. The techniques are not meant to be memorized and used by the nurse as a stereotyped approach or response. In and of themselves, they are not absolutes, and their use does not guarantee therapeutic effectiveness. They are merely the means by which the nurse conveys her ability to be therapeutic. In order for the communication process to be therapeutic, the nurse must modify and adapt the techniques to the peculiarities of the participants and the prevailing situation.

The therapeutic techniques commonly employ questions as the usual method of operation. It is important for the nurse to remember that direct questions tend to decrease communication and that indirect or open-ended questions are far more productive. In employing the skills of communication, the nurse should be careful to particularly avoid using those direct questions that elicit only a yes or no response, as these types of questions produce no feedback and tend to create an inquisitional atmosphere. However, direct questions can and should be used when specific facts are needed. Broad openings and general leads are more appropriate in that they allow the patient to take the initiative as well as provide an opportunity for him to expand on the topics under discussion. Questioning leads, using "how" and "why," also require careful consideration in their application. Too many hows and whys tend to increase feelings of inadequacy when the patient's response comes back, "I don't know." A response to a how or why question requires that an individual be able to think in a rational, procedural, organized manner and realize causes and implications.

All questions should be clear and precise. The nurse must bear in mind that responses to questions are more dependent on the form the questions take than on the person to whom the question is directed. In other words, if a question is not clear or precise, no person can be expected to respond appropriately, or clearly. Asking the patient to clarify a vague statement not only assists the nurse with her response, but shows an active interest in the patient's feelings. Therefore, the kind, the manner, and the purpose of the question become significant factors in implementing the communication practices and applying the skills of communication.

In Table 14–1 we present nine common therapeutic techniques of communication. We identify the technique, define it, indicate its purpose and provide concrete examples to demonstrate its use.

TABLE 14–1. NINE COMMON THERAPEUTIC TECHNIQUES OF COMMUNICATION

Technique	Definition	Purpose	Examples
Exploring	Obtaining all pertinent data on a particular subject or feeling.	1. To increase the level of self-perception of the participants. 2. To acquire mutually understood information. 3. To move beyond the superficial and deal with the more complex or hidden meanings of the message. 4. To encourage the sender to evaluate described material.	P: I feel sad about going but not so sad that I _____. N: What? P: I heard them talking about me in the hall. N: Tell me about the incident. P: I don't feel well today. N: What seems to be the matter? P: I want to get married to a woman who is living with another man, but I don't know . . . N: You seem unsure—you don't know what?
Clarifying	Attempting to find the meaning of the communicated message.	1. To establish mutual understanding. 2. To identify common meanings associated with terms or phrases. 3. To promote and encourage further communication between the participants. 4. To facilitate the recognition of individual differences. 5. To decrease distortions in perception. 6. To decrease the level of verbal distortions.	P: I have a pass to go home for the weekend. N: What does this mean to you? P: That nurse has pilot's eyes. N: What do you mean? P: Gone are days when things were simple. N: I'm not sure I understand what you are trying to tell me.
Reflecting	Conveying to the sender his expressed thoughts and related feelings.	1. To acknowledge to the sender that the message has been received. 2. To demonstrate to the sender that the receiver is searching for understanding of the message. 3. To enable the sender to perceive the communication as an extension of self.	P: She just burns me up! N: You sound angry. P: I finished my O.T. project. Everyone thought it was pretty good. N: You seem pleased with yourself.

TABLE 14–1. CONTINUED

Technique	Definition	Purpose	Examples
		4. To promote objectivity in determining the meaning of the message.	
Focusing	Concentrating on a specific thought or feeling regarding a particular point.	1. To draw the attention of the sender to significant data. 2. To encourage the sender to separate relevant data from irrelevant data. 3. To sustain goal-oriented communication. 4. To discourage the sender from rambling. 5. To interrupt and forestall rapid subject changes.	P: Tom is always picking on me, no matter what I do. N: Give me an example. P: They said I can't go home. N: Who are "they"?
Informing	Responding to direct questions with needed facts.	1. To share knowledge. 2. To promote understanding. 3. To make facts clear. 4. To build trust. 5. To establish confidence in and reliability of the sender.	P: What time do I go to the dentist? N: You have a one o'clock appointment. P: What about this information? Who gets to see it? N: Only me and my instructor.
Using silence	Communicating without verbalization.	1. To convey the receiver's interest, acceptance, and understanding. 2. To allow the sender to assume initiative. 3. To provide the sender with time to collect and sort out his thoughts. 4. To provide an opportunity to share with the sender his indirectly expressed feelings. 5. To emphasize a point. 6. To provide an opportunity to introduce a new idea or feeling. 7. To allow for relief from emotionally charged content.	P: My mother has been saying that she does not want me home permanently. That's not a good feeling. N: (remains silent) P: They always got me out before. I'd love to go home, that's for sure. N: (remains silent) P: I hope she lets me return. I'm scared. I don't know where I will live if I can't go home. N: (remains silent)

(continued)

TABLE 14–1. CONTINUED

Technique	Definition	Purpose	Examples
Validating	Confirming one's observations and interpretations.	1. To facilitate accurate appraisal of the sender and his communicated message. 2. To avoid making assumptions. 3. To verify cues. 4. To arrive at mutual understanding that increases rapport and establishes a basis for collaboration.	P: I didn't want to come, but my mother brought me anyhow! N: Sometimes it's difficult to do the things we have to do. P: Yeah, they're always yelling at each other and at me. N: It must be hard to keep your cool when everybody is yelling.
Evaluating	Assessing the significance of a communicated message.	1. To determine progress. 2. To acknowledge differences. 3. To provide feedback from which clarification and understanding is derived. 4. To make comparisons and exercise judgment so that the sender is better able to engage in decision-making.	P: I am getting better. N: In what ways do you feel better? P: As a child my brother was always in the limelight. Everybody noticed him. N: It must have been very difficult for you. Can you recall how you felt then?
Summarizing	Developing a concise résumé of the communicated message.	1. To facilitate recall of important points. 2. To promote clarification and achieve new understandings. 3. To maintain a point of interest. 4. To provide a basis for developing a plan of action. 5. To bring discussion of a particular subject to a conclusion.	P: That's all I have to say today. N: During the session you and I have discussed . . . (At the initiation of a session the nurse begins with summary of last session.) N: Last time we talked about some of your feelings about being here in the hospital . . .

NURSE–PATIENT INTERACTIONS

The following (situations I to III) are excerpts from nurse–patient interactions which demonstrate the use of the theraputic techniques of communication.

Situation I: Danny—Initial Visit

Danny, age 13 was referred for out-patient psychotherapy by juvenile court. His mother remained with Danny during the first session to provide the nurse with background information. On the second visit his mother stated that Danny was scared and wanted her to remain with him. During this second session Danny sat opposite the nurse, crossed his legs left over right, sat with his head down, playing with his shoestrings, and avoiding looking directly at the nurse. For the most part, he did not verbally respond to the nurse's open-ended approaches. Periods of silence were breached by the mother.

Dialogue in Interaction	Comments
Nurse: Tell me something about yourself. *(Danny gives a grunt that is followed by a pause, which lasts 1 minute.)*	A general open-ended statement is used to elicit information, to put him at ease, and to encourage him to assume the initiative.
Mother (turns to Danny): Danny, before we came you were telling me about cutting up at school and the bad influence of your friends and you wanted to know about changing schools.	
Danny: I just can't get Cs at Westwood. ***(Mother turns to nurse and talks about private schools versus public schools and says what she thinks should be done about Danny's schooling.)***	Mother is aware of Danny's discomfort and even though she too is uneasy, she tries to protect him.
Nurse (interrupts mother, turns to Danny): Danny, what do you think prevents you from getting Cs?	Direct question for focusing and exploring.
Danny: Too much fooling around!	
(Mother interjects a long explanation of the school schedule.)	
Nurse (turns to Danny's mother): I'd like Danny and me to spend the rest of the time together getting to know each other. Would you mind waiting downstairs?	Clarifying the role of nurse–therapist. Mother's presence inhibits the development of the therapeutic nurse–patient relationship.
(Mother hesitates, then nods her head and leaves the room.)	
Nurse: I asked your mother to leave because I thought you found it hard to talk with me while she was here.	Seeking validation of interpretation of Danny's behavior.
(Danny makes no verbal response.) *Nurse (after pausing)*: Danny, tell me more about yourself.	Resistance to active participation is demonstrated by Danny's nonverbal response.
(Danny makes no verbal response.) *(Nurse waits 5 minutes.)*	Silence used for the purpose of demonstrating interest and acceptance. Provides opportunity for Danny to assume the initiative.
Nurse: It takes time for stangers to get to know each other, and communicating with adults might be difficult.	Informing to promote understanding and acceptance despite negativistic behavior.

(continued)

Dialogue in Interaction	Comments
(Danny avoids looking at the nurse, sits with head down, and plays with pant legs and shoes. After waiting through 5 minutes of silence, the nurse verbalizes her observations at 2-minute intervals.)	
Nurse: You might be having trouble finding words to begin.	Reflecting to acknowledge to Danny that his behavior is understood.
(Danny grimaces.)	
Nurse: Perhaps you didn't want to come to see me, and that might be making you angry.	Reflecting and clarifying to promote continued understanding and validation of impression.
(Danny shows increased agitated movements.)	
Nurse: How do you feel about having to come for counseling?	Direct question to draw attention to the connection between behavior, feelings, and demands placed on him by the court.
(Danny shrugs his shoulders.)	
Nurse: An hour's session is a long time. I think it might help us to get better acquainted if we have two half-hour sessions per week.	Informing to encourage further communication. Evaluation to provide feedback.
(Danny shows no change in behavior.)	
Nurse: I'll contact Mr. S about your school schedule and let you know the response at the next session.	Informing to share plans for action regarding initially expressed concern.
(Still no change in Danny.)	
Nurse: Our time is up. I'll see you next Monday and Friday for a half-hour.	Informing to promote understanding.
(Danny immediately runs out of the room.)	

Danny—Fourth Session.

Danny missed his third appointment because he went to visit some friends and later told his parents that he forgot. At the fourth session, Danny reluctantly entered the office, selected a seat opposite the nurse, and acknowledged her good morning with a "Hi!"

Dialogue in Interaction	Comments
Danny: What did Mr. S have to say?	It should be noted that while Danny did not verbally respond to the nurse in the previous session and even missed a session, he immediately initiated the interview by recalling an issue raised in the last session—a definite indication that though one may not think the patient is paying any attention, every word is heard and many are remembered!
Nurse: I called him but he was busy. I left a message for him to call me back. I'm waiting for his call now. If it doesn't come today, I will call him again first thing in the morning.	Informing to share knowledge and outcome of nurse's intervention. Building trust through keeping promise.

Dialogue in Interaction	Comments
(Danny nods his head affirmatively.)	
Nurse: What did you think about the last session?	Encouraging evaluation to provide feedback.
Danny: What do you mean, what did I think?	
Nurse: What were some of your feelings about it?	Explaining to encourage Danny to take the initiative.
Danny: I'm tired. I didn't want to come today.	Danny changed the subject, apparently unable to verbalize feelings at this point. Danny remained silent for 10 minutes. Opening with, "I'm tired" is also an effort by the patient to avoid emotional content. Though it may not be necessary to pick up and discuss, the nurse must be consciously aware of what reasons might provoke this type of opening, that is, lacking of readiness by Danny to explore and share feelings.
Nurse: Tell me something about school, what you like or dislike?	Redirecting focus to his initial concern while pursuing opportunity to explore feelings in a less threatening manner.
Danny: Teachers are stupid. They yell at you.	
Nurse: Stupid? In what way? Give me some other examples in which you think teachers are stupid.	Reflecting and clarifying. Exploring.
Danny: When you cut study hall or your lunch period and they catch you.	
Nurse: How is that being stupid?	Clarifying.*
Danny (shrugs shoulders): You gotta go to the office. Sometimes they don't do nothing.	
Nurse: They don't say anything?	Reflecting.
Danny: You have to go back to where you're supposed to be.	
Nurse: And that's being stupid?	Validating.
Danny: Yeah.	
Nurse: It's sometimes hard to do the things you're supposed to do.	Reflecting.
Danny (makes no response for approximately 1 minute): Nobody likes Mr. S.	
Nurse: I wonder why?	Exploring.
Danny: He makes you do things you have to do.	
Nurse: Oh! I see.	Exploring.
Danny: Nobody in the whole school likes him.	
Nurse: That's an awful lot of people to have not liking you.	Evaluating.
(Danny is silent.)	
Nurse: Do you dislike Mr. S too?	Focusing.

*For the remainder of the interaction examples, the focus is directed toward identifying specific techniques of communication. Comments regarding content and process have been omitted. The reader is encouraged to use the omission as an opportunity to analyze, interpret, and evaluate the nurse–client communication.

Dialogue in Interaction	Comments
(More silence.)	
Nurse: What else about school do you like or dislike?	Exploring and refocusing.
Danny: Nothing!	
Nurse: It's sometimes difficult to share feelings.	Verbalizing the implied.
Danny: Yeah.	
Nurse: Today you shared with me some thoughts you have about school. Perhaps in our next session we can talk more around your feelings.	Summarizing and setting up a plan of action for the next session.

Situation II: Mr. Wyle

This second excerpt is from an actual series of interactions that took place between a student nurse and a 40-year-old white male who was diagnosed as a schizophrenic, catatonic type. The illustration is extracted from the fifth interaction the student had with this patient.

Dialogue in Interaction	Comments
Mr. Wyle: What do you want to ask?	
Student: I don't want to ask anything, Mr. Wyle. Is there something you'd like to talk about?	Informing and explaining.
Mr. Wyle: There's not much to tell, like I told you before—about getting a lawyer—both my sisters say I don't take my medicine and that's how they got me into the hospital. And I say I do take my medicine. My whole family thinks I'm crazy and I don't. Otherwise, I couldn't carry on a conversation like this.	
Student: You're telling me that you and your lawyer are trying to prove that you are capable of handling your own affairs. Am I correct?	Validating.
Mr. Wyle: Yes, that's just about the size of it.	
Student: Okay, what would you say or what could you do to prove the point that you are capable of handling your own affairs?	Focusing.
Mr. Wyle: Well, just prove it to certain people, like Dr. Kriss for one.	Exploring.
Student: And you can do this by . . .	Exploring.
Mr. Wyle: Yeah, by taking my medicines.	
Student: Before, you told me that sometimes you forget. Then your behavior changes.	Validating.
Mr. Wyle: Naw—it don't change that much!	
Student: But it does some?	Validating.
Mr. Wyle: It doesn't change at all as far as I'm concerned.	
Student: At all?	Reflecting.

Dialogue in Interaction	Comments
Mr. Wyle: Well, maybe some, but not that much to have me "stamped insane." What behavior would I have? I don't go around stealing and knocking people in the head!	
Student: You stated before that you forget what you do when you don't take you medicine.	Validating.
Mr. Wyle: Forget? I don't forget.	
Student: Wait a minute, Mr. Wyle. We seem to be getting off the track.	Focusing.
Mr. Wyle: You mean take medicine and stuff?	
Student: And what happened when you forgot it?	Exploring.
Mr. Wyle: Not much! My mother used to complain.	
Student: Complain?	Reflecting.
Mr. Wyle: Yeah, about what I did.	
Student: What did you do?	Exploring.
Mr. Wyle: She's very old, you know, and sometimes she doesn't even notice if she's giving it to me or not.	
Student: And you don't remind her?	Reflecting.
Mr. Wyle: Well, I feel I'm a little bit too old to be guided along by her hand. After all, she's 63. Personally, I hate to tell you this but I hate to be around her because she is so old. I have to realize that what she says half the time is from age.	
Student: Give me an example.	Exploring.
Mr. Wyle: Well like, she says, "Why don't you own a car?" and I said, "I don't know. I don't have the money." She said, "I'll save the money for you." And I said, "But you don't give me the freedom that it takes to drive a car." 'Cause theoretically, being in a place like this you shouldn't be able to drive a car 'cause it "stamps" you as being mentally ill. Mentally ill people shouldn't be allowed to drive a car. How could they? And endanger lives of other people.	
Student: What do you mean by "stamped mentally ill"? That seems to upset you.	Focusing. Validating.
Mr. Wyle: Why sure it does! Because I'm not mentally ill.	
Student: Could you give me a definition of being mentally ill?	Clarifying.
Mr. Wyle: Mentally ill?	
Student: Yes.	Informing.
Mr. Wyle: A mentally ill person is a person that is sick, hears voices, that goes around talking to himself, that goes around doing oddball	

(*continued*)

Dialogue in Interaction		Comments
	actions that the rest of society doesn't do . . . And has fits, and takes a catatonic fit.	
Student:	Catatonic fit?	Clarifying.
Mr. Wyle:	Yeah, you know, goes around like this (*he starts shaking, rolling his eyes, and wriggling*) and hears voices.	
Student:	Do you ever hear voices?	Direct question.
Mr. Wyle:	No, but this guy in the group he hears voices. He's got a problem, he shouldn't drive a car or be in public working.	
Student:	Do you have a problem?	Direct question.
Mr. Wyle:	Yes, I got a problem—taking this medication. Now why does she have to inject it?	
Student:	We discussed this last week, Mr. Wyle. We decided that you would have to discuss receiving injections with Dr. Kriss.	Informing.
Mr. Wyle:	Yeah, that's right. *(He rolls his eyes back.)*	
Student:	What were you thinking about just now?	Reflecting.
Mr. Wyle:	I was just wondering if I asked you, if you heard voices, would you tell me you heard them?	
Student:	Now that I know you, yes, I would tell you.	Informing.
Mr. Wyle:	Well, you're honest. I see you're honest. I'll have to think about . . . *(seemed to be concentrating)*	
(Silence for 2 minutes.)		Using silence.
Mr. Wyle:	So what you said you would risk being "stamped mentally ill" and tell someone that you heard voices, in order that they may help you understand why you heard them.	
Student:	Yes, Mr. Wyle—that is what I mean.	Validating.
Mr. Wyle:	Hmm!	
Student:	Mr. Wyle, it's almost time to end the interview for today. We talked about several things, mainly your concern about being labeled mentally ill, taking your medication, some difficulties with your mother, and about people hearing voices. Next time let's talk about each of these things in more detail.	Summarizing.

Situation III: Miss Smythe

Miss Smythe is a 43-year-old white female who was admitted to a medical floor with the diagnosis of a cerebral vascular accident. She is a Catholic, and shortly after admission, the hospital chaplain visited her and administered while she was unconscious the Sacrament of the Sick, "Last Rites." When Miss Smythe regained consciousness and was informed, she became exceedingly angry and refused to see the chaplain again. She was very concerned about her care and frequently talked about leaving the hospital, but at the same time refused to participate in her care. A student was assigned to care for Miss Smythe. The following dialogue took place during morning care.

	Dialogue in Interaction	Comments
Nurse:	Good morning, Miss Smythe. My name is Miss Rosario and I will be caring for you this morning.	Giving information. Stating purpose.
Miss Smythe:	Rosario, Rosario, that's Italian, isn't it? You're a Catholic, aren't you? I'm a Catholic, too. Do you know what the Church did to me? They gave me the Last Rites. I'm dead already and I don't know it. They knew it!	
Nurse:	You really seem upset this morning.	Reflection of feeling.
Miss Smythe:	Yes! Yes, I am! You'd be upset too if they did that to you.	
Nurse:	Tell me more about what's been happening.	Exploring to encourage verbalization of feeling.
Miss Smythe:	I told you! They gave me the Sacrament of the Dead while I was unconscious.	
Nurse:	The Sacrament of the Dead? I'm not sure what you mean.	Asking for clarification.
Miss Smythe:	You know, the last Sacrament they give you when you're dying. I'm not dead yet.	
Nurse:	The fact that you received the Sacrament must have been very frightening.	Validating impression.
(Miss Smythe	*begins to cry.)*	
(Nurse moves	*chair to bedside, sits down and remains with patient as she cries.)*	Using silence.

As a result of this outburst, the relief experienced through the tears, the support provided by the nurse's presence, and the opportunity to further verbalize and explore feelings, the patient was able to come to a better understanding of her condition. She was able to ask questions about the amount of residual paralysis, the extent of disability she could expect, and if the limitations would prevent her from returning to her job.

SUMMARY

In this chapter we have highlighted the basics of the communicative process and illustrated some of the therapeutic techniques. Some of it is skeletal: we have deliberately eliminated details, expansion of concepts, and thorough dialogues. The reader is referred to other references that explain the dynamics of communication and the therapeutic processes in depth. However, this chapter on the method, practice, and process of communications offers the essential components that help the nurse develop her communicative skills in mental health practice.

SUGGESTED READINGS

Almore, M. G. Dyadic Communication. *American Journal of Nursing*, Vol. 79, No. 6 (July, 1979), 1076–1078.

Anderson, M. L. Talking about Sex—With Less Anxiety. *Journal of Psychiatric Nursing and Mental Health Services*, Vol. 18, No. 6 (June, 1980), 10–15.

Anvil, C. A., & Silver, B. W. Therapist Self-Disclosure: When is it Appropriate? *Perspectives in Psychiatric Care*, Vol. 22, No. 2 (April–June, 1984), 57–61.

Bayer, M. Saying Goodbye through Graffiti. *American Journal of Nursing*, Vol. 80, No. 2 (February, 1980), 271.

Benjamin, A. *The Helping Interview*, 2nd ed. Boston: Houghton Mifflin, 1969.

Blondis, M. N., & Jackson, B. E. *Nonverbal Communication with Patients: Back to the Human Touch*, 2nd ed. New York: Wiley, 1982.

Bradley, J. C., & Edinberg, M. A. *Communication in the Nursing Context*. New York: Appleton-Century-Crofts, 1982.

Ceccio, J. F., & Ceccio, C. M. *Effective Communication in Nursing: Theory and Practice*. New York: Wiley, 1982.

Collins, M. *Communication in Health Care*. St. Louis: C. V. Mosby, 1977.

Cooper, J. Actions Really Do Speak Louder Than Words. *Nursing '79*, Vol. 9, No. 4 (April, 1979), 113–116, 118.

Cosper, B. How Well Do Patients Understand Hospital Jargon? *American Journal of Nursing*, Vol. 77, No. 12 (December, 1977), 1932–1934.

Dahl, B. W. Formality Versus Familiarity: Communicating with Names. *Ohio Nurses Review*, Vol. 53, No. 4 (April, 1978), 5–6.

Edwards, B. J., & Brilhart, J. K. *Communication in Nursing Practice*. St. Louis: C. V. Mosby, 1981.

Egolf, D. B., & Chester, S. L. Speechless Messages. *Nursing Digest*, Vol. 4, No. 2 (March/April, 1976), 26–29.

Fast, J. *Body Language*. New York: M. Evans and Co., 1970.

Hames, C. C., & Joseph, D. H. *Basic Concepts of Helping: A Wholistic Approach*. New York: Appleton-Century-Crofts, 1980.

Harper, R. G., Wiens, A. N., & Matarazzo, J. D. *Nonverbal Communication: The State of the Art*. New York: Wiley, 1978.

Hays, J. S., & Larson, K. *Interacting with Patients*. New York: Macmillan, 1963.

Hein, E. C. *Communication in Nursing Practice*, 2nd ed. Boston: Little, Brown, 1980.

Heineken, J. Treating the Disconfirmed Psychiatric Client. *Journal of Psychosocial Nursing and Mental Health Services*, Vol. 21, No. 1 (January, 1983), 21–25.

Jungman, L. B. When Your Feelings Get in the Way. *American Journal of Nursing*. Vol. 79. No. 6 (June, 1979), 1074–1075.

Kasch, C. R. Interpersonal Competence and Communication in the Delivery of

Nursing Care. *Advances in Nursing Science*, Vol. 6, No. 2 (January, 1984), 71–88.

Kerr, N. J. Discussion of Common Errors in Communication Made by Students in Psychiatric Nursing. *Perspectives in Psychiatric Care*, Vol. 16, No. 4 (July/August, 1978), 184–187.

Kesler, A. R. Pitfalls To Avoid in Interviewing Outpatients. *Nursing '77*, Vol. 7, No. 9 (September, 1977), 70–73.

Lancaster, J. Communication. The Anatomy of Messages. *Nursing Management*, Vol. 14, No. 9 (September, 1983), 42–45.

Lore, A. *Effective Therapeutic Communications*. Bowie, Md.: Robert J. Brady Co., 1981.

Mahon, N. E. The Relationship of Self-Disclosure, Interpersonal Dependency, and Life Changes to Loneliness in Young Adults. *Nursing Research*, Vol. 31, No. 6 (November/December, 1982), 343–347.

Marlowe, H. A., & Marcotte, A. Patient Skills: Non-Verbal Decoding. *Journal of Psychosocial Nursing and Mental Health Services*, Vol. 22, No. 4 (April, 1984), 8–11.

McMahon, Dr. J. J. *The Art of Listening To Yourself: Between You and You*. Reston, Va.: Reston, 1983.

Mercer, L. Pseudocommunication with Patients. *Nursing '80*, Vol. 10, No. 2 (February, 1980), 105–108.

Mercer, L., & O'Connor, P. *Fundamental Skills in the Nurse-Patient Relationship: A Programmed Text*. Philadelphia: Saunders, 1974.

Northhouse, P. G., & Northhouse, L. L. *Health Communications: A Handbook for Health Professionals*. Englewood Cliffs, N. J.: Prentice-Hall, 1985.

O'Brien, M. J. *Communications and Relationships in Nursing*. St. Louis: C. V. Mosby, 1974.

Orem, D. E. *Nursing: Concepts of Practice*. New York: McGraw-Hill, 1971.

Peplau, H. *Interpersonal Relations in Nursing*. New York: Putnam Publishers, 1952.

Peplau, H. Talking with Patients. *American Journal of Nursing*, Vol. 60, No. 7 (July, 1960), 964–966.

Pluckhan, M. L. *Human Communication: The Matrix of Nursing*. New York: McGraw-Hill Book Co., 1978.

Purtilo, R. *Health Professional/Patient Interaction*, 3rd ed. Philadelphia: Saunders, 1984.

Ramaekers, Sister M. J. Communication Blocks Revisited. *American Journal of Nursing*, Vol. 79, No. 6 (June, 1979), 1079–1081.

Robinson, A. M. Graffiti: Way-Out Outlet for Patients. *R.N.*, Vol. 37, No. 1 (January, 1974), 38–39.

Sayre, J. Common Errors in Communication Made by Students in Psychiatric Nursing. *Perspectives in Psychiatric Care*, Vol. 16, No. 4 (July/August, 1978), 175–183.

Scheflen, A. E. *How Behavior Means*. New York: Jason Aronson, 1974.

Smith, E. Are You Really Communicating. *American Journal of Nursing*, Vol. 77, No. 12 (December, 1977), 1966–1968.

Smith, V. W. I Can't Believe I Said That. *Nursing Outlook*, Vol. 18, No. 5 (May 1970), 51.

Smith, V. M., & Bass, T. A. *Communication for Health Professionals*. New York: Lippincott, 1979.

Strayhorn, J. M., Jr. *Talking It Out: A Guide to Effective Communication and Problem-Solving*. Champaign, Ill.: Research Press, 1977.

Talento, B., & McKeever, L. C. Improving Interviewing Techniques. *Nursing Outlook*, Vol. 31, No. 4 (July/August, 1983), 234–235.

Tobiason, S. J. B. Touching Is for Everyone. *American Journal of Nursing*, Vol. 81, No. 4 (April, 1981), 721–730.

Travelbee, J. *Interpersonal Aspects of Nursing*. Philadelphia: F. A. Davis Co., 1966.

VanDersal, W. How To Be a Good Communicator—And a Better Nurse. *Nursing '74*, Vol. 12, No. 4 (December, 1974), 57–64.

Veninga, R. Communications: A Patient's Eye View. *American Journal of Nursing*, Vol. 73, No. 2 (February, 1973), 320–322.

Veninga, R. Defensive Behavior: Causes, Effects and Cures. *Nursing Digest*, Vol. 3, No. 3 (May/June, 1975), 58–59.

Welt, S. R. Can Training Do The Job? *Journal of Psychosocial Nursing and Mental Health Services*, Vol. 22, No. 4 (April, 1984), 12–15.

Wildhaber, A. R. The Silent Patients Speak. *R.N.*, Vol. 36, No. 5 (May, 1973), 108.

Wilson, J. S. Deciphering Psychotic Communication. *Perspectives in Psychiatric Care*, Vol. 17, No. 6 (November/December, 1979), 254–256.

15

THE THERAPEUTIC NURSE–PATIENT RELATIONSHIP

LEARNING OBJECTIVES

On completion of this chapter the reader should be able to:

1. Explain rapport as the core concept in the establishment, development and maintenance of a therapeutic nurse–patient relationship.
2. Identify strategies that facilitate the interactive–interventive process.
3. Distinguish among the strategies of building trust, **acknowledging and exploring readiness**, and **setting limits**.
4. Identify specific nursing activity that demonstrates the implementation of these strategies.
5. Describe the operational phases within the interactive–interventive process.
6. Identify the therapeutic tasks to be accomplished within the orienting, working, and terminating phases of the process.
7. State impediments to the nurse–patient relationship.
8. Recognize and implement specific intervention directed toward success in the therapeutic nurse–patient relationship.

THE CORE CONCEPT

The crux of the therapeutic relationship is the systematic building of rapport. The achievement of rapport is the initial step toward an effective working therapeutic relationship. **Rapport** is a multifaceted core concept. It is:

- A mutual sharing of the participants' humanness.
- A willingness to become involved with another person.
- An openness that permits another person "to be" without inflicting penalty "for being."
- A demonstration of a receptivity that intensifies the awareness of the participants' perceptions about self and others.
- Growth toward mutual acceptance and understanding of individuality.
- The end result of one's care and concern for another–in action.

Rapport is not a tangible substance. It is a feeling state experienced between and among people, often identified as a mutual comfortableness. Its existence is implied, and its presence may be validated through observable behaviors. Rapport is that condition of a relationship that leads to an atmosphere of mutual confidence and respect. Although the establishment of rapport requires coparticipation, the nurse must assume responsibility for its initiation with clients. The nurse's attitudes and actions must be congruent and clearly demonstrate to the client her belief in and value of a humanistic and holistic approach to life and living.

THE INTERACTIVE–INTERVENTIVE PROCESS

The interactive–interventive process is similar in structure to the communication process in that it is a planned series of events composed of phases each of which must be worked through and achieved before the next can be undertaken. The phases are **orienting**, **working**, and **terminating**. Many references include another phase termed **selection phase**, which occurs prior to orientation. The rationale for including a selection phase is the belief that some patients can benefit therapeutically from a more intensive nurse–patient interaction than can others, thus requiring that the nurse make a decision with regard to who should and who should not receive therapy from her. We strongly feel, however, that all patients have a right to nursing care. The nurse–patient relationship is a therapeutic process involved in the delivery of nursing care. Therefore, *all patients have a right and all nurses have an obligation to engage* in a therapeutic relationship with every patient. We advocate that nursing judgments not be in terms of selection of patients for a therapeutic relationship but rather be directed toward the selection of specific nurse–patient goals to be accomplished through this therapeutic relationship with each client.

Orienting

Basing her actions on the nursing diagnosis and stated objectives for nursing care, the nurse initiates the orientation period of the interactive–interventive process. The purpose of this phase is to build trust in order to be ready to explore with the patient those concerns that seem to be most important to him. Although the nurse initiates the contact using a permissive approach, she also provides structure by identifying for the patient the purpose of the contact and by clarifying roles and expectations with regard to meeting place and length of time. Two major functions for the nurse during the orienting period are the observation and assessment of the patient and the creation of a therapeutic climate conducive to spontaneous verbalizations. These functions permit the nurse to collect data that will enable her to determine the patient's specific areas of difficulty in behavior and psychological functioning and thereby enable her to plan for effective nursing activity. The therapeutic tasks to be accomplished by the nurse in the orienting phase are as follows:

- Foster a feeling of security through the continued building of trust.
- Assist in the verbal expression of thoughts and feelings.
- Identify areas of inadequate functioning.
- Assess areas of strengths and weaknesses.
- Set priorities for nursing intervention.
- Assess readiness for problem-solving and decision-making.
- Initiate and set boundaries of therapeutic contract.

The outcome of the orientation phase is the establishment of a contract for care that has been negotiated between and among the participants. A **treatment contract** is an open, mutually agreed upon and clearly stated written set of expectations and responsibilities as related to the therapeutic goals. It establishes the parameters of who is responsible to whom for what, under what conditions, for what purpose, when, and why. It clearly delineates the shared objectives and goals. Such a treatment contract provides a basis for mutual understanding of the structure and process involved in the therapeutic alliance. It serves as a referent for goal-directed activity and as a basis for monitoring progress toward goal attainment.

The skeletal form of the contract is established on initial contact. This skeletal contract would address important informational and limit-setting criteria. Included in these criteria would be: meeting dates and times, as well as the expected termination date; location;

length of sessions; purpose of the therapeutic alliance; and clarification of issues surrounding confidentiality. The final contract, at the end of the orienting phase, reflects the specific goals to be pursued during the remainder of the time that the contract is in force.

The therapeutic contract is a tool for direction and control. As such, it acts as a guide for the investment of joint commitment. However, it is neither a static document nor is it engraved in stone. It is subject to evaluation and revision as goals are achieved or the needs of the client change.

Working

The nurse–patient interaction enters the second phase of the therapeutic relationship process when the patient is able to focus on the unpleasant and often painful aspects of his life. At this time, the patient demonstrates an ability to cope with the interpersonal demands of the therapeutic process. Together, the nurse and the patient concentrate on achieving the previously identified therapeutic goals. Nursing activity is directed toward increasing the normalcy of the patient's behavior. In other words, the nurse assists the patient to move toward his optimal level of functioning. The working phase is much more structured than the orienting phase. Now, the nurse assists the patient to focus on ideas, themes, emotional overtones, patterns of behavior, and coping strategies. Although structured, spontaneous interaction is encouraged, the nurse channels therapeutic communication toward the identified goals.

The therapeutic tasks to be accomplished by the nurse in the working phase are as follows:

- Increase the individual's awareness and perception of the reality associated with his particular experiences.
- Assist him in developing a realistic self-concept.
- Promote his self-confidence.
- Assist him in recognizing areas of discomfort and distress.
- Increase his ability to verbally describe his feelings.
- Assist him in his attempts to make comparisons.
- Assist him in drawing conclusions regarding the comparisons.
- Encourage him to select a realistic plan of action.
- Provide opportunities for him to implement the plan of action.
- Encourage him to evaluate the results of his behavior.
- Provide him with an opportunity for independent functioning in order for him to test out new learning and adaptive strategies.

Terminating

The last phase of the interactive–interventive process is the **terminating phase**. Termination provides the client and nurse with an opportunity to systematically review the accomplishments achieved within the working phase. Implicit within the termination phase is a mutual summarizing of the experiences shared by the participants and a crystallization of the meaning derived.

Since the therapeutic alliance is a singularly intimate and invested encounter, and since the patient frequently tends to view the therapist as a powerful force in his life, the nurse must be aware that when she engages in the process of termination, both of them need to work through and finalize this distinctly emotional and traumatic experience. The phenomenon that occurs in the termination process is generally referred to as **separation anxiety**, a type of anxiety experienced when one loses contact with a significant, nuturing other.

Termination is a gradual weaning process because termination involves a separation or loss and engenders within the participants corresponding feelings of discomfort, ambivalence, fear, anxiety, pain, or anger. The client frequently misplaces or misdirects expression of these feelings toward the therapist or the environment. Therefore, successful termination requires that the nurse address and help the client to resolve these feelings.

Termination is initiated by mutual agreement when the client demonstrates:

- Ability to care for his personal physical needs and contribute to the maintenance of his environment.
- Evidence of increased independence and ability to function without the nurse's support.
- Increased ability to be self-governing.
- Increased emotional stability over a period of time.
- Increased self-esteem.
- Ability to cope with frustration, anxiety, conflict, and hostility.

The following situation typifies some of the problems and concerns of the patient when confronted with the reality of termination.

Mrs. Jones, a 43-year-old, Caucasian female, came to a mental health clinic for complaints of general malaise and dissatisfaction with her job and her relationship with her second husband. Two children were born to the first marriage, which ended in divorce 7 years previous to her first clinic appointment. A contract was made for Mrs. Jones to participate in 12 therapy sessions. After successful therapeutic engagement the contract was extended to include three termination sessions, one every 2 weeks. Mrs. Jones missed her second termination session. During the third scheduled appointment she began to complain bitterly about dissatisfaction and fear of others "ripping her off," as she had at the beginning of therapy. She stated that her work was not appreciated, and neither would her teenage daughter's work be appreciated in an approaching sewing contest. The nurse acknowledged Mrs. Jones' concerns and feelings and assisted her in ventilating negative feelings. Mrs. Jones requested a continuation of therapy. The nurse recognized the patient's feelings about termination. Mrs. Jones was obviously experiencing separation anxiety that, in turn, produced feelings of fear, anger, frustation, and a sense of loss. These feelings were discussed with Mrs. Jones, who insisted that she needed more therapy. However, the therapist held to the original contract, and therapy was terminated. Two weeks later Mrs. Jones called the nurse to announce that her daughter had won the sewing contest, her job was going so well that she was given a merit raise, and her marital relationship was "great."

The amount of time needed to accomplish the terminating phase is dependent on the duration of the relationship, the level of independent functioning achieved, and the presence of unresolved problems. Generally, a nurse–patient relationship that has been in existence over a long period of time and has been very intense requires a longer time span before termination can be achieved. Conversely, a brief, less intense relationship requires a shorter period of time. However, there are other factors that may tend to influence the rapidity with which termination takes place. Some of these factors include premature discharge, trial visit or transfer, the nurse's change in assignment, illness of either party, the nurse's vacation, or, in the case of a student, completion of a rotation. Even though these factors may tend to speed up the terminating phase, all the steps in the process itself must be followed in order for termination to be therapeutically effective. Since the primary task of the terminating process is dissolution of the relationship, the nurse must:

- Space contacts with the patient further apart.
- Decrease the amount of interaction time.
- Establish a less intense, more relaxed atmosphere.
- Provide opportunity for the expression of painful feelings related to separation.
- Review what has been accomplished *during* the relationship.
- Focus on material that is future-oriented.
- Decline to respond to or follow-up cues that could lead to new areas of exploration.
- Provide for necessary referrals.

STRATEGIES

To facilitate the interactive–interventive process, the nurse must employ specific strategies. These strategies are designed to promote nurse–patient effectiveness as evidenced by the achievement of the mutually established goals of the relationship. They include building trust, acknowledging and utilizing readiness, and setting limits.

Building Trust

Trust and rapport go hand in hand, but trust is not necessarily a direct result of rapport. One can achieve rapport without ever achieving trust. However, in the therapeutic relationship, as the nurse develops rapport, she lays the foundation for building trust.

To trust is to believe in self and to believe in others. It implies that an individual can rely on himself or on another in all kinds of circumstances. In a relationship, trust is a mutual exchange of faith. It allows for the acceptance of another's judgment as a possible means of attaining personal satisfaction through goal achievement or problem solving. Trust occurs in different degrees and is frequently tested by the participants in interpersonal encounters. Trust is an outgrowth of a feeling of security and is evidenced by respect for life. It is also evidenced by an awareness of life and a "zest for living." It is built on faith, hope, and integrity. Moreover, the basic concepts of love, empathy, sympathy, acceptance, assurance, and helpfulness referred to in Chapter 13 serve as a foundation for the building of trust between the nurse and the client.

The building of trust involves the use of a two-phase strategy. The first phase concerns the demonstration of the nurse's confidence in self. Her confidence is in direct proportion to her personal and professional knowledge and her ability to function as an integrated person. The nurse's self-confidence is demonstrated through the presentation of the "real self" rather than the presentation of an assumed "nursing role." This does not mean that the professional roles of the nurse are not enacted in the process of building trust, but rather that the totality of the professional self functions in a holistic manner, bringing to the interactive process more than a "fragmented" or "summated" self. The roles are a direct expression of the professional self and not a cloak to be taken on or discarded at will.

The second phase is concerned with the nurse's helping the patient develop trust in himself and in others. In implementing this phase of the strategy, the nurse may have to begin at "rock bottom," at the patient's primal need stage. That is, she may have to help him to meet his dependency needs, first the physiological ones and then the psychological, social, and cultural ones. The nurse's reliability and credibility are demonstrated to the patient through nursing intervention. The interventions are directed toward alleviating problems arising from the simple, obvious activities of daily living or from the more complex, covert, and unexpressed concerns of the individual. *The primary nursing care goal is to decrease feelings of insecurity and assist in establishing feelings of security.* Once the individual feels secure in the nurse–patient relationship, he can trust. The nurse fosters the growth of this initial trusting through specific planned actions. Three major nursing interventions that promote trust are: to show respect, to be honest, and to provide consistency. Specific nursing activities that would exemplify these interventions are included in Table 15–1.

Acknowledging and Utilizing Readiness

Readiness is another aspect of the process in the development of a relationship. Readiness is an attitudinal and emotional state in which the individual is able to respond to the nurse. It is based on the urgency to satisfy instinctual emotional needs and is a demonstration of the patient's motivation to participate in the therapeutic process. There are several factors involved in the acknowledgment of the readiness. These include: a statement of intention, an identification of the ultimate goal, and a recognition of and appreciation for active participation in working toward the intended goal. The level of readiness depends upon the individual's degree of perception as well as his intellectual capacity. Exploiting the aspect of readiness is significant because it is the foundation for the development of insight. Progression of the relationship is in direct proportion to the nurse's ability to take advantage of readiness and her ability to maximize opportunities to encourage and strengthen the relationship.

In determining readiness, the nurse must also consider the patient's level of anxiety, since gross or uncontrolled anxiety inhibits the therapeutic alliance and problem solving. Nursing activity should be directed toward reducing anxiety to a manageable level. Some initial specific nursing interventions that increase anxiety are as follows:

1. Maintaining continuous contact with the patient over an extended period of time.
2. Listening attentively to the patient.

TABLE 15–1. NURSING INTERVENTIONS DESIGNED TO PROMOTE TRUST

Show Respect	Be Honest	Provide Consistency
Use the patient's name and title.	Keep promises.	Adhere to planned schedule.
Listen and give consideration to the patient's request.	Be "open and aboveboard" in words and actions.	Follow through on planned actions.
Allow for sufficient time to respond to questions.	Give reasons and explanations, especially when request cannot be met.	Adhere to set limitations.
Give clear instructions regarding procedures, policies, and activities.	Consult with patients about their preferences.	Seek opportunities to pursue and foster the nurse–patient relationship outside of the regularly scheduled interaction session.
Openly acknowledge personal limitations in knowledge and ability.	Acknowledge individual requests.	Hold self and client accountable for terms of contract.
Exhibit dependability and accountability.	Accede to requests with limits of the situation.	
	Apologize for inconveniences.	
	Preserve confidentiality.	

3. Keeping the nurse's responses to a minimum.
4. Responding clearly, briefly, and specifically.

For a more detailed description of nursing intervention directed toward the control and reduction of anxiety, the reader is referred to Chapter 21.

Resistance to engagement in the interventive–interactive process is encountered frequently by the nurse in many forms. Resistance can be inferred from such behaviors as complacency, digression, failure to keep an appointment, coming late, leaving early, or nonparticipation in the session. A demonstration of resistance means that the client is attempting to avoid pursuit of the identified therapeutic goal and maintain the status quo. In such instances the nurse must create a climate for readiness by increasing the client's level of anxiety. The heightening of anxiety is accomplished through the withdrawal of support. Withdrawal of support increases his level of discomfort and is employed to motivate him to work on his problems. This is particularly true where the patient is highly dependent, procrastinates excessively, or manipulates to avoid confronting problems or stresses.

Specific nurse interventions that increase the patient's anxiety level include the following:

1. Maintaining direct eye contact.
2. Delaying response to the patient's immediate need for gratification.
3. Ignoring superficial content by not responding.
4. Remaining silent when the patient is pressing for a personal opinion or decision from the nurse.
5. Introducing or focusing on topics that have been identified as emotionally charged.
6. Confronting the patient with an observation about his behavior.

Once the nurse's assessment identifies the client's readiness, there are certain interventive strategies that can be employed. These strategies are designed to capitalize on this readiness by helping the client to progress toward therapeutic involvement in the interactive–interventive process. We identify three strategies that can be used to facilitate readiness. These nurse strategies are: be accessible, be concerned, and provide comfort. Table 15–2 lists specific nursing activities to achieve these three nurse behaviors.

Setting Limits

Setting limits is another strategy a nurse can use to permit exploration, growth, and movement toward the development of the therapeutic nurse–patient relationship. **Setting limits** is the identification of

TABLE 15–2. NURSING INTERVENTIONS TO FACILITATE READINESS

Be Accessible	Be Concerned	Provide Comfort
Approach at frequent intervals. Designate specific times the nurse is available. Allow for flexibility in schedule. Exhibit openness and receptivity. Give undivided attention. Offer support, encouragement, and reassurance.	Display a willingness to become involved. Display warmth and spontaneity. Encourage verbalizations. Encourage an expression of positive and negative feelings. Recognize verbal and nonverbal leads, clues, or signals. Focus on expressed concerns.	State the purpose of the relationship. Provide confidentiality. Provide a private area where exploration of concerns can be pursued. State how shared material is to be used by self and other members of the health team. Clarify purpose for interactions. Give realistic and sincere responses. Allow patient to proceed at own rate. Follow through on stated goals.

boundaries both for the patient and for the nurse. It is the means by which the security of both patient and nurse are safeguarded. Setting limits is a structure that demonstrates its positive value through the reduction of anxiety. Setting limits provides a frame of reference that gives direction to choices and orientation for therapy. To be effective, setting limits must be a continuous process, consistently employed on both the verbal and the behavioral levels. Specific limits are negotiated between the nurse and the client and arise from the presenting needs of the patient. Although limits serve as guidelines for control, they may and should be periodically reevaluated.

The nurse must assume responsibility for clearly identifying limits in terms of setting time, clarifying goals and roles, and providing a place for interaction. Limits should be kept to a minimum and be consistent with the needs of the participants within the relationship. Specific nursing interventions designed to implement the setting of limits are presented in Table 15–3.

STUMBLING BLOCKS AND STEPPING STONES

The student and beginning practitioner often encounter difficulties in implementing a therapeutic nurse–patient relationship. Many times the kinds of difficulties encountered arise out of the nurse's inexperience and anxiety. Major stumbling blocks frequently experienced occur in the areas of scheduling of appointments, methodology of recording, contract violations, hesitancy about dealing with feelings,

TABLE 15–3. NURSING INTERVENTIONS TO INITIATE LIMIT SETTING

Set Time	Clarify Goals and Roles	Provide Place
Make specific appointment times.	Identify purposes and goals.	Select an appropriate place.
Be consistent in scheduling appointments.	Explore role of the participants.	Be consistent with therapy location and atmosphere.
Start and end on time.	Establish expectations.	Prevent interruptions.
Do not extend the session beyond the scheduled time.	Remain focused on relevant data.	Provide for privacy.
	Adhere to the specifics of the therapy contract.	

overreliance on stereotyped responses, and inability to maintain the relationship on a therapeutic level. These trouble spots can be avoided or at least diminished in intensity and frequency. There are ways—stepping stones—by which the inexperienced practitioner can help herself to move more easily and comfortably into the therapeutic nurse–patient relationship. In Table 15–4 stumbling blocks are expressed as "What if . . .?" Questions are answered by "Try this . . ." stepping stones.

TABLE 15–4. COMMON STUMBLING BLOCKS AND STEPPING STONES IN INITIATING AND MAINTAINING A THERAPEUTIC RELATIONSHIP

Stumbling Blocks: What if . . .	Stepping Stones: Try this . . .
1. The patient doesn't come to the session?	Locate the patient. Reschedule the appointment. Remind the patient ahead of time. Give the patient an appointment card. Review the contract with the patient.
2. The patient is habitually late?	Determine patient's orientation to time. Remind the patient of the approaching hour. Be on time and wait for the patient. Explore with the patient his reasons for lateness. Close the session on time.
3. The nurse is late or has to change the schedule time?	Notify the patient directly or through another person or by a written message. Apologize. Reschedule when appropriate.
4. The patient asks to cut the session short or change the time of the meeting?	Explore the expressed need. Reorient the patient to the time schedule as per initial contract. Reschedule when appropriate.

(continued)

TABLE 15–4. CONTINUED

Stumbling Blocks: What if . . .	Stepping Stones: Try this . . .
5. The patient abruptly leaves the session?	Ask, "Where are you going?" As the patient is leaving, say, "I will wait until . . ." (the end of the session). Remain in the room. Wait expectantly for the patient's return—do not become involved in any other activity.
6. The patient objects to the nurse's making notations?	Listen to the objections. Explain the purpose and use of note taking. Reinforce the positive concept of confidentiality. Matter-of-factly continue to record. Discontinue recording; write a summary immediately after the session.
7. The patient wants to read the notes?	Let him—he has the right.
8. The patient asks, "Who sees the notes?"	State clearly who will have access to the notes. Abide by the contract made with the patient.
9. Other members of the staff ask to see the detailed notes?	Keep the staff informed as to the patient's progress. Refuse diplomatically to show detailed notes. Inform the staff of contract confidentiality.
10. The patient asks the nurse to give the notes to his doctor or other staff?	Explore with the patient the reasons for his request. Encourage the patient to speak for himself. Offer to accompany the patient and to support his interpersonal approaches with others.
11. The patient calls the nurse by her first name?	Recall to yourself the differences between a social and a therapeutic relationship. Do not respond. Repeat your proper name and title. Explore reasons with patient. Reinforce the accepted policy used within the treatment setting.
12. The nurse wants to call the patient by his first name?	Review the differences between a social and a therapeutic relationship. Review the policy of the unit. Explore the request in light of the patient's ego identity.
13. The patient asks personal questions?	Briefly answer factual and self-evident questions. Explore with the patient his need to ask. Redirect the focus of communication toward patient.
14. The sessions are interrupted by patients or staff?	Clearly state to interrupting individual that a therapy session is in progress. Confront staff with their behavior.

TABLE 15–4. CONTINUED

Stumbling Blocks: What if . . .	Stepping Stones: Try this . . .
	Place a "Do Not Disturb" or "Therapy in Session" sign on the door.
15. The patient doesn't want to talk?	Sit quietly. Look at patient with an interested, expectant expression. Observe nonverbal behavior. Use indirect, open-ended statements at intervals, such as, "You seem to be thinking . . ." Remind the patient of the remaining time: "You still have 15 minutes."
16. The patient says, "I have nothing to say" or "I don't know"?	Rephrase the question. Learn to sit quietly, to wait, and be patient. Confront the patient in light of treatment goals as identified in the contract. Recognize and deal with your own feelings evoked by the patient's response. Remain optimistic. Continue to explore areas of interest and concern. Be persistent—don't give up.
17. The nurse uses the same responses over and over again?	Vary responses. Deal with resultant rejection. Deal with patient's anger. Deal with patient's avoidance of you. Review and analyze your notes: look for stereotyped nurse responses. look for missed cues. rephrase nurse responses. try out alternatives in next session. Be sensitive to mistakes and learn from them. Consult with instructor, head nurse, or member of the interdisciplinary team.
18. The patient tells the nurse to go away or says, "Don't bother me!"	Remain calm. Assess the patient's level of hostility. Make judgments based on the assessment and act accordingly: leave patient with a promise to return at a later time. remain and explore patient's feelings.
19. The nurse's questions upset the patient or make him more "nervous"?	Good—something's happening. Maintain focus on the topic—don't avoid it: identify the topic. help patient to recognize the need to explore the topic

(continued)

TABLE 15–4. CONTINUED

Stumbling Blocks: What if . . .	Stepping Stones: Try this . . .
	Review and analyze data to prevent: prying. pushing beyond the patient's level of readiness.
20. The nurse wishes to use self-disclosure as a therapeutic strategy?	Analyze need for engaging in self-disclosure, yours and client's. Examine advantages and disadvantages to the client. Temper self-disclosure with judgment.

SUMMARY

The nurse–patient relationship is a three-phased interactive–interventive process that includes orientation, working, and termination. The process is goal-directed and involves the patient in a collaborative effort with the nurse to identify specific concerns, explore potential solutions, and reach resolution. Rapport is essential for its initiation, while trust, readiness, and limit setting facilitate its development.

SUGGESTED READINGS

Assay, J. L., & Whetsell, I. Memorandum. *Journal of Psychiatric Nursing and Mental Health Services*, Vol. 18, No. 7 (July, 1980), 35–36.

Bammer, L. M. *The Helping Relationship: Process and Skills*, 2nd ed. Englewood Cliffs, N. J.: Prentice-Hall, 1979.

Bernstein, L., & Dana, R. H. *Interviewing and the Health Professions*. New York: Appleton-Century Crofts, 1970.

Brockoff, D. Y. What is NLP? *American Journal of Nursing*, Vol. 83, No. 7 (July, 1983), 1012–1014.

Bromley, G. E. Confrontation in Individual Psychotherapy. *Journal of Psychiatric Nursing and Mental Health Services*, Vol. 19, No. 5 (May, 1981), 15–18.

Burns, N. Realistic Goals Don't Mean Failure. *Nursing '79*, Vol. 9, No. 5 (May, 1979), 55–59.

Campaniello, J. A. The Process of Termination. *Journal of Psychiatric Nursing and Mental Health Services*, Vol. 18, No. 2 (February, 1980), 29–32.

Cole, D. Mr. Jarrett Was Ready To Give Up . . . But I Wasn't. *Nursing '78*, Vol. 8, No. 3 (March, 1978), 40–41.

Davanloo, H. (Ed.). *Short-Term Dynamic Psychotherapy*. Vol. 1. New York: Jason Aronson, 1980.

Feldman, R., Cousins, A., & Grinaldi, D. The Developmental Phases of the Nurse/Resident Relationship on an In-patient Psychiatric Unit. *Perspectives in Psychiatric Care*, Vol. 19, No. 1 (January, 1981), 31–32, 37–39.

Gahon, K. A. Problem Solving as a Therapeutic Process. *Journal of Psychiatric*

Nursing and Mental Health Services, Vol. 14, No. 11 (November, 1976), 37–39.
Garant, C. Stalls in the Therapeutic Process. *American Journal of Nursing*, Vol. 80, No. 12 (December, 1980), 2166–2169.
Goldberg C. Therapeutic Tasks: Strategies for Change. *Perspectives in Psychiatric Care*, Vol. 18, No. 4 (July/August, 1980), 156–162.
Gordy, H. E. Gift Giving: Its Effects on the Nurse-Patient Relationship. *American Journal of Nursing*, Vol. 78, No. 6 (June, 1978), 1026–1028.
Homes, C. C., & Joseph, D. H. *Basic Concepts of Helping: A Wholistic Approach*. New York: Appleton-Century-Crofts, 1980.
Hanlon, R. Contracting for Care. *American Journal of Nursing*, Vol. 84, No. 3 (March, 1984), 335.
Hardin, S. B., & Durham, J. D. First Rate. *Journal Psychosocial Nursing and Mental Health Services*, Vol. 23, No. 5 (May, 1985), 9–15.
Johnson, M. N. Self-Disclosure: A Variable in the Nurse-Client Relationship. *Journal of Psychiatric Nursing and Mental Health Services*, Vol. 18, No. 1 (January, 1980), 17–20.
Kennedy, C. W., & Garvin, B. M. The Effect of Status and Gender on Interpersonal Relationships in Nursing. *Nursing Forum*, Vol. 20, No. 3 (1981), 274–287.
Kesler, A. R. Pitfalls To Avoid in Interviewing Outpatients. *Nursing '77*, Vol. 7, No. 9 (September, 1977), 70–73.
Knowles, R. D. Building Rapport Through Neuro-Linguistic Programming. *American Journal of Nursing*, Vol. 83, No. 7 (July, 1983), 1011–1014.
Kopacz, M. S., & O'Connor, Sister C. M. Through A Glass Darkly. *American Journal of Nursing*, Vol. 75, No. 12 (December, 1975), 2159–2160.
Kottler, J. A. Promoting Self-Understanding in Counseling: A Compromise between the Insight and Action-Oriented Approaches. *Journal of Psychiatric Nursing and Mental Health Services*, Vol. 17, No. 12 (December, 1979), 18–23.
Langs, R. *Resistances and Interventions*. New York: Jason Aronson, 1981.
Loomis, M. E. Levels of Contracting. *Journal of Psychosocial Nursing and Mental Health Services*, Vol. 23, No. 3 (March, 1985), 9–14.
Lynn, L. M. Lisa and the 2:00 Miracle. *Nursing '80*, Vol. 10, No. 5 (May, 1980), 68–70.
McCann, J. Termination of the Psychotherapeutic Relationship. *Journal of Psychiatric Nursing*, Vol. 17, No. 10 (October, 1979), 37–39.
McEnany, G. W., & Tescber, B. E. Contracting For Care. *Journal of Psychosocial Nursing and Mental Health Services*, Vol. 23, No. 4 (April, 1985), 11–18.
Mooney, J. Attachment/Separation in the Nurse-Patient Relationship. *Nursing Forum*, Vol. 15, No. 3 (1976), 2959–2964.
Murphy, K. E. Use of Territoriality in Psychotherapy. *Journal of Psychiatric Nursing and Mental Health Services*, Vol. 19, No. 3 (March, 1981), 13–15.
O'Brien, M. J. *Communications and Relationships*. St. Louis: C. V. Mosby, 1974.
O'Brien, P., Caldwell, C., & Transeau, G. Destroyers: Written Treatment Contracts Can Help Cure Self-Destructive Behaviors of the Borderline Patient. *Journal of Psychosocial Nursing and Mental Health Services*, Vol. 23, No. 4 (April, 1985), 19–23.
Poole, K. Breaking the Ice. *Nursing '81*, Vol. 11, No. 2 (February, 1981), 159–161.
Provost, J. Intervention in a Schizoaffective Depressive Behavior Pattern: A Behavioral Approach. *Perspectives in Psychiatric Care*, Vol. 12, No. 2 (April/June, 1974), 86–89.

Purtilo, R. *Health Professional/Patient Interaction*. Philadelphia: Saunders, 1984.

Searight, R. Being Honest with Gary Was the Least—and the Most—We Could Do. *Nursing '80*, Vol. 10, No. 2 (February, 1980), 54–56.

Steckel, S. B. *Patient Contracting*. Norwalk, Conn.: Appleton-Century-Crofts, 1982.

Storey, B. W. The Catatonic Schizophrenic and Relationship Therapy. *Journal of Psychiatric Nursing and Mental Health Services*, Vol. 16, No. 3 (March, 1978), 46–50.

Travelbee, J. *Interpersonal Aspects of Nursing*. Philadelphia: F. A. Davis Co., 1966.

Travelbee, J. *Intervention in Psychiatric Nursing*. Philadelphia: F. A. Davis Co., 1970.

Trekas, J. It Takes 2 To Achieve Compliance. *Nursing '84*, Vol. 14, No. 9 (September, 1984), 58–59.

Welch, M. J. Using Metaphor in Psychotherapy. *Journal of Psychosocial Nursing and Mental Health Services*, Vol. 22, No. 11 (November, 1984), 13–18.

16

GROUPS

Their Purpose and Structure

LEARNING OBJECTIVES

On completion of this chapter the reader should be able to:

1. Define the term **group**.
2. State the purpose groups serve.
3. Discuss the importance of groups in life.
4. List the benefits derived from a group experience.
5. Define **group structure**.
6. Compare and contrast distinguishing features of group structure.

PURPOSE AND IMPORTANCE

The need for group association is a universal phenomenon. In all facets of personal development people are constantly seeking ways to cooperate with one another. Individuals realize that cooperative relationships are essential to the progress of human society and indeed to existence itself. Therefore, there is much seeking of and searching for new and appropriate forms of facilitating positive interaction. Groups serve such a purpose.

A **group** is a unit of society composed of two or more people in interaction. It is a dynamic entity that exists with a clearly defined and understood purpose and objective. Groups are formed to meet the social, emotional, and physical needs of individuals. The individual achieves healthy development through appropriate group life experiences throughout his entire life. Just as an individual learns about individual interpersonal relationships from his "significant other," so he learns his interpersonal group relationships from the initial primary group, his family. His family's interaction with him and with others, as a unit of society, serves as a model on which he bases other group interactions. In fact, the individual's successful development of his own satisfying life-style depends on his ability to relate well with others. Groups have power to support individual effort and accomplishment; reject behavior that does not conform to group values, norms, or expectations; foster creativity; and deal with critical issues that impede individual or group progress. Groups provide the mechanism for the resolution of interpersonal conflicts in all levels of human interaction.

When an individual moves into a group experience, he expands all aspects of his own personality. His uniqueness as an individual is enhanced by the collective presence of all other members of the group. As an individual operates within a group situation, he identifies with others, and this bond provides a reciprocal influence between the self and the group. The group is never merely a sum of its individual members or parts, but takes on an added dimension that is a composite of the diversities of the group members. But a group is more than a composite of various personalities; the reciprocal influence each member exerts on the others causes individuals to assimilate the characteristics of the group.

In Chapter 9, interpersonal relationships were identified in terms of group types: primary, secondary, and tertiary. A **group** is a joint enterprise in which mutual need gratification and interdependency exist between and among group members. Simultaneously, an individual usually belongs to at least one primary group and to one or more secondary and tertiary groups. These secondary and tertiary interpersonal group relationships are commonly referred to as **reference-group relationships**.

A child begins his group experience with birth, when he joins his parents and siblings. Together they form a primary group. During infancy and the preschool period, the family, as the initial primary group, sets the stage for the child's future group experiences. When the child begins school, his classmates and teachers make up another potential primary interpersonal group. With the broadening of the child's living experiences through introduction of new or expanded group participation, there is a proportionate increase in the range and selectivity of his relationships. There is also a visible increase in his emotional and intellectual growth. Thus, group experiences have a twofold effect in the early stages of life. First, as the child develops relationships within the group, he develops distinction as a person; and second, as the child participates in group interaction, he is in turn stimulated to explore his environment and grow further.

With preadolescence and adolescence, group participation becomes closely aligned with the physical process of maturation and the psychosocial quest for independence. At this stage of development, the allegiances, mores, attitudes, and behavioral patterns of the peer group tend to surpass and supplant family and school as the primary learning group. Peer-group involvement is an important aspect in the growth and developmental scheme of an individual's personality in that it facilitates social growth and value system integration, which in turn leads to participation in the broader spectrum of adult society.

Primary and reference groups are ever present and changing throughout the individual's life. Group experiences are essential to the psychosociocultural development of the individual. Participation in groups facilitates the maturation of relationships between the individual and society. These relationships are analogous to mechanisms the individual can use to assist in the attainment of self-actualization.

If, as stated above, group experiences are essential, how do they contribute to the development of a healthy, functioning member of society? Group experiences are beneficial in that they provide the individual with the following:

- A basis for identification with peers.
- A means by which the interpersonal needs for acceptance, recognition, and control can be met.
- The freedom "to be," that is, the ability to express self without fear of censure or retaliation, along with the freedom to be different in the presence of others.
- The freedom to choose and form a deeper and more intimate relationship with individuals within the group.

In addition, group experiences permit and provide the individual with opportunities to do the following:

- Exercise independence while remaining secure in the knowledge that dependency needs will also be met.
- Develop interpersonal skills as a participating member of society.
- Evaluate skills with respect to his ability to learn and to achieve.
- Formulate attitudes and values.
- Set goals for self.
- Experiment.

STRUCTURE

Structure refers to the organization of the group and the processes used to maintain the group and facilitate the group's achievement of its identified goal. The structure of a group describes the pattern of the interdependent relationship of each member, one to the other. The patterning of the group provides the stability for the functioning of the group. It permits the group to regulate action, identify constraints, and impose order by defining the parameters of its operation. These parameters include its composition, the status accorded to individual members, the roles assumed, the specific functions attached to identified roles, the norms and values held, the degree of flexibility present, the communication patterns used, and the degree of cohesiveness achieved.

Composition

Composition refers to membership. The composition of any group depends on the purpose of the group. Groups are composed of people who have vested interests, common concerns, and mutual needs. Groups form, merge, disintegrate, and reorganize according to their gratification of needs and realization of goals. Ideally, group composition reflects a membership sufficiently similar enough to provide the participants with mutual support, yet different enough to expose the participants to stimulation and motivation for continued active membership.

Although group composition may vary according to size, types of membership, and purpose, there are certain features of group membership and behavior that remain constant and contribute to the success of groups. These features include the individual's status within the group; the role chosen by the individual or designated by the group; the norms and values exhibited by the group; and the kind of flexibility, communication patterns, and cohesiveness maintained.

Status

Status is the prestige that an individual member holds within a group in relationship to other members. Status designates prominence within the group in relation to all other members and is bestowed on the individual by consensus of the group. It designates a person's position, influences his degree of effectiveness in carrying out his role, and increases the power he is able to exert. Status is arbitrary and subject to change. Fluctuation in status is often governed by the addition or subtraction of group members, modification of group goals, or changes in members' roles.

Role and Role Function

Role is the "part" an individual plays in group life. A role may be assigned or assumed. An **assigned** role is one which is delegated by the group to satisfy a group need, whereas the **assumed** role is taken on by the individual member to satisfy his needs. Role depends on the expectations the individual brings to the group with respect to self and the expectations for the relationship the self has with others. To accomplish a specific group task, roles may sometimes be exchanged among members. **Role functions** are those operations or activities which exemplify a given role.

Specific roles that may be found in any given group situation would most likely include the following:

Leader. The leader is a coordinator. Leadership encompasses three facets—managerial ability, technical adroitness, and expertise in human relations. The leader is that individual group member who demonstrates ability in organizing and making use of the capabilities of group members to achieve the specific tasks or goals of the group. A successful leader is able to accept and follow through on the responsibility for group performance. The leader must also demonstrate an ability to hold group members accountable for their specific tasks within the group. Other traits displayed by a successful group leader include self-directiveness, initiative, dependability, conscientiousness, adaptability, and sensitivity to group climate. Group leadership requires the ability to perform any and all functions that enable the group to achieve its goal, promote group viability, maintain and encourage people-to-people interaction, and increase interdependence among group members. Leadership may be acquired in one of two ways, either by formal appointment or through the natural selection of an emerging group.

Some specific role functions that are required of a leader are listed as follows:

- Initiating action.
- Clarifying issues.
- Focusing on goals.
- Supplying data necessary to facilitate group function.
- Mediating issues.
- Assisting in defining member roles and functions.
- Evaluating group member performance with respect to identified goals.
- Providing for encouragement and recognition of group members.
- Allowing and encouraging active participation by all members, especially those that hold minority viewpoints.
- Promoting effective patterns of communication.
- Facilitating the decision-making and problem-solving processes.
- Providing for a mechanism for accurate record keeping.
- Encouraging mutual trust, respect, and warmth.

Follower. The follower is a group member who fulfills a specific role and performs role functions in relationship to the type of group, its purpose, and its goals. Each group member contributes uniquely to the group. There are many different subroles within a given group that members can assume; however, not all of these roles are present in every group. Some of the more common roles that occur consistently in groups are described in the following list:

Diplomat—the member who makes himself responsible for maintaining group harmony. The diplomat displays a high degree of sensitivity regarding the individual needs of group members. He employs tact in the resolution of potential discord and attempts to reconcile disagreements.

Humorist—the member who makes himself responsible for releasing group tension. The humorist effectively applies exaggeration and satire to provide comic relief, which results in the dissipation of mounting anxiety, frustration, or hostility.

Liaison—the member who makes himself responsible for communicating the needs, concerns, and issues of the group to outside authorities. He is a spokesman for the group who relays clear and concise messages to and from the group.

Specialist—the member who makes himself responsible for meeting the particular requirements of the group. The specialist acts as a resource person who provides information amd access to such things as activities, commodities, donations, or funds.

Listener—the group member who makes himself responsible for "lending an ear" and acting as confidant to troubled group members. The listener demonstrates friendliness, warmth, sympathy or empathy. The listener is highly responsive to the individual needs of group members.

Talker—the group member who feels responsible for maintaining communication in the group. He makes use of every opportunity to expound on all issues and has a tendency to be repetitive. This behavior can generate agitation and negative feelings toward the talker. If left unchecked, it can produce disintegration or goal failure within the group. In other instances the talker, through his incessancy, allows other group members to daydream or lose sight of group goals.

Silent participant—the group member who assumes an inconspicuous place within the group. He functions primarily as an observer and is sensitive to the nuances present in the group. The silent participant hesitates to draw attention to himself; however, when called upon, he contributes to the total functioning of the group.

Norms and Values

Group norms are rules governing the actions of group members. They are established within the group, for the group, and are enforced by group consensus. Group norms spell out the criteria for the procedural activity of the group, such as how decisions are to be made and implemented and which member will fulfill what role. A **group value** is the shared belief of the group. Values held by the group are consciously operational and have both a moral and motivating aspect. The moral aspect enables the group to collectively assess the appropriateness or inappropriateness of either individual action within the group or the joint action of the whole group. This moral aspect offers guidelines and encouragement for specific behaviors or postures to be carried out or assumed by the group in its operations. Group values, although collectively operational for the group, may vary for a particular individual within the group. Differences in values among individual group members are generally acceptable to the group; however, differences in norms among individual members of the group are not acceptable to the group.

Flexibility

Group flexibility is the ability the group possesses to adapt and grow as a collective body. The degree of flexibility within any given group is based on the degree of understanding that each individual member has for all other members of the group. Flexibility implies that when a group encounters new experiences, new problems, or sees new dimensions to its stated goals or purpose, it can mobilize the specialized capabilities of its individual members in accomplishing the group goal. In a flexible group, each member feels free to assume the initiative or to follow.

Communication Patterns

Group communication patterns are those channels through which individual members of the group receive information pertinent to the collective functioning of the group. The communication pattern within a group is the mechanism for interpersonal interaction, that is, the way *who* says *what* to *whom* and *when*. To be effective, the communication pattern must allow for openness and honesty. An effective communication pattern provides the individual member with a feeling of security—security in the knowledge that when he sets forth his ideas and feelings and exposes his inner self to collective group inspection, he will not experience rejection, retaliation, or invalidation. Communication patterns reveal the sanctions imposed by the group on the degree of freedom individuals have to engage in self-disclosure.

Cohesiveness

Group cohesiveness is the demonstration of attraction that members have for each other in terms of kinship. It is the group working together as a collective unit and an expression of the desire to remain together as a unified whole. Group cohesion contributes to the viability and efficacy of the group. It increases the interpersonal rewards for individual members of the group by supplying gratification through recognition, approval, and support. Group cohesion promotes group mobility toward fulfilling group goals. Cohesiveness is essential to maintaining cooperativeness and continuity of group life as well as promoting its quality.

SUMMARY

A group is a collection of interdependent people who are bound together by a shared interest, common goal, or mutual need. Participation in groups facilitates maturation and assists in the movement toward self-actualization.

The manner in which a group is organized and the mechanisms used to maintain the group as it moves toward the attainment of its goal is referred to as its **structure**. The structure of a group is defined by several distinct characteristics, which include composition, status of members, roles, norms, and values, degree of flexibility, communication patterns, and cohesiveness. The purpose of the group together with its structure influence and give direction to the process and outcome of group activity.

SUGGESTED READINGS

Blumberg, A., & Galembiewski, R. T. *Learning and Change in Groups*. Clinton, Mass.: Colonial Press, 1976.

Cartwright, D., & Zander, A. *Group Dynamics*. New York: Harper & Row, 1968.

Calhoun, G., & Perrin, M. Management, Motivation and Conflict. *Topics in Clinical Nursing*, Vol. 1, No. 3 (October, 1979), 71–80.

Durald, M. M., & Hanks, D. The Evaluation of Co-Leading a Gestalt Group. *Journal of Psychiatric Nursing and Mental Health Services*, Vol. 18, No. 12 (December, 1980), 19–23.

Glasser, P., Sarri, R., & Vinter, R. *Individual Change through Small Groups*. New York: Free Press, 1974.

Hankins-McNary, L. The Use of Humor in Group Therapy. *Perspectives in Psychiatric Care*, Vol. 17, No. 5 (September/October, 1979), 228–231.

Hare, P., Borgatte, E. F., & Balec, R. F. *Small Groups—Studies in Social Interaction*. New York: Knopf, 1962.

Homans, G. C. *The Human Group*. New York: Harcourt, Brace & Co., 1950.

Jacobs, A., & Spradlin, W. *The Group as Agent of Change*. Morgantown, W. Va.: Behavioral Publications, 1974.

Johnson, D., & Johnson, F. P. *Joining Together Group Theory and Group Skills*. Englewood Cliffs, N. J.: Prentice-Hall, Inc., 1975.

Kelly, P., Ashby, P., & Coates, G. Establishing a Group. *American Journal of Nursing*, Vol. 79, No. 5 (May, 1979), 914–915.

Larson, M. L., & Williams, R. A. How To Become a Better Group Leader: Learn To Recognize the Strange Things That Happen to Some People in Groups. *Nursing 78*, Vol. 8, No. 8 (August, 1978), 65–72.

Levenstein, A. So You Want to Be a Leader? *Nursing Management*, Vol. 16, No. 3 (March, 1985), 74–75.

Merritt, R. E., Jr., & Walley, D. D. *The Group Leader's Handbook: Resources, Techniques and Survival Skills*. Champaign, Ill.: Research Press, 1977.

Mills, T. M. *The Sociology of Small Groups*. Englewood Cliffs, N. J.: Prentice-Hall, Inc., 1967.

Otto, H. A. *Group Methods to Actualize Human Potential*. Beverly Hills, Calif.: Holistic Press, 1973.

Racy, J. How a Group Grows. *American Journal of Nursing*, Vol. 69, No. 11 (November, 1969), 2396–2402.

Reichert, R. *Self-Awareness through Group Dynamics*. Dayton, Ohio: George A. Pflaum Publisher, 1970.

Rogers, C. R. *Carl Rogers on Encounter Groups*. New York: Harper & Row, 1970.

Shepherd, C. R. *Small Groups: Some Sociological Perspectives*. Scranton, Pa.: Chandler, 1964.

Slavson, S. R. *Introduction to Group Therapy*. New York: International Universities Press, 1965.

Smith, L. L. Finding Your Leadership Style in Groups. *American Journal of Nursing*, Vol. 80, No. 7 July, 1980), 1301–1303.

Theelen, H. A. *Dynamics of Groups at Work*. Chicago: University of Chicago Press, 1954.

Whitman, H. H., Gustafson, J. P., & Coleman, F. W. Leaders and Members. *American Journal of Nursing*, Vol. 79, No. 5 (May, 1979), 910–913.

Yalom, I. D. *The Theory and Practice of Group Psychotherapy*. New York: Basic Books, 1975.

17

GROUP PROCESS

LEARNING OBJECTIVES

On completion of this chapter the reader should be able to:

1. Define and distinguish between the terms **content** and **process**.
2. Compare and contrast the characteristics of effective group growth and development.
3. Distinguish between **task** and **maintenance** functions in groups.

DEFINITION AND DESCRIPTION

There are two main dimensions of group work—content and process. **Content** refers to the specific task or topic on which the group is focused. Most group members, including the leader, pay conscious and continuing attention to the content aspect of group work. The second dimension, **process**, concerns what is happening to and among the people within the group during the period of time the group is in operation. Generally, the membership pays very little attention to process even though the process greatly influences, for better or worse, the impact of the group. By definition, **group process** is the interaction between and among group members. Group process can be either healthy or unhealthy. From a healthy standpoint, group process facilitates the effective and satisfying functioning of the members and enhances their well-being. Unhealthy group process, on the other hand, tends to contribute to or reinforce the existing pathology of the members.

Specifically, **process** refers to how, what, when, where, why, and under what circumstances or conditions the group operates. Group process can be observed. It is identified through the participative and communicative patterns used by the members: the leadership style employed and the functions shared; the prevailing atmosphere or climate that occurs during each session; the demonstration of competition and cooperation in the resolution of conflict; the group's understanding of and commitment to its goals; the problem-solving and decision-making approaches and procedures used; and the norms or standards of behavior manifested.

To develop skill in implementing an effective leadership role, the leader must be able to identify the dynamics involved in group process. One way to explicate this complex and fascinating therapeutic interactive–interventive method is to make the leader aware of the need to see (observe). This method allows the leader to take stock of the group interacting (that is, to identify how these interactions impact on leadership, the subgroups, and the group as a whole) and come to recognize the positive-negative ambiance in which the members transact with one another.

To facilitate exploration there are certain questions, that is, a collection of observable data, that the leader might consider and that will assist in the identification of the process in operation. With regard to **participation**, the leader might ask: Who are the most vocal or least verbal participants? Does the pattern shift? If so, why? Who facilitates the movement of the group toward its goal? For what reason? How are the silent people treated? Is the treatment consistent? Regarding **communication**, the leader might ask herself: Is there a noticeable direction to the communication, that is, does all the communication flow from the leader to the group, or does it flow from the group to the leader? In essence, is there an observable pattern in communication flow? Is there subgrouping? Is there consistent support or disagreement among certain members? Are there inside/outside tendencies, that is, do certain people seem to be "outsiders"? Do some members leave and return? Is the communication predominantly cognitive (intellectual) or sometimes affective (feelings expressed)? When looking at leadership, the observer might ask such questions as: Do some members of the group exert more influence on the group than others? Is there any shifting in the power base? If so, what may account for this shift? Does there seem to be a leadership struggle, that is, a pull and tug between members to gain control? Between whom? Why? What is its effect on the group? On the task or outcome? What leadership styles are evident? On whose part? With what effect?

Generally speaking, there are three identifiable **leadership styles**: autocratic, democratic, and laissez-faire. **Autocratic leadership** is excessively controlling; it calls for the imposition of will on others. The autocratic leader makes decisions, demands support, evaluates others, and blocks other members from assuming the leadership role. **Democratic leadership** includes everyone in discussions and decision-making. This style of leadership allows for the open expression of ideas and feelings and seeks similar expressions from all members involved. The leader does not pass judgment on members' expressed beliefs, values, thoughts, or feelings. Democratic leadership deals with tension or conflict in a problem-solving way and invites feedback from others. **Laissez-faire leadership**, on the other hand, displays dramatic lack of involvement. This type of leadership is excessively permissive and goes along with any ideas or decisions, but lacks a commitment to follow through. The laissez-faire leadership style does not require initiative or response by the leader. The leader responds or participates mechanically or superficially and seeks to establish no guidelines for group action. The outcome of this type of leadership behavior is often chaos within the group.

In considering **group atmosphere**, the leader attempts to assess the existence of "attraction for" and "approval from" the group by its members. To make this determination, several aspects need to be addressed. Questions designed to elicit this information might include the following: What is the feeling tone of the session? Is it friendly, hostile, mixed, changing, pleasant, or concerned? Do people appear involved and interested? What behavioral indications support the interpretations made? Which member or members appear to prefer congeniality? Who provokes conflict? What is the effect of their behavior on the atmosphere? Do members work together harmoniously toward the identified goals, or do they digress and move toward tangential outcomes?

When **conflict** arises within the group, the group goal may be sabotaged. To determine the manner in which the group engages in seeking resolution to the conflict and thus preservation of the group, the leader needs to ask questions directed toward assessing the effects of the identified conflict on goal attainment. Such questions might include: On what evidence is an interpretation of conflict made? Is the conflict continuous or periodic? Under what circumstances does conflict arise? What effects does it produce on the members and on the task? How is conflict handled? Is it allowed to become personal and vindictive, thereby splitting the group, or is it acknowledged and worked through by the group, using a problem-solving approach?

The **goal** of any group represents the reason for the group's existence. The group's effectiveness depends on the clear definition and mutual understanding by the members of the group's task. In analyzing the group's movement toward achievement of goals, several questions need to be raised. Are the goals specific? Are the goals clearly stated? Do the members seek clarification? Are the stated goals embraced by all members of the group? Is resistance demonstrated toward achievement of the goals—by whom and in what way?

In looking at the type of **decision-making** exercised by the group, the leader needs to be aware that the manner in which decision-making is conducted can either foster cohesion within the group or alienate and divide group members. In the leader's observation of group operations, questions that are relevant to the type of decision-making practices employed need to be raised. For example, is there an accepted pattern for decision-making? By this we mean: Does the group engage in gathering facts, note alternatives, discuss the pros and cons, test consequences, arrive at the decision through consensus or through majority vote? Do some members tend to want to make decisions for the group? How are these individuals received? What is the effect of their reception on the self-authorized decision-maker? Is there a tendency to jump from subject to subject without reaching decisions or conclusions? If so, why?

Norms and **standards** influence the quality of communication and level of interaction between and among group members. They foster conformity and facilitate movement toward goal attainment. There are several questions the leader might ask in attempting to identify the overt and covert governance of group behavior: (1) What behaviors are consistently demonstrated by group members (such as politeness, promptness, tardiness, acceptance or nonacceptance of the designated leader) and what topics or behaviors are avoided by group members? (2) Are norms and standards explicitly stated, or are they implicit? (3) What happens if there is an occasional deviation from any of the established norms? (4) What happens if any of the norms break down completely? (5) How are norms changed or new ones adopted?

Within any group encounter, there are some variables inherent in each situation that may affect group process. The leader needs to be aware of the existence of these variables, since they may create problems for the group. These variables include the size and composition of the group membership; the time and timing of group meetings; physical facilities (such as space, acoustics, equipment, comfort); and stage of group development.

Now that we have guided the reader through the maze of questions that might be raised with respect to group process in operation, in the next segment we will address effectiveness and productivity. We hope, through this discussion, to provide the reader with a better understanding of one of the most fascinating and universally used techniques, the group.

EFFECTIVENESS AND PRODUCTIVITY

For a group of individuals to move and develop from an aggregate of people to a group of people involves certain specific tasks. These tasks are as follows: (1) to determine the purpose and goal of the group, (2) to identify the needs of the participants, (3) to determine who shall be included and how membership shall be recruited, and (4) to determine how the group shall organize itself to carry out its purpose. Effectiveness of group activity, that is, the development of a maturing, well-functioning group, gives evidence of certain characteristics. These characteristics are as follows:

1. A free and accepting group climate—makes it possible for members to easily communicate personal attitudes and feelings of a cooperative and supportive as well as a hostile nature.
2. Participation and commitment—demonstrates the involvement and movement of a majority of the group's membership toward the identified goal.
3. Movement toward the goal—indicates that hidden or personal agendas are beginning to disappear.
4. Problem solving—becomes possible as group members determine the facts, analyze these facts, formulate solutions, test out alternatives, and finally find a solution agreeable to all.
5. Consensual decision-making followed by action—becomes possible as minority and majority points of view are elicited, accepted, and understood. There is some evidence that commitment to action and ability to carry out this action are higher when consensus is reached and a majority vote overrules the minority.
6. Task output or production—becomes greater as group matures and becomes cohesive. Complexity of the task may increase as group grows.
7. Ability to utilize expertise from both inside and outside the group—increases as the group develops.
8. The ability to evaluate—uses feedback and shifts gears on both the task and maintenance levels.
9. Ability to accept limitations—increases as group becomes more cohesive and group-task-oriented.

One of the continuing problems facing the leader in group work is the ongoing attempt to maintain the group's cohesion and productivity. To do so, the leader must become aware of group structure and its related dynamics. Every group operates on two levels, the group task level and the group maintenance level. In dealing with the first level, each member readily recognizes and acknowledges the need to accomplish the assigned tasks. In meeting its need for goal attainment, the group engages in the performance of certain operations or functions directly associated with the identified task. The following functions are carried out by the group as it works toward task accomplishment:

Initiating. Making a beginning contribution to a discussion about the task.

Information seeking. Making sure that the group has all the data it needs to make a decision and that all members of the group have an equal understanding of the issue.

Information giving. Providing new or updating old information about the task.

Opinion giving. Freely sharing one's views about the task.

Elaborating. Asking another member to expand more on what has been said or picking up on the idea of another and developing it.

Coordinating. Pulling together the ideas of two or more group members.

Evaluating. Assessing ideas, not people; suggesting criteria upon which objective judgments can be made.

Preserving. Maintaining the personal integrity of each group member.

Emerging. Introducing a novel idea; stating a feeling that gives or continues the group's momentum.

Structuring. Recommending procedures that can be followed to facilitate the task.

Clarifying. Making more explicit ideas or concepts so that they are more clearly understood.

Frequently, the members are so conscious of the need to accomplish the task that they are unaware of the other level that is operating simultaneously, that is, the group maintenance level. As people work together on a task in a group, they are also doing something to and with one another. Consequently, a group consists of a constantly changing network of interactions and relationships. A group needs to have a growing awareness of itself as a group and to face the need of maintaining the relationship within it, if the task is indeed to be accomplished. The maintenance level refers to what is happening to persons within the group as the work is carried out.

These maintenance functions, when performed, will help the group build, improve, and strengthen working relationships. Performing such functions will help a group to create an emotional climate that will hold it together and make it easier for members to work cooperatively and contribute to the achievements of the goals of the group. Maintenance functions include the following:

Gatekeeping. Making sure that each member has a chance to express his views and that some members do not dominate or take control of the entire discussion.

Encouraging. Assisting the group to experiment with new approaches, change meeting methods, explore the subject in depth, consider new goals.

Harmonizing. Finding commonality to reduce polarization; constructively dealing with conflict.

Supporting. Acknowledging individual or aggregate contributions of members through positive feedback to facilitate acceptance, need gratification, and encouragement.

Consensus seeking. Resolving win–lose situations; striving for what is best for the group.

Giving and receiving feedback. Providing the group with information about its progress as a group.

Standard setting. Stating and reviewing standards set by the group for both task performance and group maintenance.

Analyzing. Helping the group to understand its process and how the process is affecting task performance.

SUMMARY

Each member is a fundamental and vital component of all group processes, and all members are equally responsible for moving the group toward completion of its task and for contributing to the total outcome of the group process. However, the leader has the responsibility for structuring and maintaining the process that takes place within the group. Effectiveness and productivity are governed by the group's overall ability to execute its task and maintenance functions.

SUGGESTED READINGS

Adrian, S. A Systematic Approach to Selecting Group Participants. *Journal of Psychiatric Nursing and Mental Health Services*, Vol. 18, No. 2 (February, 1980), 37–41.

Cartwright, D., & Zander, A. *Group Dynamics*. New York: Harper & Row, 1968.

Collison, C. R. Grappling With Group Resistance. *Journal of Psychosocial Nursing and Mental Health Services*, Vol. 22, No. 8 (August, 1984), 6–12.

Hare, P., Borgatte, E. F., & Balec, R. F. *Small Groups—Studies in Social Interaction*. New York: Knopf, 1962.

Hardin, S. B., Stratton, K., & Benton, D. The Video Connection—Group Dynamics Onscreen. *Journal of Psychosocial Nursing and Mental Health Services*, Vol. 21, No. 11 (November, 1983), 12–17, 20–21.

Hogan, R. A. *Group Psychotherapy: A Peer Centered Approach*. New York: Holt, Rinehart & Winston, 1980.

Homans, G. C. *The Human Group*. New York: Harcourt, Brace, 1950.

Loomis, M. E. *Group Process for Nurses*. St. Louis: Mosby, 1979.

Merton, R. K. The Social Nature of Leadership. *American Journal of Nursing*, Vol. 69, No. 12 (December, 1969), 2614–2618.

Racy, J. How A Group Grows. *American Journal of Nursing*, Vol. 69, No. 11 (November, 1969), 2396–2402.

Sampson, E. E., & Marthas, M. *Group Process for the Health Professions*. 2nd ed. New York: Wiley, 1981.

Shepherd, C. R. *Small Groups: Some Sociological Perspectives*. Scranton, Pa.: Chandler, 1964.

Swanson, M. G. A Check List for Group Leaders. *Perspectives in Psychiatric Care*, Vol. 3, No. 3 (1969), 120–126.

Zander, A. *Groups at Work*. San Francisco: Jossey-Bass, 1981.

Zander, A. *Making Groups Effective*. San Francisco: Jossey-Bass, 1982.

18

THE INTERACTIVE–INTERVENTIVE PROCESS IN GROUPS

LEARNING OBJECTIVES

On completion of this chapter the reader should be able to:

1. Define and distinguish between the **process** and **dynamics** of the interactive–interventive process in groups.
2. Distinguish between a social and a therapeutic group.
3. Identify types of therapy groups.
4. Identify the nurse's role and responsibility for initiating and conducting the interactive–interventive process in groups.
5. Recognize impediments to the therapeutic group process.
6. Implement specific intervention for the success of the interactive–interventive process.

DEFINITION AND PURPOSE

The interactive–interventive process conducted in small groups is commonly referred to as group therapy. **Group therapy** is a structured or semistructured process of therapeutic intervention in which the cognitive, behavioral, and emotional reactions of the individual members of the group, toward one another and toward the leader, are acknowledged and understood as projections of individual interpersonal distress. Participation in group therapy provides a reeducational experience in which the individual as a "separate self" and the group as a "collective self" are involved in a process of learning and problem solving for the purpose of dealing with the cognitive, emotional, and behavioral reactions necessary to the production of change within themselves and with the group.

There are significant differences between a social group and a therapeutic group. These differences occur in four major areas: organization, membership, composition, and use of the leadership role. A comparison between the characteristics of a social and a therapeutic group is illustrated in Table 18–1.

PROCESS

Group effectiveness is a direct result of the educational process that exists and develops between the therapist (group leader) and the group members. However, the therapist's involvement in the process is

TABLE 18–1. MAJOR DISTINGUISHING CHARACTERISTICS BETWEEN SOCIAL AND THERAPEUTIC GROUPS

Social Group	Therapeutic Group
Organization	
Casual, most often for diversional, professional, or religious activities.	Purposeful, educative, interventive, and preventative.
For a variety of reasons dependent on needs or interests.	Specific change objective in mind.
Membership	
Varies in terms of numbers, purpose, or goals.	Limited to persons experiencing some deficiency or difficulty in coping.
	Limited to those seeking therapeutic assistance.
Composition	
More likely to have a heterogeneous mixture.	Occasionally heterogeneous.
More likely to be representative of a cross-section of society.	Deliberate selection is based on specific factors such as age, sex, marital status, presenting problem, or specific needs.
Leadership Role	
Usually by election, appointment, or consensus.	Therapist is the primary group leader.
Less well defined.	Clearly structured and defined.
Flexible.	Employs specific therapeutic leadership tasks.
	Implements and guides therapeutic process.
	Emphasizes therapeutic process over the social process.

not a guarantee of success in and of itself. The therapist must cultivate certain factors in the group process that encourage and enhance change. These factors include the following:

1. *Sharing information*—the mutual exchange of relevant data that provides a basis for understanding.
2. *Hope*—the belief in self and in the process that help and comfort is available, that at the end of the tunnel there is the light of acceptance, understanding, relief, and recovery.
3. *Universality*—security in the knowledge that "my problem," feelings, and behaviors are known, felt, and shared by others. It is the idea that the self is not alone in its distress, not "so different."
4. *Altruism*—an unselfish interest in others and their well-being. It is the expression of mutual concern, support, recognition, comfort, assurance, and respect among the members of the group.
5. *Transference of primary group images and relationships*—the therapeutic group is substituted for the initial primary group, the family, and may be compared to it. This comparison and substitution permits the individual to nullify past learned group interaction and expectations and create for self a new set of experiences and expectations.
6. *Socialization*—a process in which the techniques and skills necessary for social interaction are explored, experimented with, and evaluated within the context of the group, by the group. The outcome of socialization is learning new patterns of acceptable social interaction.
7. *Ventilation*—an active verbal participation in the group process through the use of self-disclosure and self-exploration. It provides the individual member with an opportunity to test concepts, validate ideas and feelings, examine values, and reassess these in light of responses obtained from fellow group members.

GROUP DYNAMICS

Group therapy differs from individual therapy in that it more closely approximates a broader cross-section of social or emotional experiences. In addition, group therapy makes use of comprehensive social interaction. These two factors give group therapy the added benefit of providing feedback that is derived from a multiplicity of responses. Regardless of the type of group, specialized needs, or therapeutic goals, there is a mechanism of operation that consistently occurs. This mechanism is divided into four stages: group formation and organization, group interaction, group cohesion, and group dissolution.

The Stage of Group Formation and Organization

This stage is that period of time in which the therapist scrutinizes the patient population in reference to patient needs and problems that can best be served through the group process. Consideration is given to homogeneity of needs and problems, age and sex of participants, goals to be achieved, allocation of time, the member's ability and willingness to participate in the group process, and the optimal number of participants. Group formation involves a series of negotiations, the end result of which is the identification of a contract between the leader and members and between the members, each with the others.

The Stage of Group Interaction

This stage covers that period of time it takes group members to become acquainted. During this period of testing, the members behave as strangers and are cautiously polite to one another. This stage allows time for discussion of who the members are, their reasons for being in the group, and the identification of potential goals. This second stage is characterized by conflict and lack of unity. The members demonstrate distrust and covert hostility. These projected feelings are directed toward individual members as well as toward the therapist. When the membership begins to interact more openly and positively with one another, the group, together with the leader, moves into the third stage.

The Stage of Group Cohesion

Hostility and anxiety become more overt in this stage. Feelings and expressed concerns are dealt with more directly by the group. As similarities are identified and discussed, thoughts and feelings revealed, and conflicts and frustrations handled, group cohesiveness develops. As group cohesiveness increases, there is a proportionate increase in the productivity of the group. The result of increased group cohesiveness and productivity is a change in the communication pattern. No longer do individual group members speak directly to individuals; they now address themselves to the entire group. This intergroup communication pattern enhances the opportunity for emotional and social reeducation. The group is able to focus its attention on fulfilling the identified therapeutic goals.

The Stage of Group Dissolution

This stage begins as the therapeutic tasks of the group near completion. It is that period of time necessary to bring about effective dissolution of group relationships. During this stage group members face and cope with the feelings associated with loss and separation anxiety. Members freely express feelings of being abandoned, rejected, or forsaken. Effective resolution depends on the group's ability to cope with these painful expressions. Because of the developed emotional maturity of the group that results from the cohesive stage, it is now able to be mutually supportive during this crisis period and successfully complete the final therapeutic task of closure.

TYPES OF THERAPY GROUPS

Within the scope of group therapy, three points of reference can be distinguished that serve as a basis for determining the type of group therapy most effective to meet particular client needs. These points of reference include the following:

1. The theoretical framework under which the group operates.
2. The particular characteristics or nature of the group members.
3. The therapeutic task to be accomplished.

Generally, throughout the literature reference is made to various therapeutic group modalities. Table 18-2 is a synthesis and comparison of what we perceive to be three major types—**didactic-inspirational, interventive-exploratory**, and **activity**.

THE NURSE'S ROLE IN GROUP THERAPY

There are many different kinds of approaches that can be utilized in the practice of group therapy and many different types of group therapies. Each method is distinctive and has its own particular characteristics and expected sets of outcomes. Nonetheless, whatever approach the nurse–group therapist chooses, there are specific leader behaviors that are fundamental and universal. These behaviors may be viewed in terms of attitudes, abilities, and functions or tasks.

Attitudes

The leader's attitude toward group process is just as significant as her attitude toward any other aspect of practice. The attitudes conveyed dictate nurse behaviors. The positive attitudes of personal worth, integrity, open-mindedness, advocacy, hopefulness, and involvement discussed in Chapter 12 are the same positive attitudes needed by the leader in the interactive–interventive process in groups. A leadership approach based on these attitudes enables the leader to express to the group realistic, therapeutic expectations for success and change. The

TABLE 18–2. TYPES OF THERAPY GROUPS

	Didactic-Inspirational	Interventive-Exploratory	Activity
Definition	A group process that places emphasis on an educational experience designed to foster intellectual and emotional exchange while reflecting ethical, religious, or societal values.	A group process that encourages group members to verbally express and examine emotional or psychological problems within the context of their past and present individual and group interpersonal relationships.	A group process that emphasizes social interaction versus verbal interaction among group members and encourages the development of ego strengths and control.
Goal	Better adaptation to environment through education and inspiration.	Development of insight leading to adaptation, modification, or reconstruction of personality structure or behavior patterns.	Development of the socialization process; better adaptation to physical and social environment; and opportunity to test out relationships within a nonthreatening environment.
Theoretical base	Learning theory. Behavior modification. Biofeedback.	Psychoanalytic theory. Behavioral theory. Gestalt psychology. Reality therapy. Transactional analysis.	Social theory. Behavior modification. Milieu therapy. Nonverbal communication theory.
Primary therapeutic role function of leader	Provide information. Encourage discussion. Support existing coping mechanism and defenses. Persuade members to solve a specific type of problem. Promote group solidarity and comradeship.	Encourage the expression of ideas and the ventilation of feelings. Confront existing defenses. Assist in the development or modification of coping mechanisms. Offer reassurance, empathy, and feedback to group members.	Plan, organize, and coordinate social, recreational, occupational, and industrial activities. Identify and reinforce previous interests. Promote the development of new outlets.
Examples:	1. Discharge planning group 2. Recovery Incorporated 3. Alcoholics Anonymous 4. Sex education 5. Health education 6. Rap group 7. Narcotics Anonymous 8. Prenatal instruction 9. Ostomy Club 10. Dietary instruction	1. T Group 2. Encounter 3. Psychodrama 4. Family therapy 5. Intensive psychotherapy 6. Marital counseling 7. Adolescent therapy 8. Adjustment to disability of handicaps group 9. Conflict resolution 10. Crisis intervention	1. Current events group 2. Remotivational group 3. Reality orientation 4. Music therapy 5. Play therapy 6. Art therapy 7. Body building or exercise group 8. Field trips 9. Social skills 10. Self-care management

leader conveys to the group, through these attitudes, her commitment and concern. She reacts with thoughtfulness, simplicity, and honesty, demonstrating by her actions a willingness to share in the responsibilities of the group work. The leader's attitude toward the group should clearly indicate that every person within the group, without exception, is the most important person there. Whatever the individual says or does not say is significant within the context of the experiences of the group.

Abilities

The nurse must possess the skills and abilities needed by leaders of any kind of group. The leadership role in group therapy involves having role functions as a group member, but maintaining a distinct line between the patient and nonpatient role. In any initial group therapy contact, the nurse-leader is automatically identified and looked to as "leader"; however, it is the skill and ability the leader exercises that enable her to maintain the leadership role and, through it, maintain the control or direction of the group toward its therapeutic goal.

In addition, the leader needs therapeutic skills. These would include the skillful use of the therapeutic communication process; technical expertise in the maintenance and promotion of group interaction; an awareness of the dynamics of group process; the ability to interpret and integrate behavior within the context of group experiences; and the ability to intervene on behalf of individual members. Other abilities necessary for successful leadership include an awareness of self and the part self plays in the context of group interaction; recognition and resolution of the leader's own internal conflicts; and, last but not least, the capacity for empathy.

Functions or Tasks

In implementing group therapy, the leader must be aware of specific functions or tasks commensurate with the leadership role. Fulfillment of these functions with their associated tasks enables the leader to guide and direct group process. We have identified six major functions that lie within the realm of nurse responsibility. These functions are forming the groups, organizing the group, identifying recurring themes, encouraging the development of commonly shared perceptions, assessing the affective tone of the group, and evaluating group process. These functions and their associated tasks are listed as follows:

I. Formation of the group
   1. Select potential participants based on predetermined criteria.
   2. Conduct an interview with each potential participant.

3. Present to potential participants the selected purpose and goals of the group.
4. Assess ability of potential participants to meet criteria and their willingness to participate.
5. Finalize selection of group members.

II. Organization of the group
1. Select appropriate time and place.
2. Arrange for record keeping.
3. Encourage members to attend.
4. Convene the group.
5. Introduce group members.
6. Restate and clarify purpose and goals.
7. Identify limits.
8. Initiate the development of group norms and values.
9. Encourage spontaneous participation.

III. Identification of recurring themes
1. Listen skillfully.
2. Be actively involved in the developing group process.
3. Clarify verbal and nonverbal communication.
4. Investigate, explore, validate, and evaluate content.

IV. Encourage the development of commonly shared perceptions
1. Identify individual perceptions.
2. Investigate and explore possible similarities and differences.
3. Encourage and support group interface.
4. Assist and support members in their search for group consensus.

V. Assess the affective tone of the group
1. Recognize and identify and increase in the level of verbal and nonverbal activity.
2. Recognize and identify any increase in the level of psychomotor activity.
3. Identify and analyze possible and probable causes.
4. Validate interpretations with the group.
5. Intervene to exercise control either by supporting an individual member or by limit setting.

VI. Evaluation of group process
1. Monitor progress of group movement toward goal attainment.
2. Analyze and interpret data obtained from each session.
3. Redirect group effort toward goal based on progress, analysis, and interpretations made.
4. Seek collaboration or supervisory input.
5. Record progress of group according to the established system of record keeping.
6. Facilitate closure.

STUMBLING BLOCKS AND STEPPING STONES

Like the nurse-practitioner who has difficulty in initiating her role as therapist with patients on a one-to-one basis, the beginning group leader may also encounter some difficulties in the implementation of an actual therapeutic group session. Some of the common stumbling blocks the leader is likely to encounter along with some stepping stones that will assist her in dealing with these difficulties are presented in Table 18–3.

TABLE 18–3. COMMON STUMBLING BLOCKS AND STEPPING STONES ASSOCIATED WITH GROUP THERAPY

Stumbling Blocks: What if . . .	Stepping Stones: Try this . . .
1. The prospective group members demonstrate initial resistance to attending the group?	Encourage patients to verbalize their negative feelings. Listen intently. Accept expressed thoughts and feelings without judgment or criticism. Restate and clarify purpose. Suggest that the patients "give it a try."
2. All members of group try to talk at once?	Stop the interaction and regain control of group by stating, "Everyone is talking at once." Explore with the group possible causes for behavior. Encourage recognition of individual speakers. Focus attention on individuals when they speak. Review and reestablish the "ground rules."
3. One member continues after several sessions to remain silent?	Design strategies that require a verbal response from each member; for example: • ask each member for an opinion; • call on selected members, including the silent participant; • make a matter-of-fact observation about the member's silence. Ask the group to comment on the member's silence.
4. One person monopolizes the discussion?	Allow the other group members to intervene and set limits if they are able. Interrupt positively and request another group member to give an opinion about what is being said. Explore the feelings of the group when one member talks all the time.
5. A group member uses excessive profanity, causing disruption?	Exercise control and impose limits. Enforce the limits.
6. The patient is resistant to limit setting?	Remain firm—don't back down. Request the patient to leave the group until he regains self-control. Set up an individual session to explore the patient's feelings.

(*continued*)

TABLE 18–3. CONTINUED

Stumbling Blocks: What if . . .	Stepping Stones: Try this . . .
	Encourage the individual to maintain group membership.
7. A group member is verbally aggressive toward the therapist?	Set an example by maintaining your "cool." Absorb hostility. Speak in a low, even tone. Maintain eye contact if possible. Identify the angry feeling. Assist the patient to recognize his anger.
8. A group member is verbally aggressive toward another member?	Sit still and observe—avoid taking sides. Allow time for group members to exert control. Determine group feeling about the aggressiveness. Distract attention by focusing on feelings. Act as arbitrator. Deflect hostility by acting as a buffer between aggressor and group.
9. The group is not progressing?	Reevaluate data with a colleague consultant. Review with the group progress to date with respect to initial framework and stated goals. Explore with the group reasons for lack of productivity. Reaffirm group objectives and goals. Ask for suggestions from the group for reaching the goals.
10. There is a hidden agenda, i.e., issues unmet or unattended to?	Allow sufficient time for each member to express thoughts and feelings. Encourage members to rephrase the purpose and goals in their own terms. Review the stated agreed-upon goals to reduce misunderstanding. Share perceptions and request feedback.
11. A task-oriented group cannot reach a consensus?	Summarize positions or data already presented. Keep focus on immediate concern. Encourage the group to explore alternatives.
12. A member of the group is rejected by the group?	Focus attention of group away from "rejected member." Demonstrate acceptance by supporting group member's attempt to become part of the group. Give recognition to isolated member when merited. Assist the group to identify cause for group behavior toward rejected member. Reevaluate the isolated member's readiness for group participation. Consider these possible alternatives: • remove the individual from the group. • transfer him to another group.

TABLE 18–3. CONTINUED

Stumbling Blocks: What if . . .	Stepping Stones: Try this . . .
	• set up individual therapy. • confront group with the group's behavior toward the isolated member.
13. A member negatively manipulates?	Ignore the manipulative behavior. Treat disruptive behavior matter-of-factly. Restate positively expectations in relationship to group goals.
14. A member discloses highly emotionally charged data about himself?	Elicit feelings of group members about the data. Identify any changes in the membership's attitude or opinions toward the sharing person. Maintain the therapeutic objective self toward the sharing member. Remind membership that they are bound by confidentiality outside the group.
15. The group is approaching termination and the members are withdrawing?	Draw the group's attention to the observed behavior. Introduce the topic of termination and facilitate discussion about what termination means to the members. Encourage ventilation of feelings, i.e., anger, loss, fear, depression, or rejection.

SUMMARY

The interactive–interventive process in group is a therapeutic encounter that provides each member with a reeducational experience directed toward personal and interpersonal growth. The main purpose or outcome is change. The change that occurs results from the group's ability to share, offer mutual support, and provide feedback within the context of comprehensive social interaction.

The group leader is responsible for structuring and managing the process. Through careful planning, the leader develops interventions that foster group cohesiveness and maximize the therapeutic potential of the group.

SUGGESTED READINGS

Authier, J., & Gustafson, K. Group Intervention Techniques: A Practical Guide for Psychiatric Team Members. *Journal of Psychiatric and Mental Health Services*, Vol. 14, No. 7 (July, 1976), 19–22.

Birkhead, L.M. The Nurse as Leader: Group Psychotherapy With Psychotic

Patients. *Journal of Psychosocial Nursing and Mental Health Services*, Vol. 22, No. 6 (June, 1984), 24–30.

Britnell, J.C., & Mitchell, K.E. Inpatient Group Psychotherapy for the Elderly. *Journal of Psychiatric Nursing and Mental Health Services*, Vol. 19, No. 5 (May, 1981), 19–23.

Brooks, D.D. Teletherapy: or How To Use Videotape Feedback To Enhance Group Process. *Perspectives in Psychiatric Care*, Vol. 14, No. 2 (1976), 83–87.

Clark, C.C. *The Nurse as Group Leader*. New York: Springer, 1977.

Davis, A.G. Goal Attainment of Psychiatric Clients After Group Experience To Learn Social Independence Skills. *Issues in Mental Health Nursing*, Vol. 3, Nos. 1–2 (January, June, 1981), 159–184.

Ferguson, B.B. A Parent's Group. *Journal of Psychiatric Nursing and Mental Health Services*, Vol. 17, No. 12 (December, 1979), 24–27.

Friedman, W.H. *How To Do Groups*. New York: Jason Aronson, 1979.

Goldberg, C., & Stanitis, M.A. The Enhancement of Self-Esteem through the Communication Process in Group Therapy. *The Journal of Psychiatric Nursing and Mental Health Services*, Vol. 5, No. 12 (December, 1977), 5–8.

Hagar, R. Evaluation of Group Psychotherapy—A Question of Values. *Journal of Psychiatric Nursing and Mental Health Services*, Vol. 16, No. 12 (December, 1978), 26, 31–33.

Krumm, S., Vannatta, P. & Sanders, J. A Group for Teaching Chemotherapy. *American Journal of Nursing*, Vol. 79, No. 5 (May, 1979), 916.

Lancaster, J. Activity Groups as Therapy. *American Journal of Nursing*, Vol. 76, No. 6 (June, 1976), 947–949.

Larkin, A.R. What's a Medication Group? *Journal of Psychosocial Nursing and Mental Health Services*, Vol. 20, No. 2 (February, 1982), 35–37.

Marram, G.D. *The Group Approach in Nursing Practice*. St. Louis: Mosby, 1973.

Pelletier, L.R. Interpersonal Communications Task Group. *Journal of Psychosocial Nursing and Mental Health Services*, Vol. 21, No. 9 (September, 1983), 32–36.

Rogers, C. Carl Rogers Describes His Way of Facilitating Encounter Groups. *American Journal of Nursing*, Vol. 71, No. 2 (February, 1971), 275–279.

Scheidman, J. Remotivation without Labels. *Journal of Psychiatric and Mental Health Services*, Vol. 14, No. 7 (July, 1976), 41–42.

Shaffer, J.B., & Galinsky, D.M. *Models of Group Therapy and Sensitivity Training*. Englewood Cliffs, N.J.: Prentice-Hall, Inc., 1974

Silbert, D.T. Human Sexuality Growth Groups. *Journal of Psychiatric Nursing and Mental Health Services*, Vol. 19, No. 2 (February, 1981), 31–34.

Slavson, S.R. *Dynamics of Group Psychotherapy*. New York: Jason Aronson, 1979.

Slimmer, L.W. Use of the Nursing Process To Facilitate Group Therapy. *Journal of Psychiatric Nursing and Mental Health Services*, Vol. 16, No. 2 (February, 1978), 42–44.

Yalom, I.D. *The Theory and Practice of Group Psychotherapy*. New York: Basic Books, 1975.

Yearwood, A.C., & Hess, S.K. How Can a Patient Change in 28 Days? *American Journal of Nursing*, Vol. 79, No. 8 (August, 1979), 1436–1438.

19

STRATEGIES FOR PLANNING EFFECTIVE NURSING CARE

LEARNING OBJECTIVES

On completion of this chapter the reader should be able to:

1. Define a **nursing care plan.**
2. Identify broad nursing care goals applicable to any client in any practice care setting.
3. Describe the scope and use of the nursing care plan and its relationship to the nursing process.
4. Identify the rules of thumb in developing an efficient and effective nursing care plan.

INTRODUCTION

To create a dynamic nursing care plan, time, involvement, judgment, and coordination are necessary. **Time** to observe the patient, interact with him, confer with colleagues, review initial admission information, and keep abreast of progress. **Involvement** to implement the assessment process, evaluate planned interventions, and develop new strategies based on the changing needs of the patient. **Coordination** to maximize the effectiveness of the health team to act on the readiness displayed by the patient. **Judgment** to be aware of the patient's ability to be involved, recognize the level of patient functioning, be able to intervene at that level, and establish and rank priorities.

When confronted with developing a nursing care plan for patients with differing, medical psychiatric diagnoses, students appear surprised and then disconcerted because the overall goals for care appear to be repetitious. For example, helping the patient to develop a realistic and positive self-concept can apply to both the patient with an anxiety disorder and the patient with schizophrenia. This repetition occurs because all people operate under the same basic human need system. The uniqueness of the care plan evolves as the nurse completes her assessment, identifies the degree which needs are not being met, establishes a nursing diagnosis, identifies the priorities that exist for the particular patient, and determines the therapeutic interventions necessary to assist the patient toward optimal functioning.

The setting of realistic objectives for patient care depends on two factors: the extent of the problem as identified through a nursing diagnosis, and the capacity of the individual to move toward healthy adjustment. In other words, goals for nursing care may not change, but the emphasis, approach, and interventions do change.

Some of the broad nursing care goals that are applicable to all patients in distress, regardless of diagnostic category or practice setting, are listed as follows:

1. To prepare the individual and his family for a hospital experience that meets their needs.
2. To create and maintain an environment that reflects an attitude of honesty, support, and genuine concern for patient needs.
3. To help the patient attain and maintain his optimal physical health and mental stability.
4. To help the patient develop a realistic and positive self-concept from which healthy feelings of self-esteem and self-respect can emerge.
5. To increase feelings of security through a climate that demonstrates acceptance of the individual and fosters a feeling of belonging.
6. To cultivate and support an atmosphere which makes use of the individual's assets and encourages him to maximize his potential for change.
7. To identify, explore, and demonstrate to the individual satisfactory and effective ways of establishing and maintaining interpersonal relationships.
8. To assist the patient by recognizing the degree of anxiety, frustration, and stress he experiences and by providing him

with opportunities to learn effective problem-solving methods to deal with crises.

9. To assist the patient to set realistic goals that result in gratification and enable him to function to the level of independence his potential capabilities permit.
10. To develop the concept that life is appreciated and enjoyed through self-directed behavior and that an individual is responsible for maintaining self-directed behavior not only in personal and interpersonal situations, but also in work and leisure activities.
11. To provide continuing support, reassurance, and teaching to the patient and his family.
12. To prepare the patient and his family to make the transition from the hospital environment to the community.

Often when a student or a new practitioner enters a psychiatric practice setting for the first time, her anxiety increases. As a result, she sometimes displays an inability to assess patient concerns, formulate nursing diagnoses, set realistic goals, apply principles, and develop methods that result in the effective delivery of competent, qualified nursing care. Frequently, she asks questions like: "Now that I'm here, what do I do?" "How do I find out?" and "How do I go about it?" In order to respond to these and similar questions and to assist the student to make the transition from a general practice setting to a psychiatric practice setting, we remind the nurse that psychiatric nursing, like all other fields of nursing care, requires order and the setting of priorities. To achieve this end, the nurse must develop a knowledgeable and functional nursing care plan utilizing a problem-solving approach.

A NURSING CARE PLAN: WHAT IS IT? WHAT DOES IT DO?

A **nursing care plan** is a written outline, a logical, orderly, systematized assessment and identification of the patient's nursing diagnoses, objectives for care, and the methods and strategies for achieving the objectives. It is the nursing process in operation. A nursing care plan enables the nurse to establish order, set priorities, and develop goals (Table 19–1).

STRATEGIES

Nursing care plans do not materialize out of thin air. A considerable amount of time, effort, and thought goes into the construction of a

TABLE 19-1. NURSING CARE PLAN—DEFINITION AND PURPOSE

What is it?	What does it do?
1. A means of individualizing care.	Allows the nurse to adapt basic nursing interventions. Promotes flexibility in accordance with the unique response from each patient within the context of his total experience.
2. A mechanism to assist the patient to solve his problems or concerns.	Provides the patient with the opportunity to actively participate in the planning and implementation of his own care.
3. A mechanism for systematic communication.	Provides to those who will administer the actual care, specific, necessary, and detailed information. Promotes consistency and continuity of care. Provides a safeguard against a possible breakdown in communication among staff members.
4. A tool for assisting the coordination of total patient care.	Allows the nurse to plan and collaborate with colleagues and those in other disciplines.
5. A basis for the evaluation of patient care.	Provides the nurse with a point of reference in determining whether or not the expected outcomes were achieved. Identifies the degree to which the plan was effective, thereby creating a basis for realistic, deliberative change.

workable and effective nursing care plan. We have identified some basic strategies for designing nursing care plans. They are outlined in Figure 19-1 and discussed in the following paragraphs. We consider these strategies to be fundamental to the sound development of a care plan. These strategies, if followed, will result in a practical guide that will be meaningful and satisfying to both patient and nurse.

The first strategy is that the nurse must use problem solving as a prerequisite for patient care. **Problem solving** consists of the identification of a problem, the orderly collection and examination of data related to the problem, the formulation of one or more possible solutions, the implementation of a selected solution, and the evaluation of the results. It is a practical, efficient, and effective tool. Its use as a method of operation has to become so routine that it is second nature for the nurse to use it to intervene on behalf of the patient. Its major benefit to the nurse is that it helps to maintain objectivity because it provides a method by which the nurse can organize the information she has about the patient as well as identify the information she still needs to obtain.

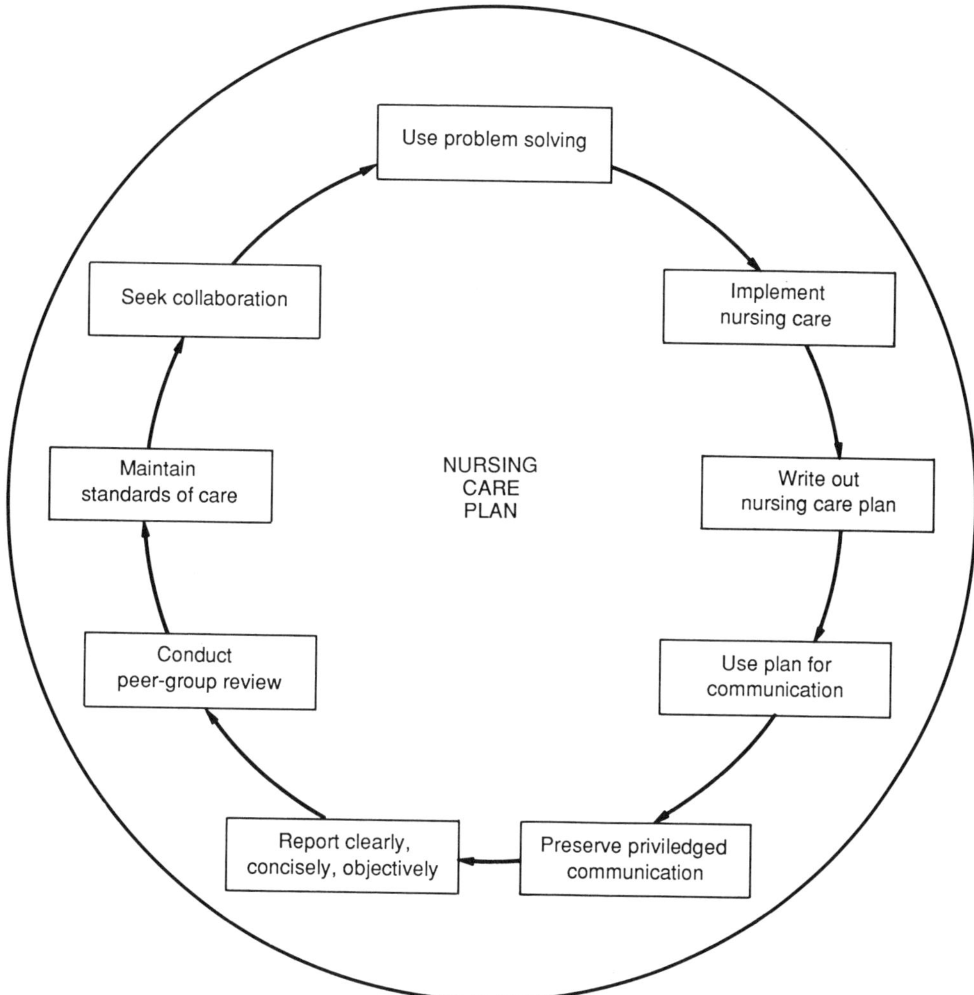

Figure 19–1. Strategies for Designing Nursing Care Plans

The second strategy is that the nurse implements the nursing process. This means that the nurse engages in a deliberative rather than intuitive set of actions designed to create an organized framework for the delivery of care to the client.

The Nursing Process

Nurses demonstrate accountability and responsibility to clients through the **nursing process**; a mechanism that can be used to evaluate nursing effectiveness. There are five major components within the nursing process. These are **assessing**, **analyzing–synthesizing**, **planning**, **implementing**, and **evaluating**.

Assessment. Nursing assessment is a process whereby the nurse examines the client in his totality in an effort to determine the significance or value of subjective and objective data that have been collected regarding the client and his concerns. The client can be an individual, family, group, or community. The parameters of the assessment criteria may change for an individual or group, but the process remains the same. The process involves interaction, observation, and measurement in order to derive a comprehensive and accurate set of data.

As applied to an individual client, assessment requires that the nurse collects all available data from such sources as the client; his family and significant others; medical, social, and developmental records; psychological findings; laboratory reports; and contributions from other disciplines. In fact, any and all sources are used that may provide relevant data.

It is important to note that the process of assessment is not haphazard. The process and specificity of the kind and type of data required is governed by (1) the philosophy of the nurse, (2) the theoretical framework from which the nurse practices, and (3) the type of client. The end result of assessment is a complete client profile. This profile provides the nurse with basic information with regard to the client's life-style, physical care needs, emotional needs, need for education, and health care goals.

Analysis–Synthesis. Analysis–synthesis is a dual process of breakdown and reintegration of data. Together, analysis and synthesis are used to interpret and give meaning to the collected data. **Analysis** involves the categorization of the subjective and objective data. Analysis is used to determine existing patterns and to identify gaps in the data base. **Synthesis** is the reorganizing and uniting of the pieces to form a meaningful whole.

This step in the nursing process is influenced by the nurse's knowledge base and her ability to utilize the cognitive skills of objectivity, critical thinking, and decision-making along with inductive and deductive reasoning. Objectivity provides for accuracy in interpreting client data; critical thinking requires the sifting of data in an attempt to generate ideas about what the data may mean. Decision-making is discriminative thinking that requires deliberation and judgment in the selection of a particular action. Deductive and inductive reasoning are used to process information, that is, to make inferences and draw conclusions from the presenting data, which result in the formulation of a nursing diagnosis.

The **nursing diagnosis** is a summary statement(s) or judgment(s) made by the nurse about the data gathered and prioritized during the assessment process. Each statement identifies an actual, potential, or possible patient problem that requires nursing intervention in order to be solved. A nursing diagnosis describes the client's health status with respect to his activities and life-style. In effect, it is a statement of the client's behavioral response to an existing condition or situation in living.

Since the 1960s, the profession has recognized that nursing diagnoses serve as the beginning scientific basis for nursing practice. The North American Nursing Diagnosis Association (NANDA) has developed a list of diagnoses that it has recommended for testing in clinical practice. This list is acknowledged as incomplete, especially with respect to those diagnoses that would have relevance for the practice of psychiatric–mental health nursing. Table 19–2 contains a list of approved nursing diagnoses from the Fifth Conference of NANDA. Those diagnoses that have specific reference to psychiatric–mental health nursing have been identified by an asterisk.

The development of nursing diagnoses is an ongoing process. The current diagnoses listed are being used both as they have been formulated and with user modifications. The Association hopes that, as practitioners implement their use, feedback regarding applicability will be forthcoming to guide future revisions.

Planning. The third step in the nursing process is planning. **Planning** is the identification of specific objectives and the designing of interventions needed to accomplish them. Planning includes prioritizing the nursing diagnoses according to presenting needs. In addition, it also involves the identification of interventions reflecting the levels of preventive care that promote, restore, and maintain health.

The **objectives** are long- and short-term outcome statements of client achievement written in behavioral language. Short-term objectives are tentative, dynamic, and reflect the changes in the needs of the client while long-term objectives are stated as the ultimate expectations of client response with respect to the nursing diagnoses. Objectives are mutually derived through collaboration and consultation between the client and his supportive network and the nurse.

Interventions are prescriptive nursing orders. They detail who, what, when, where, and under what circumstances specific roles and functions of the nurse are to be enacted. Interventions assist the client to achieve the identified objectives.

Implementing. Implementing is operationalizing the plan. It is putting into action interventive techniques and strategies to achieve the stated objectives. In this phase of the nursing process, the nurse applies the scientific knowledge and theoretical framework in carrying

TABLE 19–2. NURSING DIAGNOSES APPROVED BY THE NORTH AMERICAN NURSING DIAGNOSES ASSOCIATION

Activity intolerance
Activity intolerance, potential
Airway clearance, ineffective
*Anxiety
Bowel elimination, alteration in: constipation
Bowel elimination, alteration in: diarrhea
Bowel elimination, alteration in: incontinence
Breathing pattern, ineffective
Cardiac output, alteration in: decreased
Comfort, alteration in: pain
*Communication, impaired: verbal
*Coping, family: potential for growth
*Coping, ineffective family: compromised
*Coping, ineffective family: disabling
*Coping, ineffective individual
*Diversional activity, deficit
*Family process, alteration in
*Fear
Fluid volume, alteration in: excess
Fluid volume deficit, actual (1)
Fluid volume deficit, actual (2)
Fluid volume deficit, potential
Gas exchange, impaired
*Grieving, anticipatory
*Grieving, dysfunctional
Health maintenance, alteration in
Home maintenance management, impaired
Injury, potential for
*Knowledge deficit (specify)
Mobility, impaired physical
*Noncompliance (specify)
Nutrition, alteration in: less than body requirements
Nutrition, alteration in: more than body requirements
Nutrition, alteration in: potential for more than body requirements
Oral mucous membrane, alteration in
Parenting, alteration in: actual or potential
*Powerlessness
Rape trauma syndrome
*Self-care deficit: feeding, bathing/hygiene, dressing/grooming, toileting
*Self-concept, disturbance in: body image, self-esteem, role performance, personal identity
*Sensory-perceptual alteration: visual, auditory, kinesthetic, gustatory, tactile, olfactory
*Sexual dysfunction
Skin integrity, impairment of: actual
Skin integrity, impairment of: potential
Sleep pattern disturbance
*Social isolation
*Spiritual distress
*Thought processes, alteration in
Tissue perfusion, alteration in: cerebral, cardiopulmonary, renal, gastrointestinal, peripheral
Urinary elimination, alteration in patterns
*Violence, potential for: self-directed or directed at others

*May be applicable to clients with psychiatric disorders.

From Kim, M.J., McFarland, G.K., & McLane, A: Classification of Nursing Diagnoses: Proceedings of the Fifth National Conference. St. Louis: Mosby, 1984. Reprinted with permission.

out prescriptive orders. As interventions are executed, the nurse observes client responses and adds any new or changing information to the data base.

Evaluating. The final step in the nursing process is evaluation. **Evaluation** is based on feedback and is concerned with outcomes projected by the interventions. Evaluation focuses on the changes in the client's behavior and health status. The evaluation may result in revision of the nursing diagnosis, modification of objectives, or changes in the interventions.

In summary, the nursing process then sets the stage for the delivery of care. In designing the nursing care plan, this second strategy enables the nurse to meet client needs in a logical, systematized fashion and also provides the basis for effecting standards of care, identifying predictable outcomes, as well as stimulating opportunities for clinical research.

The third strategy is that the nurse must write out the nursing care plan. Problem-solving and the nursing process have little impact on patient care until the outcomes of these actions become a written reality. The written nursing care plan is a basic form of communication concerning the care of the patient. Satisfactory, efficient, and relevant nursing care cannot be provided unless those assigned and held accountable for that care know what to do, when to do it, who is to do it, and what are the expected results. The written plan also permits the nurse to evaluate her approach and to introduce the necessary modifications to the original plan as nursing diagnoses become resolved, the goals and objectives are met, and the focus changes. A written nursing care plan provides for three important factors in patient care: **consistency**, **continuity**, and **coordination**. Thus, the written nursing care plan provides the nurse and all other staff members with a point of reference.

The fourth strategy is that the nurse must use the nursing care plan as an effective means of communication. To implement this strategy requires that the care plan forms the hub for shared information. For example, the care plan is the primary tool for giving report at the change of shift; for monitoring client progress; for sharing information with the interdisciplinary team; and for making referrals. Thus the nurse facilitates communication between herself and the client, between herself and her peers, and among other professionals.

This leads to the *fifth important strategy which is the nurse's obligation to preserve the patient's right to privileged communication.* This strategy means that the nurse takes all necessary measures to provide for confidentiality. These measures apply to records and record keeping, to written and verbal communication, and to the selection of the appropriate place and time to convey to other members of the health team private information about the patient. The nurse has a moral and ethical responsibility to insure that what the patient reveals to her is handled in a professional manner. Consent from the patient must be secured verbally, in writing, or both, before any information can be shared. It also means that nurses cannot exclude the patient from pertinent information concerning himself. The patient has a right to know such things as his temperature, test results, the names of medications prescribed for him, and treatment procedures to which he is being subjected. Currently there is much in the literature regarding the rights of patients. And, in fact, the importance of safeguarding patients' rights has resulted in a national movement that has sponsored legislation and a revision of probate court actions in many states. For the patient to provide "informed consent," he must have basic knowledge of what treatment entails and the expected outcome of that treatment. The patient has the right of access to any and all records that are kept on him. No one else but those immediately involved with health care delivery to him have the right of access to such information. The emphasis placed on confidentiality and the patient's right of access to information neither automatically absolves the nurse from exercising professional, ethical judgment regarding the amount and depth of information to be provided or withheld, nor permits her the "right" to make arbitrary choices.

Our *sixth strategy is that the nurse must report in a clear, concise, objective manner*. In the reporting process, the nurse assumes a liaison role between the patient and other care providers. As such, the nurse transmits significant information regarding the appearance, behavior, and conversation of the patient. This information adds to the existing data base and serves as another mechanism for continuing systematic communication among members of the health team. The report should contain only that information which is absolutely necessary for the ongoing care of the patient. In order to achieve this type of reporting, extraneous material such as personal opinions, value judgments, hypothetical speculations, and irrelevant, subjective comments must be eliminated. One benefit of objective reporting is enhancement of patient care because the mind of the reader or listener is free to look at the problem or situation without the introduction of subjective bias.

Strategy seven is that the nurse must engage in peer-group review. **Peer-group review** is a process in which the individual nurse, along with her nurse colleagues, assess and evaluate the quality of care that has been provided a particular patient. This review should be carried out according to established hospital criteria and the official American Nurses' Association Standards of Practice. The expected outcome of peer-group review is twofold: (1) assistance to the nurse in improving her practice and (2) holding the nurse accountable for that practice. Both of these outcomes insure that the patient is the recipient of the best possible care. It is directly related to the assurance of the quality of that care.

The eighth strategy is that the nurse is obliged to develop, exercise and maintain standards of care. The standards of care we refer to are those developed by the Congress for Nursing Practice of the American Nurses' Association (see Chapter 1). Everyone is not required to carry out procedures in an identical manner, but everyone is required to safeguard and adhere to the scientific principles on which the procedures are based. In addition, these standards require that the nurse not shortchange the patient and his care because of time, load, money or expediency. It means that the nurse takes time with the patient and, relates to the patient in such a way that he does not feel he is a burden or that his needs are less important than those of the patient across the hall. Adherence to standards for care manifests the nurse's appreciation for the dignity and worth of the person and also expresses the nurse's accountability for the delivery of effective patient care.

Strategy number nine is that the nurse must collaborate. **Collaboration** means the nurse actively seeks to share her knowledge and expertise. It implies that the nurse acknowledges and seeks to include the expertise peculiar to other members of the health team in carrying out the total treatment program of the patient. It means that the nurse volunteers pertinent information about the patient's progress and concerns to members of other involved disciplines. Collaboration benefits the nurse in that it allows her to seek consultation for the purpose of clarification and validation of her own nursing observations, assessments, and interventions and evaluation.

SUMMARY

Nursing care requires order and priority setting. These strategies are general prerequisites that the nurse needs to develop order and to set priorities in planning a sound, practical approach to the implementation of effective nursing care. Again, we reemphasize that some approaches and nursing care practices cut across all fields of practice, and each specialty area of practice must also operate on these. The uniqueness found in each specialty results primarily from the specific area of focus and the manifested needs of the patient. The constant is the framework, the nursing process, and the principles that govern its implementation and operation. What vary are the presenting concerns of the patient, the major symptoms associated with the problem, specific methods of intervention available, and the way in which the nurse implements and utilizes the potential of the creative therapeutic self.

The planning of effective nursing care requires the utilization of the nursing process in the construction of a written care plan. For us, nursing care goals remain constant. Individualization occurs and is determined by identifying each patient's unmet needs and selecting those goals that are applicable to him. These goals are subject to change as problems become resolved or as new needs arise. The nursing care plan makes explicit to all health care personnel nursing's contribution to the totality of patient care. Furthermore, the care plan serves as the written record of contract between the nurse and the patient and also as a means of holding the nurse responsible and accountable for her practice.

To formulate and implement a practical and usable nursing care plan, we have identified nine basic strategies that we consider essential. These strategies are: use problem-solving; implement the nursing process; translate the designed plan to a written format; use the written plan to facilitate communication; preserve privileged communication; report change, or effectiveness, or outcomes clearly, concisely, and objectively; evaluate outcomes through peer-group review; maintain nursing care standards; and lastly, seek collaboration to clarify and verify patient's progress or continued concerns. The outcome of the application of these strategies is an operational nursing care plan that has optimal potential for meeting patient needs and resolving patient problems. In Chapter 26 these strategies are applied in detail in what we consider an optimal, effective, and meaningful nursing care plan.

SUGGESTED READINGS

Atkinson, L. D., & Murray, M. E. *Understanding the Nursing Process.* New York: Macmillan, 1980.

Brooks, E. R. The Starting Point. *Nursing Management*, Vol. 14, No. 6 (1983), 35–37.

Carpenito, L. J. *Nursing Diagnosis: Application to Practice.* Philadelphia: Lippincott, 1983.

Costello, S., & Summers, B. Y. Documenting Patient Care: Getting It All Together. *Nursing Management*, Vol. 16, No. 6 (June, 1985), 31–32, 34.

Crispin, A. L. Nursing—A Role in Multidisciplinary Treatment Planning. *Journal of Psychiatric Nursing and Mental Health Services*, Vol. 18, No. 4 (April, 1980), 14–16.

Farrell, J. The Human Side of Assessment. *Nursing '80*, Vol. 10, No. 4 (April, 1980), 74–75.

Forman, M. Building a Better Nursing Care Plan. *American Journal of Nursing*, Vol. 79, No. 6 (June, 1979), 1086–1087.

Gay, P. Get It In Writing. *Nursing Management*, Vol. 14, No. 3 (March, 1983), 32–35.

Gebbie, K. M. Nursing Diagnosis: What It Is and Why Does It Exist. *Topics in Clinical Nursing*, Vol. 5, No. 4 (January, 1984), 1–9.

Gordon, M., Sweeney, M. A., & McKeehan, K. Nursing Diagnosis: Looking at Its Use in the Clinical Area. *American Journal of Nursing*, Vol. 80, No. 4 (April, 1980), 672–674.

Gray, J. W., & Aldred, H. Care Plans in Long-Term Facilities. *American Journal of Nursing*, Vol. 80, No. 11 (November, 1980), 2054-2057.

Hauser, M. J., & Feinberg, D. Problem Solving Revisited. *Journal of Psychiatric Nursing and Mental Health Services*, Vol. 15, No. 10 (October, 1977), 13–17.

Herje, P. A. Hows and Whys of Patient Contracting. *Nurse Educator*, Vol. 5, No. 1 (January/February, 1980), 30–34.

Jones, P. S. An Adaptation Model for Nursing Practice. *American Journal of Nursing*, Vol. 78, No. 11 (November, 1978), 1900-1906.

Kim, M. J., McFarland, G. K., & McLane, A. M., (eds.). *Pocket Guide to Nursing Diagnosis.* St. Louis: C. V. Mosby, 1984.

Lacey, L. A. Caution: Hospitalization Without Nursing Care Planning May Be Hazardous To Your Health! *Nursing Forum,* Vol. 21, No. 1 (1984), 24–27.

Lamonica, E. L. *The Nursing Process: A Humanistic Approach.* Menlo Park, Calif.: Addison-Wesley, 1979.

Langford, T. Establishing a Nursing Contract. *Nursing Outlook,* Vol. 26, No. 6 (June, 1978), 386–388.

Martin, E. J., & Finneran, M. R. A Teaching Design: Standards of Practice as a Basis for Peer Review. *Perspectives in Psychiatric Care,* Vol. 18, No. 6 (November/December, 1980), 242–248.

O'Sullivan, A. L. Privileged Communication. *American Journal of Nursing,* Vol. 80, No. 5 (May, 1980), 947–950.

Price, M. R. Nursing Diagnosis: Making a Concept Come Alive. *American Journal of Nursing,* Vol. 80, No. 4 (April, 1980), 668–671.

Putzier, D. J., & Padrick, K. P. Nursing Diagnosis: A Component of Nursing Process and Decision-Making. *Topics in Clinical Nursing,* Vol. 5, No. 4 (January, 1984), 21–29.

Reynolds, J. I. Assessing Your Patient's Mental Status. *Nursing '79,* Vol. 9, No. 8 (August, 1979), 26–33.

Schmadl, J. C. Quality Assurance: Examination of the Concept. *Nursing Outlook,* Vol. 27, No. 7 (July, 1979), 462–466.

Stuart, M. et al. The Nursing Care Plan: A Communications System That Really Works. *Nursing '78,* Vol. 8, No. 8 (August, 1978), 28–33.

Vasey, E. K. Writing Your Patient's Care Plan . . . Effectively. *Nursing '79,* Vol. 9, No. 4 (April, 1979), 67-71.

Vengroski, S. M., & Saarman, L. Peer Review in Quality Assurance. *American Journal of Nursing,* Vol. 78, No. 12 (December, 1978), 2094–2096.

Webb, T. E., Adams, M. R., & VanDevere, C. A. Listening Reliably To Psychosocial Concerns, of Youth. *Journal of Psychosocial Nursing and Mental Health Services,* Vol. 21, No. 6 (June, 1983), 25–28.

Wilson, H. S., & Plumly S., Diagnostic Labeling: The Rotten Apple Stigma. *Journal of Psychosocial Nursing and Mental Health Services,* Vol. 24, No. 10 (October, 1984), 7–10.

Woody, A. F., et al. Do Patients Learn What Nurses Say They Teach. *Nursing Management,* Vol. 15, No. 12 (December, 1984), 26–29.

Yura, H. & Walsh, M. B. *The Nursing Process: Assessing, Planning, Implementing, Evaluating.* 3rd ed. New York: Appleton-Century-Crofts, 1978.

Zangari, M. E., & Duffy, P. Contracting with Patients in Day-to-Day Practice. *American Journal of Nursing,* Vol. 80, No. 3 (March, 1980), 451–455.

VI

NURSING INTERVENTION

The Core of Professional Nursing Practice

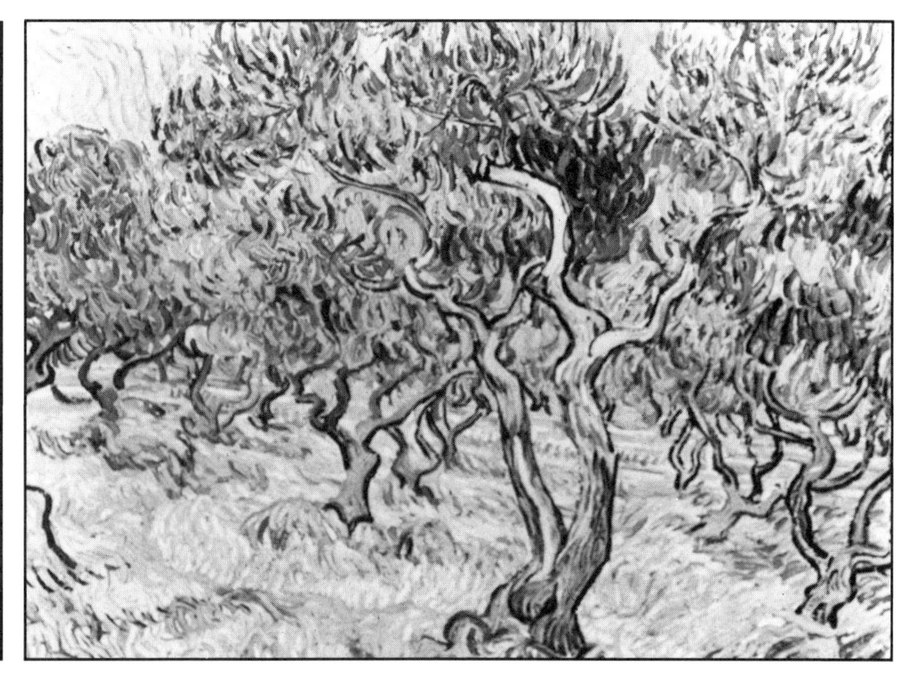

20

NURSING INTERVENTION FOR PATIENTS EXPERIENCING THOUGHT DISTORTIONS

LEARNING OBJECTIVES

On completion of this chapter the reader should be able to:

1. Identify the four major areas of disruption in the thought process.
2. Distinguish among each of the identified problems.
3. Identify specific nursing interventions for each of the problem areas.
4. Understand the rationale on which each intervention is based.
5. State specific concepts and principles underlying nursing intervention for clients experiencing thought disorders.

INTRODUCTION

The mind is a multisensory data bank of a million moments of "now." Thought is a functioning process of the brain that regulates the barometer of daily living experiences. It is the filtering and processing mechanism for the integration of inputs from the micro and macro environments. At the same time, the thought process is the output center of the brain; through speech, behavior, and body language the thought process overtly announces the physical and emotional status of the individual to others and the environs.

This chapter is concerned with nursing interventions for patients experiencing distortions in the thought process. Using NANDA's diagnostic classification system, we identify four common distortions requiring intervention: disorientation, inability to follow directions, inability to focus on reality, and illogical and unreasonable sequences of thought perception. These distortions are the presenting problem of defining characteristic. The underlying dynamics associated with each of the identified distortions become the etiologic segment of the full diagnostic statement. Thus, a sample nursing diagnostic statement reflective of a thought distortion might read: Thought Processes, Alterations in, in relation to aging as evidenced by disorientation.

> The primary nursing care goal for patients with a nursing diagnosis of Thought Processes, Alterations in, is reorientation to reality.

The specific long- and short-term behavioral objectives are derived from the data base and resulting patient profile. Therefore, the interventions detailed within this chapter are directed toward the primary goal and are not described with the specificity required by the uniqueness presented within each patient's care situation.

The concepts and principles underlying our discussion in this chapter are listed below. These have value and application in guiding the formulation of nursing interventions on behalf of and in cooperation with a person experiencing disruption in cognitive functioning.

1. All behavior has meaning.
2. Reality can produce pleasure as well as pain.
3. Too much or too little sensory input reduces the client's capacity and ability to adapt.
4. Environmental conditions and surroundings have impact on receptivity and can either enhance or detract from reality orientation.
5. Heightened levels of anxiety decrease the individual's ability to accurately perceive and assess situations and circumstances.
6. Reduction in the level of anxiety increases potential and receptivity to learning new patterns of behavior.
7. Exaggeration of normal adaptations is employed to protect the self from pain.

8. An increase in the number or variety of alternative coping mechanisms increases the individual's potential for successful adaptation to life and living.
9. Identification of logical thought sequences and ability to engage in abstract thinking provide a basis for assessing where an individual is in relation to "normal."
10. Healthy perception occurs when what the individual perceives corresponds to what is actually present.
11. Integration of sensory perception promotes a balance of positive psychic forces within the individual.
12. Focusing on immediate events heightens awareness and promotes reorientation to reality.
13. Familiar routines and people contribute to security.
14. Breaks or interruptions in established routines destroy the client's sense of security and well-being.
15. Satisfying relationships are an important factor in the maintenance of psychological equilibrium.
16. Introduction of new material (such as a hospital ward regime) must be done simply and gradually.
17. Repetition is a necessary reinforcer to promote behavioral change.
18. Selection of and participation in activities should be based on familiar life experiences and patterns.
19. Competitive experiences tend to increase the intensity of the presenting problem as well as increase the client's vulnerability to feelings of inadequacy and worthlessness.
20. Intellectual level, sociocultural background, and value system must be identified and incorporated when planning care.
21. An individual's self-worth, self-esteem, and integrity are enhanced by acceptance, respect, and concern for his well-being.
22. Family or significant others need reassurance, guidance, and support to deal with possible feelings of frustration, inadequacy, and potential guilt and rejection.

DISORIENTATION

Disorientation is specifically described as a disruption in an individual's cognitive and perceptual ability to sustain awareness of self with respect to surroundings. The most frequent manifestations of disorientation occur in relationship to the dimensions of time, place, and person. Disorientation to time is demonstrated when an individual has difficulty in remembering, keeping track of, or interpreting the current date, time of day, month, year, and season. In addition, distortions in time perception and associations may be exhibited through a lack of awareness of the passage of time, that is, the individual experiences a disruption in time sequencing. Thus, the patient is unable to state clearly how long and in which order events have taken place. This disturbance in temporal continuity is most frequently the initial cue to the nurse that the patient is experiencing loss of orientation.

As disorientation to time progresses and becomes increasingly acute, disorientation to place often follows. Behavior manifestations associated with disorientation to place include an inability to locate or identify new places (surroundings); difficulty in finding or recognizing previously familiar sites; or a failure to identify one's own place of residence or location. As the patient becomes disoriented to his surroundings, he also becomes increasingly more suspicious, agitated, and hostile.

When disorientation to person is experienced, the individual displays difficulty in identifying the people within the immediate environment, particularly new faces. In addition to the lack of recognition, there may also be an inability to comprehend and appreciate interrelationships between self and others, as well as loss of self-identity. When an individual experiences this latter phenomenon, he is unable to state who he is, where he comes from, and the purpose for which he finds himself in his present surroundings.

As indicated by the sequencing of content, disorientation can occur on a progressively deteriorating continuum ranging from mild confusion to the most severe manifestation— loss of personal identity. For the nurse this means that within the assessment process, she must pay attention to etiological factors in order to determine the client's ability to function. This attention to cause is critical if realistic objectives are to be set.

Disruptions in orientation frequently produce a concomitant and corresponding wide range of emotional responses. This spectrum of emotional responses has a direct impact on the patient's ability to maintain an adequately independent or optimal level of functioning in his daily life. Significant emotional responses that are most likely to occur, most often occur, and contribute to the individual's deterioration in intrapersonal and interpersonal relations are: heightened levels of anxiety as the needs for safety and security are threatened; frustration when the individual identifies a perceived conflict between what is and what should be; fear that arises out of the individual's perception of invasion of personal spaces; anger when others appear to disregard what the individual acknowledges as his reality; rage when attempts are made to refocus and reorient; and lastly, hostility that arises out of the individual's attempt to cope with an "alien world."

To promote and maintain a therapeutic atmosphere conducive to reorientation, the nurse should approach the patient in a calm, nonthreatening, composed manner. This approach is conveyed through control of facial expression and body posture. The nurse is careful that her expression does not mirror surprise, fear, or laughter at any statement or set of behaviors exhibited by the patient. Instead, her attitude is one of assurance, hopefulness, and helpfulness.

Specific interventions that have been found to be effective in dealing with the problem of disorientation are included in Table 20–1. They are divided according to the three dimensions of time, place, and person.

TABLE 20–1. DISORIENTATION—INTERVENTION AND RATIONALE

Time	
Intervention	***Rationale***
Make available to the patient a clock, a calendar, a daily newspaper, and *current* magazines.	To establish continuous, consistent, ready feedback.
Provide access to radio or television and evaluate the patient's interpretation of the broadcasted material.	To help the patient remain active and alert through use of visual and auditory stimuli.
Refer to specific dates, times, and events. For example: "Mr. Jones, it is noon—time for lunch"; "Mrs. Jones, it is 2 o'clock—time for you to take your pill."	To orient the patient to time sequences.
Encourage staff, other patients, and family members to talk about time-related activity.	To provide security, diminish anxiety, and reinforce continuous time input.
Provide access to and encourage patient's participation in current community or hospital activities and functions, such as baseball or football games, a Christmas party, July 4th picnic, or trips to restaurants or shopping centers.	To establish associations between time and activity and to prevent further deterioration and disorientation.
Check frequently and know the whereabouts of the patient at all times.	To provide protection and safety for the patient.
Maintain a consistent time schedule.	To provide a sense of security and to establish time reference points.
Give the patient a copy of his daily schedule.	To increase his feeling of self-worth and to provide him with a frame of reference.
Assist in helping client to order recent events according to time sequence.	To provide verbal feedback and reinforcement of continuous time input.
Place	
Intervention	***Rationale***
Tell the patient where he is: identify the hospital, ward, and room number; repeat all information as needed.	To decrease anxiety, to increase awareness, and to promote a feeling of security.
Show the patient a picture of the hospital or supply the patient with a hospital brochure.	To reinforce verbal statements regarding whereabouts.

(*continued*)

TABLE 20–1. CONTINUED

Place	
Intervention	***Rationale***
Have the patient explore and investigate his room and ward setting.	To maximize contact with reality through the use of sensory perception.
Designate the patient's room with a nameplate on the door.	To decrease frustration and to provide a means of increasing independent functioning.
Label frequently used rooms with names/pictures/ symbols to represent their function (e.g., toilet).	To promote orientation to surroundings through visual reinforcement and to foster independence.
Explain sounds the patient might hear, for example, the closing of the elevator door, carts being wheeled through the hall, and the paging and ward intercommunication system.	To decrease fear responses and to prevent mounting levels of anxiety.
Identify personnel by title: nurse, physician, nursing assistant.	To establish points of reference in reality.
Accompany the patient when he leaves the ward.	To provide protection and safety for the patient.
Provide for night lights.	To assist with visual orientation.
Maintain in familiar surroundings.	To facilitate highest level of functioning.

Person	
Intervention	***Rationale***
Address the patient by name and title.	To reestablish and reinforce identity.
Instruct staff, patients, and visitors to address the patient by name and state their own name, title, and relationship to him.	To prevent confusion, to reinforce reality, and to establish a pattern of consistency.
Permit the patient to keep personal possessions such as clothes, books, pictures, or significant mementos.	To maintain a sense of personal identity in an atmosphere that is alien to the patient.
Label clothing and possessions with the patient's name.	To establish a point of reference for the patient and to prevent others from encroaching on the patient's identity.
Provide the patient with and encourage him to carry an identification card.	To provide a tangible means of identification.
Explore with the patient his perception of self and reinforce reality when appropriate.	To correct misinterpretations and to provide consensual validation and feedback.
Plan and implement a consistent approach.	To decrease threat to security, thereby reducing anxiety resulting from change.

INABILITY TO FOLLOW DIRECTIONS

Inability to follow directions is a cognitive dysfunction in which the individual experiences a blockage of or interference with the reception of communicated messages, resulting in misinterpretation and misunderstanding. Characteristically, the individual who manifests this inaccurate interpretation of stimuli and resultant cognitive dysfunction displays confusion, appears constantly preoccupied, exhibits a faulty or fragmented memory pattern, and exhibits markedly increased feelings of fear and hostility along with a decrease in overall stimulus reception and response. In addition, there are two paradoxical patient responses that need to be called to the nurse's attention—withdrawal and aggression. In the case of withdrawal, the patient is isolating himself from potential threats while in the case of aggression, the patient is using a preservation tactic to prevent perceived harm.

Patients who frequently display the inability to follow directions are those who may be described as being depressed, psychotic, organic, or who have been hospitalized for a long period of time and are referred to as having institutional chronicity. Cultivation of an unhurried, patient, reassuring approach by the nurse along with the adoption of the positive, empathetic attitudes of personal worth, hopefulness, and involvement are perhaps the most effective basis for intervention needed to assist the patient in sorting out the real from the unreal.

Specific interventions found to be effective in dealing with the inability to follow directions are shown in Table 20–2.

TABLE 20–2. INABILITY TO FOLLOW DIRECTIONS—INTERVENTION AND RATIONALE

Intervention	Rationale
Use simple, concrete language when talking with the patient.	To reduce the possibility of misinterpretation and confusion.
Be direct.	To present clear messages.
Speak clearly in a quiet, well-modulated tone.	To decrease distortions and to promote a feeling of comfort.
Repeat for the patient instructions or information as often as needed.	To insure that the patient has heard and understood and to decrease the patient's frustration.
Ask the patient to restate instructions or information.	To correct misinterpretations immediately.
Observe the patient's behavior.	To determine effectiveness of instructions.
Remind and reorient the patient with respect to the usual daily routines.	To reduce confusion and to help the patient develop a pattern for daily living.
Provide the patient with needed instructions immediately prior to any procedure or activity.	To decrease anxiety and to contribute toward the successful completion of the activity.
Provide instructions in simple, serial steps.	To facilitate accomplishment and to protect self-esteem.
Write out instructions or schedules as needed.	To provide the patient with a handy reference.
Encourage the patient to ask questions.	To assist the patient in clarification of thoughts.
Label clearly and legibly such areas as the bathroom, the lounge, the physician's office, and the patient's room.	To promote environmental awareness and a sense of security for the patient.
Utilize past patterns for recall.	To minimize new learning necessary for compliance.
Limit sensory input.	To decrease the amount of stimuli (distractors).

(continued)

TABLE 20–2. CONTINUED

Intervention	Rationale
Limit choices.	To decrease frustration.
Provide adequate lighting in halls, bathrooms, etc.	To minimize confusion, thereby reducing fear and promoting security.
Make frequent rounds at night.	To provide reassurance, comfort, and safety.
Make use of volunteers to sit with the patient when staff are not available.	To provide comfort, to promote a sense of security, and to convey concern.
Make sure areas such as the medication room or the cleaning and supply cupboards are inaccessible to the patient.	To promote safety.
Make frequent, *brief* contacts throughout the day.	To maintain the patient's contact with reality; to provide reassurance and demonstrate concern.
Provide a night light for the patient's room.	To provide safety and to reduce visual, environmental distortions.

INABILITY TO FOCUS ON REALITY

The inability to focus on reality is excessive reliance on the use of automatic defensive operations as a primary mode of adaptation in order to avoid, eliminate, distort or manipulate current living experiences that are either consciously or unconsciously perceived by the individual as a threat to biological or psychological integrity. This clinical problem can be identified in those individuals who manifest circumstantiality and flight of ideas in order to avoid the threat reality holds for them. Because this avoidance results in movement away from reality, the patient will usually display marked anxiety, distrust, and fear of becoming involved. Behavioral manifestations include: suspiciousness of other people—their intent toward him and the accompanying fear of possible harm by them; distortions or exaggerations of what exists; isolation, agitation, hostility, anger, and identity crisis; and confused, incoherent speech patterns. The nurse should use an approach that is slow, deliberate, and cautiously friendly. Her attitude should be one of subdued warmth, integrity, and openmindedness. These attitudes are displayed through the presentation of the nurse as an individual who wishes to be helpful and to make known the facts, and who is willing to be available but does not force communication. Rather, the nurse, after assuming the initiative, steps back and waits for the patient to take the lead.

Specific interventions the nurse might adopt to facilitate the goal of reality reorientation for those patients who display an inability to focus on reality are shown in Table 20–3.

TABLE 20–3. INABILITY TO FOCUS ON REALITY—INTERVENTION AND RATIONALE

Intervention	Rationale
Verbally express recognition to the patient of his loss of contact with reality.	To assure the patient that his problem is known and acknowledged by those providing care.
Encourage the patient to be actively involved in current activities.	To increase the patient's contact with reality and to decrease the fear of involvement with others.
Demonstrate interest in the patient's physical well-being.	To establish trust and to indicate concern.
Redirect patient's anger into appropriate channels such as work or recreational activities that require the expenditure of physical energy.	To promote socially acceptable behavior and to decrease the possibility of inappropriate acting out.
Control the patient's environment with respect to noise, lights, people, and activities.	To decrease the environmental distractions that tend to stimulate inappropriate responses.
Limit activity in which competition is a significant factor.	To reduce stress, anxiety, hostility, and frustration.
Provide simple tasks.	To allow for successful completion and so increase the patient's feeling of self-worth.
Give merited recognition.	To build self-esteem and to increase trust and rapport with the nurse.
Maintain spatial distance between the nurse and the patient.	To promote comfort, to provide maneuvering room, and to decrease anxiety.
Keep promises.	To promote trust and to reduce fear.
Be honest and open.	To facilitate communication and to promote trust.
Supply needed facts.	To increase understanding and to prevent distortions and doubts.
Invite, not demand, patient response.	To allow the patient to move at his own pace.
Interrupt and refocus meaningless communication and purposeless activity.	To reestablish contact with reality.
Present and discuss alternatives.	To assist the patient to find and use more effective methods of adaptation.
Confront inappropriate and unacceptable behavior.	To help the patient to recognize the inappropriateness of his behavior.
Ask the patient to make realistic commitments.	To help the patient assume responsibility for his behavior.
Hold the patient accountable for fulfillment of commitments.	To maintain and reinforce reality expectations of responsible behavior.

ILLOGICAL AND UNREASONABLE SEQUENCE OF THOUGHT PERCEPTION

Illogical and unreasonable sequence of thought perception is a cognitive dysfunction in which the individual exhibits false or unrealistic verbal and behavioral manifestations resulting from distorted or exaggerated sensory perception. The individual is responding to the distorted or exaggerated sensory integration from within the context of the preconscious and unconscious mind. This means the reason this distortion or exaggeration occurs is that the individual has experienced overwhelming distress or a traumatic event causing suppression of reality and producing a blockage of reality because of associations. In the client's effort to ward off the traumatic event, he escapes into the illogical and unreasonable thought perception. Thus, the person's total reality is known only to himself, and based on this, his everyday living pattern is enacted from a distorted base. The layperson's term for the individual who responds and functions almost totally from an illogical and unreasonable sequence of thought perception is "crazy." The reader should keep in mind that the previously described clinical problems of disorientation, inability to follow directions, and inability to focus on reality are often conditions within the normal context of everyday living that can be and often are socially tolerated and viewed as "egocentricities." However, illogical and unreasonable thought perception in its most acute form is viewed as deviance from the norm.

In addition, illogical and unreasonable thought perception also may be found in persons whose ideas tend to be rigid, repetitive, and excessively personalized. Consequently, there is a marked decrease in the person's ability to communicate because of this rigidity, misinterpretation, and personally subjective responses. The patient is able to verbalize, but the meaning and intent of the message are not always readily apparent since their significance is known only to the patient. Because of the incoherent speech and lack of ability to be understood, the patient experiences frustration, anxiety, suspicion, rejection, and isolation. In order to assist the patient in achieving contact with reality and decreased distortion, the nurse must understand the dynamics of thought disorders and approach the patient with persistent effort and consistent acceptance. The nurse must approach the patient in a nonthreatening manner and with the attitudes of advocacy and therapeutic involvement. Specific interventions found to be effective in dealing with the clinical problem of illogical and unreasonable sequence of thought perception are included in Table 20–4.

TABLE 20–4. ILLOGICAL AND UNREASONABLE SEQUENCE OF THOUGHT PERCEPTION—INTERVENTION AND RATIONALE

Intervention	Rationale
Initiate frequent, regular contacts with the patient.	To provide contact with reality and to promote trust.
Remain with the patient despite silence, inappropriate behavior, or ineffective communication.	To express unconditional acceptance, interest, and concern.
Remain expectant and focus attention on the patient.	To convey interest, attention, and respect for the patient.

TABLE 20–4. CONTINUED

Intervention	Rationale
Listen carefully to the patient.	To pick up cues from the patient that will assist the nurse in the decoding of messages.
Pay attention to details and avoid speaking in generalities.	To reinforce reality by separating the real from the unreal.
Verify interpretations.	To assist the patient in the use of consensual validation for the establishment of a reality orientation.
Clarify patient's use of the generalized "they."	To make communication explicit.
Identify and clarify with the patient differences between his thoughts, feelings, and behavior.	To assist the patient in sorting out discrepancies in these areas.
Tell the patient that his message is not understood or followed.	To act as a "sounding board" for reality feedback.
Question illogical thinking.	To interrupt the progression of illogical thought and to reorient the patient to reality.
Set limits on and openly discourage "crazy talk."	To discourage the patient's preoccupation with fantasy.
Refrain from responding to the "crazy talk" as if the meaning were clearly understood.	To prevent falsification of reality with resulting loss of trust.
Refocus communication on the present.	To restore psychological equilibrium.
Confront the patient with his thoughts and encourage him to make judgments regarding them.	To help the patient sort out the real from the unreal.
Create situations in which the patient is likely to experience success.	To provide new, corrective, satisfying experiences to replace negative attitudes about self.
Respect requests.	To develop trust, convey respect, and to maintain integrity.
Prevent physiological and psychological overstimulation by such actions as temperature control, maintenance of nutrition, and reduction in self-threat situations.	To provide comfort, safety, and protection.
Provide explanations for changes in daily routine.	To prevent hostility and to increase trust.
Observe the patient and identify behavior that indicates specific pattern responses to illogical thinking.	To develop a base for planning effective intervention.
Prevent and protect the patient from inaccurate sensory perceptions by such actions as the initiation of immediate contact with the patient, reduction of personal and environmental hazards, and physical removal of the patient from the stress situation.	To provide safety, security, comfort, and reduction in anxiety for the patient.
Interrupt disturbed thinking process through the use of simple daily activities.	To maintain reality orientation and to decrease preoccupation with fantasy.
Provide a time and place in which the patient may remain quiet and undisturbed.	To reduce environmental stress.
Focus on the healthy aspects of the patient's personality.	To make use of patient's assets in order to increase his functioning.

TABLE 20–5. EVALUATION CRITERIA—THOUGHT PROCESSES, ALTERATIONS IN

Evidenced of Alteration	Evaluation Criteria
Disorientation	Is oriented to time, place, and person: Identifies self. Distinguishes between self and others. Responds to name when addressed. Keeps appointments. Differentiates activities according to passage of time. Can move about in environment as needed. States where he is.
Inability to follow direction	Follows directions: Remembers instructions. Repeats information accurately. Carries out specified actions or tasks. Receptive to messages. Understands messages. Verbalizes comfortableness. Alert and calm. Decreased expressions indicative of fear or hostility.
Inability to focus on reality	Focuses on reality: Organized and purposeful in action. Displays a readiness to engage in the interactive process. Participates in social interaction. Diminished reliance on automatic coping devices. Evidences increased problem-solving ability. Attends to specifics. Places events in proper perspective. Verbalizes expressions of trust, feelings of security, and confidence in self or others. Coherent speech patterns.
Illogical and unreasonable sequence of thought	Perceives accurately: Organized and purposeful in action. Ceases to experience or express hallucinations, delusions, or illusions. Manifests verbal and behavioral congruency. Participates in purposeful activities. Relates to others. Seeks out others. Demonstrates flexibility and openness to differing points of view. Expresses subjective statements indicating the presence of personal integrity and self-worth.

EVALUATION

A list of projected outcomes for each of the problems discussed in this chapter is found in Table 20–5. The evaluation criteria are based on the primary nursing care goal–reorientation to reality. This listing is general in scope and is intended to serve only as an example. It is important for the reader to note that outcome criteria are derived through the identification of the optimal expectations to be achieved with each individual patient.

SUMMARY

We have selected to address in this chapter four of the major cognitive problems encountered by nurses in their clinical practice with clients who experience disturbances or distortions in their thought processes—disorientation, inability to follow directions, inability to focus on reality, and illogical and unreasonable sequence of thought perception.

We have identified the primary treatment aim as reorientation to life and living—reality. Further, we have provided a brief definition and overview of each clinical problem and have presented to the reader essential concepts and principles upon which specific nursing interventions were developed. Moreover, we have included a section on evaluation that details in part those criteria the nurse may find useful as she engages in assessing the client's responses to nursing interventions.

We caution the reader to note that there exists no easy path or shortcut method to accomplishing optimal therapeutic goals. Effective nursing practice demands use of the nursing process in a consistent, concerted, empathetic, and dynamic manner. As the nurse incorporates the interventive strategies detailed in this chapter and becomes more skillful in the use of the therapeutic self, she will then be able to begin to add contructively, in an organized and systematized manner, to the foundation of formalized nursing theory.

SUGGESTED READINGS

Adams, M., et al. Psychological Response in Critical Care Units. *American Journal of Nursing*, Vol. 78, No. 9 (September, 1978), 1504–1512.

Alford, D. M. Expanding Older Persons' Belief Systems. *Topics in Clinical Nursing*, Vol. 3, No. 4 (January, 1982), 35–44.

Arnold, H. M. Working with Schizophrenic Patients. Four A's: A Guide to One-to-One Relationships. *American Journal of Nursing*, Vol. 76, No. 6 (June, 1976), 941–943.

Bozian, M. W., & Clark, H. M. Counteracting Sensory Changes in the Aging. *American Journal of Nursing*, Vol. 80, No. 3 (March, 1980), 473–476.

Burns, D. D. *Feeling Good*. New York: New American Library, 1981.

Clark, B. What To Do When Your Patient Lets Slip His Grip on Reality. *Nursing '84*, Vol. 14, No. 7 (July, 1984), 50–55.

Cook, J. Interpreting and Decoding Autistic Communication. *Perspectives in Psychiatric Care*, Vol. 9, No. 1 (1971), 24–29.

Davidhizar, R., Gunden, E., & Wehlage, D. Recognizing and Caring for the Delirious Patient. *Journal of Psychiatric Nursing and Mental Health Services*, Vol. 16, No. 5 (May, 1978), 38–41.

Dodd, M. J. Assessing Mental Status. *American Journal of Nursing*. Vol. 78, No. 9 (September, 1978). 1500–1503.

Field, W. E. Hearing Voices. *Journal of Psychosocial Nursing and Mental Health Services*, Vol. 23, No. 1 (January, 1985), 9–14.

Hirschfeld, M. J. The Cognitively Impaired Older Adult. *American Journal of Nursing*, Vol. 76, No. 12 (December, 1976), 1981–1984.

Knowles, R. D. Control Your Thoughts. *American Journal of Nursing*, Vol. 81, No. 2 (February, 1981), 353.

Knowles, R. D. Disrupting Irrational Thought. *American Journal of Nursing*, Vol. 81, No. 4 (April, 1981), 735.

Kroner, K. Dealing with a Confused Patient. *Nursing '79*, Vol. 9, No. 11 (November, 1979), 71–79.

La Monica, E. L. *The Humanistic Nursing Process*. Monterey, Calif.: Wadsworth Health Sciences Division, 1985.

Lore, A. Supporting the Hospitalized Elderly Patient. *American Journal of Nursing*, Vol. 79, No. 3 (March, 1979), 496–499

McFarland, G., & Wasli, E. *Nursing Diagnoses and Process in Psychiatric Mental Health Nursing*. Philadelphia: Lippincott, 1986.

Meyd, C. J. Acute Brain Trauma. *American Journal of Nursing*, Vol. 78, No. 1 (January, 1979), 40–44.

Montmeny, R. Perception. *Journal of Psychiatric Nursing and Mental Health Services*, Vol, 18, No. 6 (June, 1980), 22–27.

Rodman, M. J. Controlling Acute and Chronic Schizophrenia. *R.N.*, Vol. 41 (April, 1978), 75–83.

Schwartzman, S. T. The Hallucinating Patient and Nursing Intervention. *Journal of Psychiatric Nursing and Mental Health Services*, Vol. 13, No. 6 (November/December, 1976), 23–28, 33–36.

Tolbert, B. M. Reality Orientation and Remotivation in a Long-Term-Care Facility. *Nursing and Health Care*, Vol. 5 No. 1 (January, 1984), 40–44.

Trockman, G. Caring for the Confused or Delirious Patient. *American Journal of Nursing*, Vol. 78, No. 9 (September, 1978), 1495–1499.

Wilkinson, O. Out of Touch with Reality. *American Journal of Nursing*, Vol. 78, No. 9 (September, 1978), 1492–1494.

21

NURSING INTERVENTION FOR PATIENTS EXPERIENCING FEELING DISTURBANCES

LEARNING OBJECTIVES

On completion of this chapter the reader should be able to:

1. Identify the seven major areas of disturbed feelings.
2. Distinguish among each of the identified feeling states.
3. Identify specific nursing interventions for each emotional state.
4. State the rationale for each of the interventive techniques.
5. Apply specific concepts and principles underlying nursing intervention for clients experiencing disturbed feelings.

INTRODUCTION

The seven major areas of disturbed feeling selected for inclusion within this chapter are anxiety, fear, anger, loneliness, grief, pain, and guilt. Each represents a *real* and *human* feeling. They are called into being as an individual's affective response to crises, threats, or seemingly uncontrollable situations. It is when these subjective responses become intensified, exaggerated, or prolonged that pathology develops. These disturbances may occur for two reasons: as a result of the individual's inability to distinguish the appropriateness or inappropriateness of the response, or as a result of the individual's growing dependence on the same response as a mode of adjustment or adaptation to *all* situations regardless of similarities or differences.

To date, NANDA has approached the classification of feelings disturbances by isolating specific feelings such as anxiety or anger and making each a specific diagnostic category. However, we think that a diagnostic category could exist for affective disturbances as a whole similiar to the NANDA category of detailed alterations in thought processes. Thus, the major diagnostic classification could be **feeling disturbances**, using the specific feeling as the designated defining characteristic. The etiological portion of the diagnostic statement would continue to refer to underlying dynamics. An example of such a diagnostic statement might read: *Feeling disturbance related to a threat to self-esteem as evidenced by anxiety.*

> The primary nursing care goal is to sustain the patient during periods of discomfort while assisting him to learn new methods of adaptation and coping.

The specific long- and short-term behaviorial objectives evolve from the data base and resulting patient profile. Thus, the interventions detailed within this chapter are directed toward the primary nursing care goal rather than the specificity required by the uniqueness presented within each patient's care situation.

The concepts and principles underlying our discussion in this chapter are listed below. These have value and application in guiding the formulation of nursing interventions on behalf of and in cooperation with a person experiencing disturbances in the affective areas of functioning.

1. Feelings are essential to survival.
2. Feelings are subjective phenomena that are only inferred from behavior.
3. Feelings can be transmitted interpersonally.
4. Exaggerated feelings interfere with normal functioning, generate negative behavior, and increase the level of discomfort.
5. Avoidance of feelings leads to a constricted, uncreative, and unrealistic mode of life and living.
6. Mind and body function in concert with each other.
7. Cultural variables influence affective responses.

8. Anxiety is unavoidable.
9. Anxiety narrows or prejudices perception, interferes with learning, and produces clinical symptomatology.
10. Fear is a learned response.
11. Social isolation is indicative of a disruption in the early stages of the developmental process.
12. Investment in warm, satisfying relationships increases vulnerability to painful experiences.
13. Perception of pain is influenced by the physical and psychological equilibrium of an individual.
14. Methods of defensive functioning are minimized or reduced when an individual believes that he has been heard and understood.
15. A genuine expression of caring promotes positive feelings.
16. Awareness of feelings is the first step toward effective intervention.
17. Effective intervention requires the rechanneling of psychic energy in a constructive manner.
18. Listening promotes sharing; sharing of feelings lessens pain and discomfort.
19. Altered feeling states can be affected positively by the use of cognitive-behavioral approaches, resulting in decreased intensity or reduction of clinical pathology.
20. Effective learning involves working through feelings about currently held attitudes and beliefs as well as the new values being considered.
21. The demonstration of effective learning is measured by positive modification of behavior.
22. Acquisition of new or modified attitudes and values occurs gradually over time.
23. Conflict resolution is not effective if care providers attempt to impose personal values or beliefs on clients.
24. Motivation is greatest when the need is recognized and the proposed change meets the need.
25. Positive, satisfying experiences can be used to correct or modify developmental and maturational deficits.

ANXIETY

Anxiety is a feeling state in which the individual experiences a pervasive, vague, intense sensation of apprehension or impending disaster. It is manifested as a disproportionate reaction to life events. Anxiety is caused either by threats to an individual's self-system or by threats to his biological integrity. This means that any situation that places the individual in jeopardy, either emotionally or physically, produces a feeling of "dis-ease," which, in turn, results in a concomitant disruption in the individual's ability to function. Because of the variations in the levels of anxiety experienced and because of its pervasiveness, the individual feels a wide range of subjective responses. These responses range from a generalized sensation of uncomfortableness to a state of panic. For review of the concept of anxiety, the reader is directed to Chapter 7.

The most effective approach the nurse can assume in dealing with this type of distorted apprehension is one of thoughtful, calm objectivity. The nurse can best accomplish this approach through the expression of genuine concern for the patient and his well-being; by minimizing environmental stresses that may add to or increase the patient's level of anxiety; and by supporting and encouraging his ability to resolve the anxiety-provoking issues together with her. This nursing intervention requires that the nurse's attitude convey to the patient her sense of his personal worth along with her advocacy and hopefulness.

Specific nursing interventions found to be effective in dealing with the clinical problem of anxiety are included in Table 21–1.

TABLE 21–1. ANXIETY—INTERVENTION AND RATIONALE

Intervention	Rationale
Acknowledge the presence of anxiety.	To determine where the patient is; to determine the degree which the patient's level of functioning is impaired; and to identify what approach will serve in the best interest of the patient.
Recognize behavior patterns that indicate signs of mounting anxiety.	To establish a basis for the planning of individualized care and to prevent the anxiety from becoming more diffused.
Identify and explore anxiety provoking issues.	To establish causations and to set priorities.
Listen willingly.	To provide relief and to convey unqualified acceptance.
Assist the patient to identify what he thought or felt prior to the onset of anxiety.	To help discover the cause of the triggering event.
Discuss expectations and the differences between expectations and outcomes.	To assist the patient to identify discrepancies between expectations and "real" outcomes.
Explore details of similar experiences.	To establish the sequence of events in the development of the patient's anxiety.
Encourage the patient to identify his anxiety as anxiety.	To develop awareness in the patient.
Explore what mechanisms, if any, produced relief in the past.	To develop awareness and to evaluate effectiveness of the mechanism.
Explore possible alternatives with the patient.	To identify potential successful coping mechanisms.

TABLE 21–1. CONTINUED

Intervention	Rationale
Investigate somatic complaints: check vital signs, make physical assessments, and report findings to the physician.	To rule out and avoid overlooking the possibility of the presence of physical illness and to maintain and strengthen the bond of trust between the nurse and the patient.
Inform the patient of test results.	To maintain the nurse's integrity and to provide relief and reassurance for the patient.
Deter the patient from dwelling on physical symptomatology.	To provide the patient with relief by moving focus of attention from self and symptoms.
Refrain from asking the patient how he feels.	To discourage dwelling on the problem.
Provide patient with a full schedule of daily activities.	To involve the patient and thereby decrease the amount of time for introspection and obsessive preoccupation.
Base activity program around old or known interests.	To prevent adding stress and to insure success.
Provide suitable outlets for "working off" excess energy: cleaning the unit, running errands, and assisting with routine activities.	To create a feeling of usefulness and to provide a means by which the nurse can give merited praise to strengthen the ego.
Adhere to schedules and to patient's requests promptly.	To prevent anxiety from mounting and to convey the nurse's genuine concern.
Stay with the patient when anxiety is mounting, even if it means pacing the corridor with him.	To convey acceptance and to make use of any opportunity that might become available to reduce anxiety and to help the patient become more comfortable.
Assess the patient's need for medication and dispense if indicated.	To provide relief from overwhelming anxiety.

FEAR

Fear is an emotional response to an immediate, known, exaggerated, external, definite or perceived danger that threatens. Fear is an emotion of avoidance, an escape from danger, real or imagined. It may be either rational or irrational and is always unpleasant, restrictive, and contagious. Fear is a universal, primary feeling state. It is an alarm reaction and a learned response that derives much of its significance from cultural attitudes and beliefs as well as from unconscious associations. Fear is experienced as a lack of power or inability to handle disruptions or unexpected alterations in life situations that result in feelings of helplessness and powerlessness. Its presence triggers adaptive responses designed to protect the individual from harm.

We have identified five major categories under which specific fears may be grouped. Expressions of specific fears can be classified according to those that relate to:

1. The loss of survival.
2. Being hurt or hurting others, either physically or psychologically.
3. Losing control over self or situations.
4. Being rejected, that is, losing approval of significant others.
5. Total isolation.

Each of these categories is attributed to violations of the basic human intrapersonal and interpersonal needs for safety and security; power and control; and affection, approval, or belonging.

As a result, the individual engages in methods of protective functioning in an attempt to restore equilibrium. Therefore, to assist the patient toward restoration of equilibrium, the nurse should approach the patient with quiet, positive objectivity and self-confidence. The nurse must support the patient in the use of his usual coping and problem-solving mechanisms while assisting him to learn more satisfying and effective alternatives. The attitudes most needed to implement therapeutic interventions are those of open-mindedness and assurance.

Specific interventions found to be effective in dealing with the clinical problem of fear are shown in Table 21–2.

TABLE 21–2. FEAR—INTERVENTION AND RATIONALE

Intervention	Rationale
Remain with the patient when he is verbally expressing fear or displaying fear response behavior.	To provide protection and support.
Encourage the patient to express his awareness of danger.	To increase the patient's recognition and to establish causation.
Reconstruct with the patient previously identified fear-producing situations.	To establish causes, sequence, and responses.
Examine with the patient his responses to the stated danger.	To determine effectiveness of responses.
Support and encourage the patient to vary his responses to the identified danger.	To assist the patient to discover effective adjustment techniques that reduce fear.
Reduce or minimize identified environmental threats that produce fear; for example, if the patient expresses fear of people, assign him to a private room; assign the same staff member to provide nursing care, and introduce new people one at a time.	To provide protection and support and to allow for adaptation and adjustment.
Keep anxiety-producing situations to a minimum; proceed slowly, reduce the number of choices, and avoid confrontations.	To prevent the transformation of anxiety into fear.
Focus a portion of each interaction on areas of capability rather than on areas of dysfunction.	To maximize the patient's assets and to create an atmosphere of acceptance.

TABLE 21–2. CONTINUED

Intervention	Rationale
Give concrete assistance in the management of everyday affairs that tend to be fear-producing, such as budget planning, job hunting, or child caring.	To demonstrate tangible evidence of the nurse's interest in providing immediate relief and to allow the patient freedom to work on more abstract or general problems.
Promote relaxation through environmental and interpersonal means such as using soft lights, and music, avoiding surprises, and speaking in quiet tones.	To reduce fear-provoking environmental and interpersonal stimuli and to provide soothing stimuli.
Expose the patient gradually to any fear stimulus.	To desensitize the patient to fear stimuli and to promote successful adaptive responses.

ANGER

Anger is a disruptive emotion indicative of displeasure, frustration, and conflict. It is a compensatory, aggressive response used by the individual to prevent feelings of helplessness and hopelessness from becoming overwhelming. Anger is often perceived as a short-lived response because it is too uncomfortable for the individual to tolerate. Since it is experienced as intense feeling, its presence compels action. The action demanded is for dissipation of the anger, and the response is to act out, suppress, or repress the anger. If the individual deals with anger through the use of automatic coping devices, there is a danger that this mode of adaptation will become a chronic, habitual way of life that may result in symptom formation.

Anger is neither good nor bad, but should be recognized simply as a necessary stimulus for change. Anger occurs when the individual perceives damage to his self-respect or perceives that somehow he has failed in his attempt to exert control over self, situations, objects, or others within his immediate environment. The immediate intensity of the response evoked by the perceived damage or failure precludes recognition of alternative choices. Thus, the individual generally fails to engage in adaptive responses that will permit maintenance of his independence and self-respect or ward off unpleasant outcomes. However, anger can be used to gain clarity and to obtain release from unproductive, ineffective behavior patterns once the intensity of the response has been reduced.

The expression of this feeling is manifested in a variety of ways—some subtle and some measurably overt. Covert or indirect expressions can be seen in such verbal comments as, "I'm disappointed," "I'm blue" or "I'm down in the dumps," and in such nonverbal actions as procrastination, forgetting, or inability to concentrate. The overt expression of anger, either direct or in a modified form, is displayed through irritation, verbal threats, and name calling, the eruption of violence in the form of striking out, or in the development of physical symptomatology (as displayed in ulcerative colitis).

Because of the client's need to minimize threats or to regain control, the nurse must assist him to recognize his anger, identify its cause, and develop socially acceptable methods for its dissipation. Furthermore, when anger is at its peak, the nurse must respect the physical space needed by the patient. To facilitate interventive techniques, the nurse must approach the patient in a nonthreatening, nonjudgmental, and calmly confident manner. The most helpful attitudes the nurse needs to cultivate when working with a patient who is angry are those of integrity and personal worth.

Specific nursing interventions found to be effective in managing the clinical problem of anger are included in Table 21–3.

TABLE 21–3. ANGER—INTERVENTION AND RATIONALE

Intervention	Rationale
Observe the patient's behavior for signs of anger.	To identify and assess the patient and to safeguard the patient through early recognition and intervention.
Ask direct questions relating to observations, such as: "Are you angry?" and "Do you feel angry?"	To provide validation for observations and to assist the patient to recognize the presence of anger.
Rephrase question if patient denies or represses, for example: "You look upset" and "You sound distressed."	To clarify and verify observations regarding behavior and to facilitate recognition of anger.
Focus the patient's communication on a description of his feelings, such as: "What do you mean when you say you are sad?" and "Tell me more about being disappointed . . . frustrated . . . depressed."	To encourage expression of feelings and to prevent avoidance or denial of felt anger.
Explore with the patient feelings associated with the anger, such as guilt, humiliation, dependency, and fear.	To elicit the emotional recognition and acceptance of anger.
Identify causative factors.	To assist the patient to understand the reason for his anger.
Determine with the patient if the cause is realistic.	To evaluate the legitimacy of the anger.
Explore with the patient his methods of dealing with anger.	To assist the patient in making a connection between the expressed feeling and the displayed behavior.
Explore with the patient alternatives that are interpersonally and socially acceptable; for example, ask, "What could you do when the nurse keeps you waiting for your medications, causing you to be late for your appointment with the doctor?"	To assist the patient in using the problem-solving approach to develop an acceptable means of dealing with legitimate anger.

TABLE 21–3. CONTINUED

Intervention	Rationale
Provide socially acceptable activities for the displacement of energy associated with angry feelings, such as physical exercise, weaving, typing, and playing the piano.	To channel the expression of anger constructively, to foster feelings of accomplishment, and to increase self-worth.
Maintain your "cool" by refraining from resorting to retaliatory behavior.	To preserve integrity for the patient and the nurse and to prevent the situation from getting out of control.
Allow the patient a "cooling-down" period before exploring precipitating factors.	To assist in the development of control.
Intervene and separate those patients who are mutually antagonistic.	To set limits and to provide a safe, comfortable environment.
Set positive expectations and explain rules and regulations.	To forestall the development of or the increase in intensity of the anger.
Hold the patient accountable for destructive acts.	To assist the patient in the development of responsible behavior.
Meet requests, complaints, and demands with thoughtfulness, respect, and open-mindedness.	To demonstrate acceptance of the patient, to provide an avenue for reasonability and to support the patient's feelings of self-worth.

LONELINESS

Loneliness is a severe, painful, subjective state in which the individual feels that no one cares and that he does not belong. The lonely individual perceives himself as being deprived of intimate relationships with other human beings as well as not having an opportunity to share his thoughts, feelings, achievements, and life with significant others. It is a pervasive and painful experience that is perhaps more frightening than the feeling of anxiety. It is a state in which past relationships are almost entirely forgotten as well as one in which the future holds no promise. In essence, loneliness is experienced as an almost complete negation of being with an inability to feel, to care, or to love.

Because of the perceived deficit of intimacy in relationships, the patient who experiences loneliness often underestimates abilities, underrates or decries achievements, and loses motivation necessary to problem-solving and decision-making. Since the lonely individual is unable to experience the "give and take" of loving, communication and sharing are dramatically decreased. This lack of essential ability inhibits the development of therapeutic rapport.

The lonely individual's adjustment and adaptation to life and living are characterized by feelings of depression, dejection, despair, and desolation. The behavior this individual displays reveals an almost total lack of caring for self and others. Some specific behaviors that indicate this lack of caring include moodiness; self-depreciating acts; morbid preoccupation with death; suicidal ruminations or gestures; or complete social isolation and withdrawal from reality.

In developing a therapeutic environment for the patient displaying the problem of loneliness, it is imperative that the nurse's approach be one that actively seeks out the patient, demonstrates genuine warmth, and reflects loving concern. The attitudes the nurse cultivates to achieve this approach are those of hopefulness and involvement.

Specific interventions found to be effective in dealing with the clinical problem of loneliness are included in Table 21–4.

TABLE 21–4. LONELINESS—INTERVENTION AND RATIONALE

Intervention	Rationale
Seek out the patient and spend time with him on a regularly scheduled basis.	To demonstrate concern and to let the patient know that he is not alone—he can rely on you.
Acknowledge the patient's feeling of loneliness.	To convey empathy and understanding.
Discuss the meaning of loneliness for the patient.	To determine what loneliness means to the patient and how he experiences it.
Plan a regular schedule for the patient.	To prevent social isolation and to maintain contact with reality.
Expect attendance and involvement at scheduled activities.	To create within the individual the idea that motivation comes from within the self.
Discuss with the patient his feelings regarding involvement in activity.	To determine his level of involvement and its effectiveness in alleviating loneliness and to provide an opportunity to reinforce belonging and self-worth.
Encourage involvement in group activities.	To foster a sense of belonging and identity.
Respond to requests immediately—avoid delays.	To prevent interpretation of delay as rejection and proof of the patient's worthlessness.
Reinforce the patient's identity; for example, address him by name or personally invite him to attend the church service of his choice.	To maintain contact with reality and to establish feelings of personal worth.
Touch the patient—pat him on the shoulder, lay a hand on his wrist or arm.	To indicate presence and to convey a feeling of genuine warmth and a sense of sharing.
Assign the patient to useful, important tasks, for example, passing out lunch trays, helping sort clean laundry, taking responsibility for the care of the ward plants or pets.	To instill a sense of usefulness and productivity and to provide a basis for legitimate praise.
Give merited praise.	To provide recognition for the successful completion of activities.
Select occupational or recreational activities that are familiar to the patient and at which he is known to be successful.	To limit the possibility of failure and to provide an avenue for social intercourse.
Encourage the patient to ventilate his feelings.	To relieve tension and to foster self-worth through acceptance.

TABLE 21–4. CONTINUED

Intervention	Rationale
Focus the patient's communication on the present and the future.	To keep the patient oriented to reality and to prevent preoccupation with past problems.
Encourage the patient to be socially assertive, that is, to develop and broaden his sphere of social activity.	To develop a sense of success in social communication, sharing, and intimacy.

GRIEF

Grief is an emotional state experienced by the individual following severe loss or prolonged deprivation. It occurs when an individual experiences the loss of a person, treasured object, or part of the physical self. In grief there is a loss of love, a marked decrease in the sense of being needed, a feeling of abandonment, and a decrease in the level of self-esteem and self-worth.

Grief is a common human experience that involves a process of separation, the purpose of which is to overcome and adapt to the stress produced by the actual or potential loss. It causes a temporary impairment in the individual's capacity to function. Resolution involves stress, pain, and suffering and can be either healthy and uncomplicated or morbid and pathological. In other words, there is no painless escape from grief, since pathology is inevitable if the process of resolution is delayed, becomes fixed, or is interrupted and abandoned.

Grief is complicated by guilt and depression. Therefore, it is essential to the interventive technique to understand that guilt and depression are not the primary diagnoses. When the individual is suffering from severe loss or prolonged deprivation, he generally seeks to deny the causes or to minimize the effect they have on him so that he will not have to deal with the resultant emotional issues.

The subjective experiences associated with grief can be described as existing on a continuum. It begins with the socially accepted "normal grief behavior" following the loss of a loved one, such as crying, frequent forgetfulness, or temporary loss of time spans, and proceeds toward a severe, overpowering depression that can become pathologic in its manifestations, such as suicidal attempts, becoming reclusive, increasing malfunctioning on the job, and even loss of contact with reality. In her practice the nurse may encounter the entire spectrum of the grief and mourning continuum, but it is only when the individual has become so overwhelmed that the nurse is requested, or deems it necessary to intervene on behalf of the patient.

The approach the nurse will find most effective in dealing with grief and mourning is one that is calm, objective, unhurried, flexible, concerned, empathetic, and consistent. She must recognize and acknowledge the significance that the lost person, object, or part of the self has for the individual. Furthermore, the nurse must also be aware of the extent of interdependence that existed between the lost object, person, or part of the self and the survivor as well as the effect of the loss on the individual's personal integrated framework of functioning. The attitudes needed to implement intervention and this approach are those of personal worth, advocacy, and hopefulness.

Specific nursing interventions found to be effective in dealing with grief are identified in Table 21–5.

TABLE 21–5. GRIEF—INTERVENTION AND RATIONALE

Intervention	Rationale
Organize and plan a schedule for the patient until the patient displays an ability to take over the planning and organizing process.	To meet dependency needs.
Consult the patient about the plans.	To encourage involvement.
Encourage participation in activities of daily living.	To maintain contact with reality and to prevent regression.
Limit available choices.	To reduce stress.
Give directions and instructions; repeat as necessary.	To surmount the communication barrier produced by decreased perceptual awareness.
Encourage the patient to verbalize feelings associated with loss.	To assist the patient in developing an awareness of predominant feelings.
Discuss feelings of ambivalence, disappointment, resentment, anger, relief or guilt.	To promote the patient's understanding of self.
Remain with the patient despite his lack of ability to verbalize.	To demonstrate to the patient unconditional acceptance.
Break silence periodically with positive, nonthreatening statements of fact, such as: "Five minutes have gone by; I will be with you for fifteen more minutes" or "I'll be here tomorrow."	To establish a sense of "thereness" and "relatedness" with the patient.
Allow time for responses when communicating with the patient.	To accommodate the patient's distortions in perception and delayed response time.
Listen patiently to repetitious verbalizations of guilt or self-blame.	To demonstrate to the patient nonjudgmental acceptance.
Interrupt monologues and refocus on feelings.	To penetrate the defensive shield of superficial communication.
Remain with the patient during nonverbal ventilation of feelings such as crying, sobbing, screaming, and introspective staring.	To offer empathetic support.
Assist the patient to find meaning in his loss through his personal framework of philosophy and value systems.	To offer support, encouragement, and hope.

TABLE 21–5. CONTINUED

Intervention	Rationale
Provide an opportunity for visitation from the clergy.	To sustain the patient in his religious beliefs and to enable him to grow spiritually.
Give special attention to physical needs: oral hygiene, physical cleanliness, appropriate dress, and general attractiveness in appearance.	To demonstrate care and concern of the nurse, to prevent halitosis, to stimulate taste buds, to encourage appetite, to insure protection against climatic changes, to promote self-concept and to encourage general physical well-being.
Provide a balanced diet of frequent, small feedings and assist with eating by giving verbal encouragement, cutting up food, or feeding the patient.	To meet the nutritional needs of the patient and to prevent weight loss.
Make meal times an attractive and pleasurable experience by determining likes and dislikes, having relatives bring favorite foods from home, adding warm, bright colors to place settings, and sitting with the patient while he is eating.	To stimulate appetite, to promote socialization, and to increase feelings of self-worth.
Provide physical exercise.	To maintain the patient's normal physiological processes such as circulation, elimination, and nutrition.
Promote rest and sleep by providing warm milk or a hot tub at bedtime, remaining with the patient until he is asleep, checking periodically for wakefulness, and remaining with the patient to determine the cause of sleeplessness or to administer prescribed hypnotics.	To prevent loss of rest and to promote the patient's physical and emotional comfort.
Assign small repetitive tasks.	To relieve feelings of guilt.
Observe for clues indicative of suicidal behavior such as verbal statements in which the patient says "good-bye" instead of "good night," or when the patient indicates that everything will be fine tomorrow.	To safeguard the patient from self-destructive behavior.
Alert *all* staff members to suicide potential.	To decrease potential of environmental hazards and to provide safety and security for the patient.

PAIN

Pain is an emotional phenomenon of the mind, and, as such, it is a highly individualized subjective experience. Pain is *real*. Pain is *hurt*. And pain is suffering, anguish, and agony. It can be experienced emotionally, physically, psychologically, and spiritually. There is dull pain, excruciating pain, throbbing pain, tormenting pain, searing pain, and the pain associated with embarrassment, as in a social faux pas. The list of adjectives used to describe pain and its intensity are almost endless. But words can hardly capture the true substance of pain, for, unlike other emotional states, pain is undeniably a particularly unique and individualized sensation. What one individual may experience as painful may not be painful for another. Each individual's threshold of pain varies according to his philosophical framework, his value system, or his interpretations regarding the cause of pain. Thus pain is valued, feared, accepted, denied, or fought. An individual can interpret a painful experience as a challenge, as a punishment, as an enemy, as a warning, or as a learning experience.

In identifying, assessing, and designing therapeutic interventions directed toward the relief of pain, the nurse must fully recognize that the client and not the nurse is the expert. Thus, the nurse's approach should be one of sympathetic, empathetic personal warmth. The attitudes needed by the nurse to carry out this intervention are those of open-mindedness, advocacy, and involvement.

Specific nursing interventions found to be effective in dealing with the clinical problem of pain are included in Table 21–6.

TABLE 21–6. PAIN—INTERVENTION AND RATIONALE

Intervention	Rationale
Explore with the patient the meaning of pain to and for him from a physical, psychological, social, and spiritual viewpoint.	To acknowledge the experienced discomfort; to demonstrate interest and concern for the patient's well-being; to support endeavors to find meaning in suffering.
Investigate with the patient experiences producing pain.	To increase the patient's awareness regarding cause and effect.
Listen attentively to the patient's expressions of feelings relating to pain.	To demonstrate sympathetic and empathetic concern; to develop understanding; to alleviate distress.
Explore with the patient those coping mechanisms used to deal with pain.	To determine the effectiveness of the patient's coping mechanisms.
Seek to involve patient's social support system in pain management.	To share information for the purpose of providing the patient with relief and to incorporate external supports.
Involve the patient in identifying alternative coping mechanisms for pain relief.	To demonstrate trust in patient's ability to take charge and to act positively to control pain.
Assist the patient to choose an alternative coping mechanism(s).	To initiate and facilitate change in adaptation.
Teach the patient skills relevant to the identified alternative coping devices chosen.	To share information for the purpose of providing relief and restoration of equilibrium.
Create opportunities to test learned coping strategies within the context of a structured environment.	To safeguard the patient while encouraging independent functioning.
Evaluate with the patient the effectiveness of the strategy on pain reduction or control.	To provide feedback and opportunity for modification in order to promote highest level of functioning.

TABLE 21–6. CONTINUED

Intervention	Rationale
Support continued use of effective strategies.	To promote the patient's physical and emotional comfort.
Plan with the client for periodic reevaluation.	To maintain equilibrium and faster continued growth.

GUILT

Guilt is a pathological feeling state in which the individual projects resentment where there is conscious realization that the self has done wrong by violating some valued ethical, moral, or religious principle. It occurs when the self acknowledges conflict between what is and what should be, and it is disproportionate and unreasonable to the perceived wrong. Guilt is produced when good intentions go astray or are left unrealized, or when effort to maintain the status quo is thwarted. Thus, guilt can be described as a "hanging-on phenomenon" because the individual is trapped by immobility.

Guilt is therefore a destructive feeling, since the immobility prevents the person from either letting go or seeking resolution so that movement toward self-actualization can continue. It can be equated with an erosion process that eats away at an individual's self-concept, leaving the individual with lowered self-esteem, self-worth, and personal integrity. Added to this sense of personal devaluation is a corresponding obsession to expiate or make restitution for a perceived wrong. Guilt is also accompanied by an overwhelming apprehensiveness or fear that something terrible will happen to the self. There is a firm conviction that retribution will occur and will result in a loss of well-being and security. In its most severe form, the deterioration of the self-concept characteristic of guilt eventuates into a feeling of complete annihilation of self as evidenced in clinical depression.

Although guilt is subjective in nature, stems primarily from unresolved conflict, and is viewed by the self as condemnation of the self, there is an additional aspect involved. This aspect deals with the concern the self has for its public image. The "guilty self" has a secret; is burdened by this secret and believes that, if shared or made known to significant others, the self would be forever alienated from others. The self fears exposure that may result in shame. The loss of regard for the public self creates within the person a sense of resentment. The resentment festers and reinforces the immobilization.

A healthy person tends to function in a manner that declares the self to be free of the conventional restraints of the society. This means that the individual operates with a sense of detachment that signifies independence and self-governance. The healthy individual looks within for the guiding values and rules by which to live. Thus, reason and judgment are employed in order to arrive at a self-defined value system rather than adopting an imposed or introjected value system. The values held by the person result because the individual both feels and believes them to be worthwhile. When the healthy person breaks his code of ethics, *guilt does not result.* The healthy person feels *pain*—pain resulting from the fact that the self has inflicted hurt on someone else. The healthy person does not act out of a sense of guilt but rather out of a sense of concern or love. The person acts morally, not because he is afraid that the self will be punished, but because it makes the self happier and more satisfied to do so.

Guilt, then, is a pathological feeling that occurs when the self introjects the values of society or authority figures without regard to self-determination. Understanding the dynamics involved in the development of guilt is therefore important for the nurse because much of the intervention depends on the clarification of the value system the patient holds.

Resolution of guilt is not easily achieved because it demands an almost complete reorganization of beliefs and value system. Thus, resolution requires prolonged time and continuous effort. Probably the highest level of achievement that the nurse can expect to attain with the patient is a reduction of the immediate effects produced by guilt, a restoration of equilibrium prior to the onset of guilt, and the patient's commitment to the pursuit of investigating and learning alternative coping mechanisms for reducing, avoiding, or ameliorating the effects of guilt.

The most effective approach the nurse can assume in dealing with patients manifesting guilt is one of thoughtful, nonjudgmental confrontation accompanied by calm objectivity. The nurse can best achieve this approach through demonstrating genuine concern, fostering opportunities for self-appraisal, and encouraging the patient to assume responsibility for actions without resorting to dependence on rationalization or projection. Nursing intervention requires that the nurse's attitude conveys to the patient her sense of his personal worth.

Specific nursing interventions found to be effective in dealing with the clinical problem of guilt are included in Table 21–7.

TABLE 21–7. GUILT—INTERVENTION AND RATIONALE

Intervention	Rationale
Maintain a climate of neutrality.	To foster an atmosphere conducive to trust and sharing.
Encourage the open expression of feelings.	To provide temporary relief through sharing and to convey acceptance of the person.

TABLE 21–7. CONTINUED

Intervention	Rationale
Accept disclosures in a matter-of-fact way.	To demonstrate objectivity and concern without critical judgment.
Identify with the patient situations that evoke the feeling of guilt.	To assist the patient to recognize the connection between the feeling and the event.
Explore with the patient the beliefs and values connected with the identified events.	To assist the patient to determine the basis on which decisions to act or not to act were made.
Discuss the difference between "should" and "could."	To help the patient distinguish between reasonable and unreasonable expectations for self.
Engage the patient in exercises or role-playing activities that are designed to focus on the assumptions of responsibility for actions.	To stimulate patient's awareness of self and perceptions.
Evaluate with the client the results of the exercises.	To provide feedback.
Set limits on negative self-expression.	To reinforce positive self-concept and increase self-esteem.
Encourage the patient to accept consequences of action without devaluation of self.	To interrupt the pattern of alienation of self from others.
Create opportunities for earning merited praises.	To foster self-esteem.

EVALUATION

A list of projected outcomes for each of the feelings discussed in this chapter is found in Table 21–8. The evaluation criteria are based on the primary nursing care goal: to sustain the patient during periods of discomfort while assisting him to learn new methods of adaptation or coping. This listing is general in scope and is intended to serve only as an example. It is important for the reader to note that outcome criteria are derived through the identification of the optimal expectations to be achieved with each patient.

TABLE 21–8. EVALUATION CRITERIA—FEELING DISTURBANCE

Feeling Disturbance	Evaluation Criteria
Anxiety	Reduces or resolves anxiety: Acknowledges presence of anxiety. Initiates anxiety-reducing strategies. Reports comfortableness with self or others. Differentiates anxiety from other feelings. Focuses communication on others. Demonstrates problem-solving skills. Participates in social activities. Eliminates negative self-talk.

(continued)

TABLE 21–8. CONTINUED

Feeling Disturbance	Evaluation Criteria
Fear	Is free from fear: Ceases to verbalize expectation of danger. Evidences decreased preparation for flight or fight. Evidences decreased psychomotor activity. Identifies source of danger. Avoids danger through use of learned coping strategies. Returns to physiological equilibrium.
Anger	Expresses anger appropriately: Identifies source. Determines justification such as realistic vs. unrealistic. Verbalizes anger. Deals with anger in a socially acceptable manner. Ceases to threaten harm to self or others. Decreases aggressive acts (overt, covert.)
Loneliness	Establishes social network: Resumes contact with significant others. Establishes new relationships. Explores community resources. Expresses interest in people and activities. Verbalizes a sense of belonging. Shares thoughts and feelings with others. Cares for self. Verbalizes positive comments about self.
Grief	Resolves grief: Attends to self-care needs. Engages in social interaction. Resumes role performance and functioning. Discusses future plans. Discusses loss openly. Places loss in perspective.
Pain	Relieves pain: Reports level of comfort. Uses learned coping mechanisms to seek relief. Verbalizes methods that provide relief. Avoids pain-producing situations.
Guilt	Accepts self: Makes realistic appraisal of self. Speaks positively of self. Displays a range of positive feelings such as joy, happiness, well-being, and satisfaction. Engages in purposeful activities. Shares self with others. Clarifies values and beliefs. States realistic expectations for self.

SUMMARY

In this chapter we have presented seven of the most universal and significant human feelings that are most likely to be subjected to distortion. These feelings are those which the nurse will most frequently encounter in her daily practice, whether the practice is within the setting of a psychiatric facility, an out-patient clinic, or a medical-surgical unit of a general hospital. Because of the constant need to deal with these feelings, it is essential that the nurse identify, acknowledge, and understand the various manifestations of anxiety, fear, anger, loneliness, grief, pain, and guilt as they move from the accepted and tolerable norm to the severe and traumatizing level of pathology. It is only within the context of knowledge complemented by empathy, understanding, care, and concern that the nurse can make effective therapeutic interventions on behalf of the patient.

SUGGESTED READINGS

Benson, L. *Images, Heroes, and Self Perceptions.* Englewood Cliffs, N. J.: Prentice-Hall, 1974.

Boguslawski, M. Therapeutic Touch: A Facilitator of Pain Relief. *Topics in Clinical Nursing,* Vol. 2, No. 1 (April, 1980), 27–38.

Cowles, K. V. Life, Death and Personhood. *Nursing Outlook,* Vol. 22, No. 3 (May/June, 1984), 168–172.

Cronin, D. *Anxiety, Depression, and Phobias: How To Understand and Deal with Them.* Englewood Cliffs, N. J.: Prentice-Hall, 1982.

Davitz, J. R., & Davitz, L. L. *Inferences of Patient's Pain and Psychological Distress: Studies of Nursing Behaviors.* New York: Springer, 1981.

DeCrosta, T. Relieving Pain: Four Noninvasive Ways You Should Know More About. *Nursing Life,* Vol. 4, No. 2 (March/April, 1984), 28–33.

Doenges, M., & Moorehouse, M. *Nurse's Pocket Guide: Nursing Diagnoses with Interventions.* Philadelphia: F. A. Davis, 1985.

Dubree, M., & Vogelpohl, R. When Hope Dies—So Might the Patient. *American Journal of Nursing,* Vol. 80, No. 11 (November, 1980), 2046–2049.

Ferszt, G. G., & Taylor, P. B. The Patient's Right To Cry. *Nursing 84,* Vol. 14, No. 3 (March, 1984), 65–66, 68.

Francis, G. M. Loneliness: The Syndrome. *Issues in Mental Health Nursing,* Vol. 3, Nos. 1–2 (January–June, 1981), 1–6.

Gluck, M. M. Group Therapy in a Pain Management Program. *Journal of Psychiatric Nursing and Mental Health Services,* Vol. 18, No. 11 (November, 1980), 21–25.

Gluck, M. M. Learning a Therapeutic Verbal Response to Anger. *Journal of Psychiatric Nursing and Mental Health Services,* Vol. 19, No. 3 (March, 1981), 9–11.

Hafin, B. R., & Brog, M. J. *Emotional Survival.* Englewood Cliffs, N. J.: Prentice-Hall, 1983.

Hashizume, S. She Asked: Am I Going Crazy? *Nursing '75,* Vol. 5, No. 2 (February, 1975), 12–15.

Hauser, M. J. Bereavement Outcome For Widows. *Journal of Psychosocial Nursing and Mental Health Services,* Vol. 21, No. 9 (September, 1983), 22–31.

Hauser, M. J., & Feinberg, D. R. An Operational Approach to the Delayed Grief and Mourning Process. *Journal of Psychiatric Nursing and Mental Health Services,* Vol. 14, No. 7 (July, 1976), 29–35.

Herberner, G. F. How To Control Anger-Your Own and Others. *Nursing Life,* Vol. 2 No. 6 (November/December, 1982), 42–45.

Holderby, R. A., & McNulty, E. G. Feelings . . . Feelings: How To Make a Rational Response to Emotional Behavior. *Nursing '79,* Vol. 9, No. 10 (October, 1979), 39–43.

Jacox, A. K. Assessing Pain. *American Journal of Nursing,* Vol. 79, No. 5 (May, 1979), 895–900.

Johnson-Soderberg, S. Grief Themes. *Advances in Nursing Science,* Vol. 3, No. 4 (July, 1981), 15–26.

Kim, S. Pain: Theory, Research and Nursing Practice. *Advances in Nursing Science,* Vol. 2, No. 2 (January, 1980), 43–59.

Kirschling, J. M., & Pierce, P. K. Nursing and the Terminally Ill: Beliefs, Attitudes and Perceptions of Practitioners. *Issues in Mental Health Nursing,* Vol. 4, No. 4 (1982), 275–286.

Klepser, M. J. How Long Does Grief Go On? *American Journal of Nursing,* Vol. 78, No. 3 (March, 1978), 420–422.

Knowles, R. D. Affirmations. *American Journal of Nursing,* Vol. 82, No. 4 (April, 1982), 615.

Knowles, R. D. Dealing with Feelings: Handling Depression by Identifying Anger. *American Journal of Nursing,* Vol. 8, No. 5 (May, 1981), 968.

Knowles, R. D. Dealing with Feelings: Handling Depression through Positive Reinforcement. *American Journal of Nursing,* Vol. 81, No. 7 (July, 1981), 1353.

Knowles, R. D. Handling Anger: Responding vs. Reacting. *American Journal of Nursing,* Vol. 81, No. 12 (December, 1981), 2196.

Knowles, R. D. Positive Self Talk. *American Journal of Nursing,* Vol. 81, No. 3 (March, 1981), 35–36.

Knowles, R. D. Preventing Anger. *American Journal of Nursing,* Vol. 82, No. 1 (January, 1982), 118.

Koch, J. When Children Meet Death. *Psychology Today* (August, 1977), 64–67.

Kovalesky, A. That Night in the Neonate Nursery. *American Journal of Nursing,* Vol. 78, No. 3 (March, 1978), 414–416.

Kowalski, E. L. A Lost Life-Style. *American Journal of Nursing,* Vol. 78, No. 3 (March, 1978), 418–420.

Kowalski, K. The Impact of Chronic Grief. *American Journal of Nursing,* Vol. 85, No. 4 (April, 1985), 398–399.

Kreidler, M. Meaning in Suffering. *International Nursing Review* Vol. 31, No. 65 (1984), 174–176.

Limandri, B. J., & Boyle, D. W. Instilling Hope. *American Journal of Nursing,* Vol. 78, No. 1 (January, 1978), 78–80.

Luckman, J. & Sarenson, K. What Patients' Actions Tell You About Their Feelings, Fears and Needs. *Nursing '75*, Vol. 5, No. 2 (February, 1975), 54–61.

Madow, L. *Anger: How To Recognize and Cope with It.* New York: Charles Scribner's Sons, 1972.

Mahon, N. E. Developmental Changes and Loneliness During Adolescence. *Topics in Clinical Nursing*, Vol. 5, No. 1 (April, 1983), 66–76.

Mandel, H. R. Nurses Feelings about Working with the Dying. *American Journal of Nursing*, Vol. 81, No. 6 (June, 1981), 1194–1197.

McLaughlin M. F. Grief: Who Helps the Living? *American Journal of Nursing* Vol. 78, No. 3 (March, 1978), 422–423.

Meir, J. Loneliness. *Psychology Today*, Vol. 19, No. 7 (July, 1985) 28–33.

Misner, S. J. Using Art Therapy Techniques in Staff and Patient Education. *Nursing Outlook*, Vol. 27, No. 8 (August, 1979), 536–537.

Moustakas, C. E. *Portraits of Loneliness and Love.* Englewood Cliffs, N. J.: Prentice-Hall, 1974.

Odell, S. H. Someone is Lonely. *Issues in Mental Health Nursing*, Vol. 3, Nos. 1–2 (January–June, 1981), 7–12.

Peplau, L., & Perlman, D. (Eds.). *Loneliness: A Sourcebook of Current Theory, Research and Therapy.* New York: John Wiley & Sons, 1982.

Pestalozzi, A. For Those Who Are About To Die. *Nursing Management*, Vol. 16, No. 1 (January, 1985), 20–21.

Preddy, E. Leave Me Alone. *Nursing '75*, Vol. 5, No. 1 (January, 1975), 13–15.

Rearick, T., et al. Gaining Insight into Fear. *Nursing '78*, Vol. 8, No. 4 (April, 1978) 46–51.

Rosenfeld, A. H. Depression: Dispelling Despair. *Psychology Today*, Vol. 19, No. 6 (June, 1985), 28–34.

Ross, H. Societal/Cultural Views Regarding Death and Dying. *Topics in Clinical Nursing*, Vol. 4, No. 2 (July, 1982), 1–16.

Self, P. R. 4 Steps for Helping a Patient Alleviate Anger. *Nursing '80*, Vol. 10, No. 12 (December, 1980).

Shealy, C. N. Holistic Management of Chronic Pain. *Topics in Clinical Nursing*, Vol. 2, No. 1 (April, 1980), 1–8.

Stark, E. Breaking the Pain Habit. *Psychology Today*, Vol. 19, No. 5 (May, 1985), 31–36.

Steerman, L. T. A Review of Clinical Biofeedback. *American Journal of Nursing*, Vol. 75, No. 11 (November, 1975), 2006–2009.

Stowers, S. J. Nurses Cry, Too. *Nursing Management*, Vol. 14, No. 4 (April, 1983), 53–64.

Strauss, A., Fagerhaugh, S. Y. & Glaser, L. Pain—An Organizational-Work-Interactional Perspective. *Nursing Outlook*, Vol. 22, No. 9 (September, 1974), 560–566.

Swanson, A. R. Communicating with Depressed Persons. *Perspectives in Psychiatric Care*, Vol. 13, No. 2 (1975), 63–67.

Tavris, C. Feeling Angry? Letting Off Steam May Not Help. *Nursing Life*, Vol. 4, No. 5 (September/October, 1984), 58–61.

Thompson, L. Sensory Deprivation: A Personal Experience. *American Journal of Nursing*, Vol. 73, No. 2 (February, 1973), 266–268.

Thomsan, G. Fear, Anger, Sadness. *Transactional Analysis Journal*, Vol. 13, No. 1 (January, 1983), 20–24.

Tiger, L. Optimism: The Biological Roots of Hope. *Psychology Today,* Vol. 12, No. 8 (January, 1979), 18–26, 29–30, 33.

Welch, D. Anticipatory Grief Reactions in Family Members. *Issues in Mental Health Nursing,* Vol. 4, No. 2 (April–June, 1982), 149–158.

Westercamp. T. M. Suicide. *American Journal of Nursing,* Vol. 75, No. 2 (February, 1975) 260–262.

White, C. L. Nurse Counseling with a Depressed Patient. *American Journal of Nursing,* Vol. 78, No. 3 (March, 1978), 436–439.

Wolf, Z. R. Pain Theories: An Overview. *Topics in Clinical Nursing,* Vol. 2, No. 1 (April, 1980), 9–18.

22

NURSING INTERVENTION FOR PATIENTS EXPERIENCING BEHAVIORAL DISRUPTIONS

LEARNING OBJECTIVES

On completion of this chapter the reader should be able to:

1. Identify, define, and describe the nine types of disruptive behavior.
2. Distinguish between each of the identified behaviors.
3. Apply specific concepts and principles underlying nursing intervention for clients experiencing disruptive behavior.
4. Identify specific nursing interventions for the behaviors discussed.
5. State the rationale for each of the interventive techniques.

INTRODUCTION

In the practice of psychiatric–mental health nursing, the nurse encounters many forms of behavior associated with psychiatric disorders, emotional disturbances, stress, crises, and conflict. These behaviors differ both in mode and degree according to the patient, his circumstances, life experiences, and life-style. In addition, we cannot overlook the influences of culture, environment, and family history that may contribute to and influence the patient's system of belief and coping devices. All these factors when taken together lend themselves to the development of individualized pathological behavioral manifestations.

Of no small consequence, therefore, is the fact that nursing staff in institutional or hospital settings are consistently being confronted with a spectrum of behaviors that are classified vaguely as "management problems." Therefore, it is vital that the nurse learn about and understand the dynamics of such behaviors, select and apply methods of appropriate and successful interventions, and understand the rationale behind the use of such interventive techniques. Such knowledge creates the best ambiance for the therapeutic community, minimizes friction between patients of varying personalities, and maximizes the utilization of professional staff time toward the treatment of the whole patient.

According to the current classification system adopted by NANDA, two distinct behaviors have been identified: Social Isolation; and Violence, Potential for. While these specific diagnoses may indeed be appropriate, there appears to be a need to address other behavioral manifestations as well.

In an attempt to close this gap, we identify nine major, common disruptions in behavior. They are: negativistic, regressive, aggressive, manipulative, self-destructive, hyperactive, compulsive, addictive, and suspicious behaviors. From our standpoint, Social Isolation becomes one aspect of regressive behavior, while Violence, Potential for, is subsumed as an aspect of aggressive behavior.

We have elected to use the same approach presented in the preceeding chapter by adopting the term **behavioral disruption** as the overall diagnostic category and identifying the specific presenting behavior as the defining characteristic. The etiology continues to reflect the underlying dynamics. Thus, a sample nursing diagnostic statement addressing behavioral disruptions might read: *Behavioral disruption related to a distorted attitudinal and belief system as evidenced by negativistic behavior.*

> The primary nursing care goal for patients experiencing behavioral disruptions is to bring about a change in behavior resulting in more healthy functioning.

The specific long- and short-term objectives evolve from the data base and resulting patient profile. Furthermore, the reader should note that the interventions detailed within this chapter are directed toward the primary nursing care goal rather than the specificity required by the uniqueness found within each patient's care situation.

The concepts and principles underlying our discussion in this chapter are listed below. These have value and application in guiding the formulation of nursing interventions on behalf of and in conjunction with an individual experiencing disruptions in behavior.

1. Man creates his own world, and assuming responsibility for choices made, indicates movement toward self-actualization.
2. Behavior occurs in response to stimuli.
3. All behavior has meaning.
4. Behavior can be changed or modified.
5. Nonverbal behavior is a more significant indicator of feeling than verbal behavior.
6. Ongoing self-evaluation acts as a deterrent to maladaptive behavior.
7. Feeling secure reduces the need for maladaptive behavior.
8. Early life experiences determine behavioral responses to stress, anxiety, fear, frustration, loss, pain, and conflict as well as other threats to the self-system.
9. The learning of socially acceptable behavior is facilitated through the use of a structured setting that provides opportunities for gradual increases in independent choices and functioning.
10. Cognitive and affective distortions of self, others, and the environment increase the potential for behavioral deviance.
11. Behavioral deviance produces alienation of the self from others.
12. Behaving and evaluating behavior are culturally defined.
13. Culture influences the type of aggressive behavior displayed.
14. Appropriate verbal expression decreases aggressive behavior.
15. Use of security operations promotes feelings of well-being and conversely decreases levels of anxiety and feelings of frustration.
16. Consistency is important in setting and reinforcing limits.
17. Application of external controls may be needed to meet clients' needs for safety and security.
18. Resistance to change is diminished through acceptance, consistency, and clear communications.
19. Clients learn new behaviors through identification with care providers.
20. Retaliatory behavior on the part of the care provider can be avoided when the care provider recognizes and accepts the patient's emotional outbursts as an expression of perceived threat to his self-system and not as an aggressive act directed against the care provider per se.

NEGATIVISTIC BEHAVIOR

Negativistic behavior is obstinance—resistance to what is deemed socially right, reasonable, and acceptable. Negativistic behavior is an outward portrayal of an individual's perception of the self as unworthy and inadequate. The individual holds the belief that he is a failure despite evidence to the contrary. As a result, he rejects the self. The view of himself with respect to his surroundings, that is, the way he operates within his own social context, is correspondingly poor. From this distorted attitudinal and belief system, the individual sees any obstacle to goal attainment as a reflection of his own inadequacy in coping and by his actions programs himself for failure. The individual is firmly convinced that the future presents limited opportunities for change or amelioration, thus fulfilling his own self-defeating prophecy.

Negativistic behavior is conveyed through actions that are in opposition to general expectations. For example, the individual demonstrates an inability to comply. This inability is displayed through such behavioral actions and attitudes as procrastination, passivity, silence, blatant refusal, avoidance, or denial.

To meet the needs of a patient displaying negativistic behavior, the nurse should adopt a calm, consistent, accepting, nonjudgmental, nonpunitive approach while attempting to understand the dynamics underlying negativistic behavior. The attitudes the nurse must cultivate in order to carry out this type of approach are those of open-mindedness, hopefulness, and advocacy.

Specific nursing interventions found to be effective in dealing with the clinical problem of negativistic behavior are located in Table 22–1.

TABLE 22–1. NEGATIVISTIC BEHAVIOR—INTERVENTION AND RATIONALE

Interventions	Rationale
Present and explain expectations.	To set realistic goals and to limit the direction negative behavior can take.
Eliminate the possibility of negative choices; for example, since the expectation is that the patient will attend occupational therapy, the choices presented to the patient are for him either to attend alone or to be escorted by a member of the staff.	To discourage negative responses, to encourage the development of responsible behavior, and to prevent deterioration or loss of essential behaviors necessary for living.
Identify with the patient the manner in which he expresses negativistic behavior.	To establish the patient's awareness of behaviors requiring change.
Identify positive reinforcers.	To determine what rewards to select for the patient in order to make the behavioral change contract effective.

TABLE 22–1. CONTINUED

Interventions	Rationale
Draw up a behavioral change contract with the patient including a daily activity schedule; a list of behaviors to be changed; choices allowed, if any; rewards for fulfilling contracted expectations; and penalties for default.	To clearly identify, for the patient, staff expectations; to verbally reinforce positive responses; and to encourage self-motivation.
Present patient and all concerned staff with a copy of the contract.	To act as a positive reminder for the patient and to promote consistency of approach among staff.
Coordinate all staff efforts on behalf of the patient.	To promote a unified approach and to reinforce consistent application of the contract.
Inform and elicit support of significant others who relate to the patient.	To provide consistency; to assist concerned others to develop understanding of the patient and an awareness of the treatment program; and to promote acceptance of the patient.
Closely monitor the patient's progress.	To assess the degree to which the patient is involved; to evaluate the effectiveness of the contract; and to establish a data base for further intervention.
Record observations accurately.	To facilitate the process of change.
Reassess and evaluate the contract periodically with patient and staff.	To determine progress and establish basis for renegotiation of contract.
Renegotiate contract as needed.	To provide care and treatment according to patient's needs and progress toward goal.
Effect consistent, persistent approaches to the patient.	To demonstrate acceptance; establish rapport; build trust; and increase the patient's feeling of security.
Assist the patient to verbalize feelings about his negativistic behavior; for example, if the patient refuses to participate in a routine daily activity, say, "You seem to resent having to make your bed today"; if the patient is silent during interactions, say, "Perhaps there is something that is difficult for you to discuss."	To indicate to the patient the nurse's interest and concern as to why he is behaving as he does and to interrupt negative behavior patterns.

REGRESSIVE BEHAVIOR

Regressive behavior is a selective, defensive operation in which the individual resorts to earlier, less complex patterns of behavior. It is a defensive method of functioning engaged in by the individual in order to satisfy needs for safety and security. Regressive behavior is also employed as an outlet for labile emotions. The use of regressive behavior allows the individual to avoid the unpleasant discomfort of reality. It is a retreat to safety that over time stifles the potential for future maturational growth. As a response mechanism, it is most often employed when the individual is unable to meet expectations imposed on the self by the self or others. It is also deployed when the individual is faced with unresolved conflict or experiences unmet dependency needs. In this latter instance, the dynamics in any stress situation result in the expression of childlike helplessness, which, in turn, evokes caring from others. The caring expressed by others decreases discomfort, provides a sense of security, and reduces feelings of helplessness.

Regressive behavior can be observed in normal healthy adults in the pursuit of everyday living. For example, regressive behavior is evidenced through the spontaneous "horseplay" observed at picnics, the antics observed at the annual office Christmas party, or the playful romping of parents with small children. These kinds of regressive behaviors are time-limited. By time-limited we imply that the individual is capable of resuming his usual pattern of interacting, including the assumption of responsibility commensurate with his role functions. The maladaptive use of regressive behavior occurs when those behaviors that were prevalent and were considered appropriate during childhood are sustained over time and become a habitual response mode of adaptation.

Regressive behavior seldom permeates all areas of an individual's personality structure; even the most severely regressed patient retains some potential for the development of adequate coping devices necessary for the maintenance of survival. Some examples of regressive behavior that illustrate the extent to which the individual can be incapacitated are egocentricity or preoccupation with self, tantrums, pouting, refusal to communicate or to participate in the ordinary activities of daily living, daydreams, hallucinations, delusions, isolation, or the assumption of a fetal position. The type of nursing approach needed to care for individuals with regressive behavior is one that is warm, persistent, patient, and nonthreatening. To achieve this approach the nurse's attitude must be one of personal worth, involvement, and hopefulness.

Specific nursing interventions found to be effective in dealing with the clinical problem of regressive behavior are included in Table 22–2.

TABLE 22–2. REGRESSIVE BEHAVIOR—INTERVENTION AND RATIONALE

Intervention	Rationale
Initiate short, frequent contacts with the patient.	To convey interest and concern and to emphasize to the patient the attitude that he has personal worth.
Remain with the patient for designated periods of time.	To establish rapport and trust.

TABLE 22–2. CONTINUED

Intervention	Rationale
Maintain the focus of attention on the patient during periods of contact: look at the patient; address him by name; and direct communication specifically toward him.	To reemphasize personal worth.
Use simple language, specific words, and short sentences.	To prevent misunderstanding and misinterpretation of reality and to promote better understanding of the communicated messages.
Speak quietly, distinctly, and directly to the patient.	To decrease potential anxiety and to prevent loss of interest and understanding due to the patient's limited attention span.
Be honest and open with the patient; for example, keep promises; provide necessary information; give easy-to-follow directions and explanations for procedures.	To establish trust, to facilitate communication, and to offer him a reassuring, anxiety-free interpersonal contact.
Give merited praise and recognition based on specific, accurate observations such as, "I see you're wearing your new dress today," "You made your bed already," or "You finished your project in O.T."	To help the patient to rebuild his self-esteem.
Allow the patient to be as dependent as he needs to be; for example, if patient is mute, encourage him but don't demand a verbal response; if patient refuses to eat, prepare and serve food attractively, encourage and assist with food intake, feed if necessary; if the patient is incontinent, provide clean clothes and bedding and institute a toileting schedule.	To meet dependency needs; to guard against excessive anxiety and reinforcing feelings of rejection or subjection while preventing further ego disintegration; and to maintain a nonjudgmental, nonpunitive approach.
Observe the patient for signs and symptoms of physical illness.	To promote health and prevent illness.
Allow the patient sufficient time to respond.	To demonstrate willingness to proceed at the patient's own pace.
Encourage the patient to gradually assume initiative.	To assist the patient to move toward reality.
Gradually increase the complexity and scope of the patient's decision-making.	To reinforce reality and to encourage responsible, independent functioning.
Gradually increase exposure to people and environmental changes.	To keep the level of anxiety to a minimum.
Introduce the patient to simple, routine, familiar activities.	To reach out to the patient and to reintroduce reality in a nonthreatening and potentially anxiety-free atmosphere.
Encourage and assist the patient to carry out activities.	To increase self-esteem; to reinforce the bond of trust; and to use the activity as a focus for interpersonal communication.
Plan and initiate an uncomplicated, structured daily routine.	To provide a basis for maintaining contact with reality.
Deal with the patient on an adult level—avoid nicknames, slang, street language, or crude language.	To demonstrate respect, to increase self-esteem, and to convey a sense of personal worth.

(*continued*)

TABLE 22–2. CONTINUED

Intervention	Rationale
Control environmental conditions such as lighting, temperature, noise, and contacts with other people.	To provide the correct amount of stimuli needed by the patient and to prevent him from becoming dominated by the environment, that is, from becoming institutionalized.
Foster realism in daily living by having the patient wear his own personal clothing and eat with the proper utensils, and promote conversation in the dining room.	To increase contact with reality; to promote socially acceptable behavior; and to increase socialization.
Observe the patient for behavior pattern responses to environmental, interpersonal, and intrapsychic situations.	To gather information for planning future interventions and to increase knowledge about and understanding of the patient.
Recognize mounting tensions based on known behavioral responses.	To facilitate the planning of successful intervention on behalf of the patient.
Intervene before regression becomes more rigid or severe.	To interrupt the regressive pattern and refocus the patient on reality.
Accept the patient's need to test the nurse's integrity, reliability, care, concern, and degree of involvement.	To foster trust, develop rapport, and increase the patient's self-concept.
Identify "testing measures" used by the patient.	To increase knowledge and understanding about the patient.
Recognize situations in which "testing" is prevalent.	To plan intervention.
Respond to the patient who is testing by acknowledgment and confrontation, a search for causation and a reevaluation of the approach to the patient.	To reinforce reality; to promote realistic security operations; and to set limits on unacceptable behavior.

AGGRESSIVE BEHAVIOR

Aggressive behavior is forceful self-assertion that tends to be destructive in nature. Aggressive behavior is attack behavior that evokes retaliatory or defensive responses. The individual resorts to aggressive behavior when he perceives there is no other form of adaptation available to him. Aggressive behavior arises out of frustration or overstimulation. The particular mode of expression for aggressive behavior is learned during early stages of development. The social sanctions for specific aggressive acts are shaped by role identification with significant others and by cultural determinants within the social system.

The patient displaying aggressive behavior is hypersensitive, resentful, and believes that he is subjected to control and domination by circumstances or people. The overriding emotional response is anger that is discharged openly and directly or subtly and indirectly toward the physical or interpersonal environment. An issue that holds particular significance for clinical management of aggressive behavior relates to the form of release used by the patient within the setting. The socially acceptable form for release of aggression must be such that it does not violate the rights of others and can be used by the patient after discharge from the hospital.

The kind of therapeutic atmosphere needed by patients who display aggressive behavior is one in which the nurse takes a calm, quiet, firm, structured, accepting approach. To create such an atmosphere, the nurse must cultivate the attitudes of open-mindedness and integrity.

Specific nursing interventions found to be effective in dealing with the clinical problem of aggressive behavior are found in Table 22–3.

TABLE 22–3. AGGRESSIVE BEHAVIOR—INTERVENTION AND RATIONALE

Intervention	Rationale
Initiate frequent, regularly scheduled contacts.	To demonstrate acceptance of the patient regardless of his behavior.
Maintain spatial distance between self and patient.	To prevent the patient from feeling overpowered or dominated by the presence of "authority."
Provide clear, concise explanations for all rules and regulations.	To set control through definition of limits and to set positive expectations for responsible behavior.
Minimize external stimuli.	To prevent eruption of aberrant behavior.
Use a positive approach—make suggestions rather than give commands; invite participation rather than make demands; redirect action rather than imposing external controls.	To foster the building of trust and to emphasize integrity and reliability of the nurse.
Be honest and open in communications.	To reduce fear, anxiety, and helplessness in order to lessen the patient's sense of staff domination.
Remain rational and dependable.	To convey sincerity and security, thus promoting the patient's feelings of security and trust; to avoid power struggles.
Listen to complaints and attempt to identify their legitimacy.	To give recognition to the patient in order to increase his sense of integrity.
Respond positively to reasonable demands and requests.	To reemphasize the patient's sense of personal worth and minimize the patient's potential loss of control.
Absorb verbal expressions of anger, resentment, bitterness, belittling, or sarcasm.	To demonstrate acceptance of the individual regardless of behavior.
Define with the patient the extent of the problem.	To convey interest in the patient and to assist him to develop awareness regarding behavior, thereby reestablishing contact with reality.
Elicit patient's feelings regarding the problem behavior.	To bring feelings into awareness that coping mechanisms can be developed.
Identify the precipitating cause of aggressive behavior with the patient.	To determine the purpose of the patient's behavior so that the best method of intervention can be chosen.

(continued)

TABLE 22–3. CONTINUED

Intervention	Rationale
Devise and explore alternative behavioral responses.	To assist the patient to develop socially acceptable patterns of behaving.
Provide distraction and channel aggressive behavior through mildly competitive games like cards, checkers, chess; constructive tasks; and challenging activities at which the patient is known to be proficient.	To provide socially acceptable outlets for the expression of aggressive behavior; to foster self-esteem; and to promote feelings of accomplishment and independence.
Apply external controls (as a last resort) such as direct verbal commands ("Stop yelling!"); impose consequences for unmet expectations ("If you don't stop banging the table, you'll have to go back to your room"); and exert direct physical control by using medicinal or mechanical restraints.	To provide protection and control for the patient until such time as he is able to exert self-control.

MANIPULATIVE BEHAVIOR

Manipulative behavior is control behavior. Through manipulative behavior, an individual uses others to meet his own needs or to achieve his goals. Manipulative behavior is used to disguise the individual's underlying feelings of inadequacy, inferiority, and unworthiness. Its use by the individual is an attempt to protect himself against failure or frustration and to gain power over another. This maladaptive behavior has a depersonalizing effect on others and tends to evoke strong negative feelings on the part of the respondent. These negative feelings are conveyed through dislike, disbelief, rejection, retaliation, or punishment. Such responses tend to reinforce the individual's dependency, increase his anxiety, and foster continued use of and reliance on manipulative behavior as a mode of adaptation.

One of the frequently overlooked effects of the patient's manipulative behavior is the engendering of negativism and parallel manipulative behavior by the staff. Often the staff reacts to the manipulative, angry patient, with his incessant demands, unrealistic expectations of the staff, and endless complaints against the institution and the care given by assuming that the patient's behavior and verbal expressions are a direct, personal affront. Consequently, the staff singles out the manipulative patient as "a troublemaker," "a chronic complainer," "an inappropriate admission," and employs other derogatory terms that result in subconscious sabotage of treatment interventions and lack of interest in patient-care outcomes.

The self and subsequent understanding of the self, as discussed in Chapter 12, are of fundamental importance when approaching the manipulative patient. The approach best suited for creating a therapeutic environment for individuals with manipulative behavior is one that is firm, kind, consistent, matter-of-fact, and realistic. It is vitally important to the therapeutic process and the successful treatment of the manipulative patient that a consistent team approach be rendered on a 24-hour basis. This necessitates that the nurse must be clear, concise, and complete in her report to others regarding modifications of the patient's behavior and additions to or deletions from the original treatment approach, and must share the contributions made by other disciplines in the implementation and evaluation of the treatment contract. The significant attitudes necessary for the implementation of this approach are integrity, open-mindedness, and personal worth.

Specific nursing interventions found to be effective in dealing with the clinical problem of manipulative behavior are found in Table 22–4.

TABLE 22–4. MANIPULATIVE BEHAVIOR—INTERVENTION AND RATIONALE

Intervention	Rationale
Observe the particular way the patient's manipulative behavior is manifest.	To provide information needed for appropriate intervention.
Observe the reactions of self and others to the manipulative behavior.	To prevent other patients, the nurses, or other team members from becoming trapped by the manipulative behavior.
Identify feelings engendered within the nurse by the manipulative behavior.	To create awareness and self-understanding so that appropriate, therapeutic interruption of the manipulative cycle can be effected.
Recognize instances in which the patient is using manipulative behavior.	To avoid being used as a tool by the patient and to promote the patient's awareness of his behavior.
Refrain from responding or being "taken in" by manipulative behavior such as teasing, personal remarks designed to flatter or embarrass, and vulgar language or risqué jokes.	To prevent the continuation of the manipulative pattern and to prevent reinforcement of the patient's negative view of self.
Identify limits for the patient that the staff is willing to accept.	To formulate positive expectations and prevent "unconscious sabotage" of the therapeutic plan by the patient or the staff.
Explain to the patient, first, positive expectations, and second, the extent of the limits.	To overcome the pattern of failure and decrease frustration.
Recognize the patient's repeated attempts at testing limits.	To develop self-awareness, promote understanding, and to interrupt the patient's manipulative pattern.
Implement consistency and elicit the cooperation of all team members.	To interrupt the manipulative behavior pattern, reduce anxiety, and increase the patient's potential for cooperating with the therapeutic regime.

(*continued*)

TABLE 22–4. CONTINUED

Intervention	Rationale
Provide continuity of approach, expectations, and limits on a 24-hour basis.	To increase the patient's awareness and need for consistent controls on his own behavior and to assist the patient to learn to delay immediate need gratification.
Listen and respond openly, directly, and honestly without expressing anger, disappointment, or disgust.	To build the individual's healthy concept of self and what is acceptable, social behavior.
Assist the patient to learn to use the problem-solving approach in his relationship with others.	To help the patient to learn self-control and to accept the concepts of cooperation, collaboration, and compromise.

SELF-DESTRUCTIVE BEHAVIOR

Self-destructive behavior is revengeful, angry self-punishment. Self-destructive behavior is carried out by those individuals who believe they have failed to live up to the ideals and expectations they have set up for themselves or believe others require of them. They experience this pseudofailure in terms of radically lowered self-esteem and pervasive, personal inadequacy. They express their feelings in terms of uncertainty, helplessness, hopelessness, and vitriolic self-criticism. Underlying self-destructive behavior are tremendous feelings of anger, disappointment, resentment, and hostility. Through the self-destructive behavior, the individual attempts to strike out against and eradicate that part of the self that is so unpleasant, unrewarding, impotent, and ineffective. The self-destructive individual is so preoccupied with retaliation against the self and others that he is unable to formulate effective, satisfying interpersonal ties or glean satisfaction from any achievements.

Self-destructive acts include such behaviors as continuous scratching or picking at self; a seeming ignorance or unawareness of environmental hazards; repeated accidents, illness, and injuries; high alcohol or drug consumption; and suicidal thoughts or attempts. This type of behavior may create within the observer a feeling of dislike, disgust, repulsion, and rejection. This response on the part of staff occurs because the physical sight of self-inflicted injury is in itself distressing and because of the possible feelings of personal threat such acts provoke.

The 20th century will be noted for the prevalence of depression. It permeates every segment of civilized society, irrespective of class, race, or culture. Nursing personnel within institutions, hospitals, and other patient care facilities are constantly confronted with the problem of intervening, managing, and delivering interventive techniques for patients manifesting self-destructive behaviors. In Chapter 11 we dealt with depression, its symptomatology and dynamics. The reader will find that reviewing this chapter will be informative and helpful in understanding the self-destructive patient.

The creation of a therapeutic atmosphere must include an approach that is gentle, warm, and accepting. The attitudes necessary to implement this approach are hopefulness, personal worth, and involvement.

Specific nursing interventions found to be effective in dealing with the clinical problem of self-destructive behavior are included in Table 22–5.

TABLE 22–5. SELF-DESTRUCTIVE BEHAVIOR—INTERVENTION AND RATIONALE

Intervention	Rationale
Review family and personal history.	To make assessment of suicide potential.
Assess suicide potential.	To alert the health team and determine the immediate goal for intervention.
Listen carefully to delusional or hallucinatory content.	To pick up cues regarding increases in the level and intensity of anxiety or fear.
Listen to verbal communication for possible threats, plans, or decisions about death or dying.	To demonstrate interest and concern and to gather data for immediate crisis intervention.
Observe patient behavior closely for changes in mood, appetite, drives, levels of energy, or concentration.	To provide data with which to evaluate suicide potential and plan necessary intervention.
Make rounds at frequent, irregular intervals, particularly during the night, toward early morning, at change of shift, or during "busy times" for unit personnel.	To prevent, interfere with, or interrupt any destructive behavior.
Assign patient to a room close to the nurse's station.	To increase accessibility to the patient and opportunities for observation.
Maintain distance and interaction between patients exhibiting similar behaviors.	To prevent these patients from reinforcing one another's self-destructive behavior.
Decrease environmental hazards such as sharp instruments, cleaning supplies, belts, cords, electrical equipment, or drugs.	To provide safety and protection for the patient and to provide reassurance that someone cares and that the staff will not permit him to be self-destructive.
Plan for and assign the patient to menial but useful tasks—scrubbing sinks in the bathroom, scouring ashtrays, cleaning water fountains, emptying trash cans.	To relieve guilt, satisfy the need for "punishment," and to provide opportunity for increase in self-esteem through accomplishment of necessary and worthwhile activity.
Limit possibilities of body contact when engaging in recreational, occupational, or work activities.	To prevent the displacement of anger or hostility onto others in the immediate environment; to decrease the potential for impulsive acting out; and to prevent bodily injury to others.

(*continued*)

TABLE 22–5. CONTINUED

Intervention	Rationale
Redirect expressions of anger or hostility into acceptable channels; for example, bowling, typing, playing the piano, tearing strips of cloth to be used in weaving or as fillers for stuffed toys or pillows.	To prevent the negative feelings from being directed towards self or objects and to encourage and reinforce the use of alternatives to destructive behavior.
Insure that the patient is not left alone.	To decrease the patient's feelings that no one cares, to minimize the opportunities for destructive behavior; and to provide an opportunity for close observation without hovering.
Seek out the patient at frequent intervals and then gradually introduce him to others.	To develop closeness with the patient; to demonstrate to the patient respect for his importance as a person; and to supply opportunities for the development of potentially meaningful interpersonal relationships without overwhelming him.
Be sincere and honest with the patient: "We will not permit you to harm yourself" or "Yes, we are interested in where you are and what you are doing."	To demonstrate respect, acceptance and a sincere appreciation for his personal worth.
Design and implement with the patient a "busy" schedule.	To keep the patient occupied and to prevent preoccupation with self-destructive thoughts or behavior.
Alert all personnel to the patient's self-destructive behavior.	To minimize hazards, to promote safety, and to provide continuity of concerned care.
Implement definite limits or restrictions on mobility or whereabouts; for example, accompany the patient to all off-ward activity, assign one member of the staff to be responsible for close unobtrusive observation, or supervise the patient's use of potentially hazardous equipment.	To decrease the patient's potential accessibility to environmental hazards.
Permit the patient to verbalize suicidal threats; do not ignore them; do not argue with the patient about them; and take his statements seriously.	To establish trust; to recognize the importance of the intent; and to determine the time when protective action is most needed.
Encourage the patient to make simple decisions according to his capabilities, such as what to wear or eat, whether to watch TV or play cards.	To foster a sense of accomplishment and self-control and to exercise independent functioning.
Make all other decisions for the patient.	To eliminate overwhelming anxiety and thereby reduce the patient's need to engage in self-destructive behavior as the only avenue of escape.
Remain calm, unimpressed but not indifferent to self-destructive activity.	To provide a feeling of security; to minimize the patient's fear and guilt; and to reduce the possibility of successful completion of the suicidal act.
Convey warmth and interest in the patient but not in the suicidal act or threat; for example: "You've hurt yourself; it must be painful; let me help you."	To demonstrate acceptance of the person, to display a nonjudgmental attitude toward the person, and to convey concern and understanding.

TABLE 22–5. CONTINUED

Intervention	Rationale
Avoid angry, critical comments that might be interpreted by the patient as a dare, threat, or "calling his bluff"; for example, "Don't you know that dose wouldn't have killed you?" and "You severed a vein, not an artery."	To prevent reinforcement of guilt and further decrease in self-esteem.
Interrupt self-destructive acts by placing a protective arm about the patient and suggesting that he talk the situation over; diverting attention from the suicidal act toward something else; or making an appeal to reason or persuading him to postpone his suicidal action.	To prevent death, to allow time for interpersonal techniques to be employed, and to determine underlying causative factors for the particular self-destructive behavior.
Pay attention to physical needs by encouraging adequate nutritional intake; observing response to drug therapy; closely observing patient's ingestion of medication; promoting adequate rest and sleep; and preventing fatigue.	To promote and maintain physiological functioning.

HYPERACTIVE BEHAVIOR

Hyperactive behavior is exaggerated, irrational, excessive response to stimuli. The hyperactive individual reacts impulsively and forcefully to people, places, and things. Hyperactivity is an attempt on the part of the individual to exercise control and dominance over the environment. Furthermore, this individual is unable to focus or concentrate. Symptomatically, this means that the patient makes loose associations or displays a short attention span. The inability to concentrate precludes effective listening and communication. In addition, his pattern of speech is often fragmented and nonsequential, which indicates the stream of stimuli that he is evidently internalizing and to which he is outwardly responding. Hyperactivity is overcompensatory behavior used to mask the individual's feelings of inferiority, inadequacy, and inability to perform and to relate meaningfully to others. The hyperactive individual is angry, fearful, and in a constant state of threat. This hyperactivity is demonstrated through accelerated psychomotor activity, increase in physical prowess, and hyperventilation. The hyperactive individual is easily irritated and excited and given to wide mood swings, capriciousness, distractibility, and destructiveness.

A quiet, firm, kind, persuasive approach is most effective in dealing with hyperactive behavior. The attitudes most needed by the nurse to implement the approach are advocacy, open-mindedness, and personal worth.

Specific nursing interventions found to be effective in dealing with the clinical problem of hyperactive behavior are included in Table 22–6.

TABLE 22–6. HYPERACTIVE BEHAVIOR—INTERVENTION AND RATIONALE

Intervention	Rationale
Provide a subdued environment; remove unnecessary furniture; take pictures off walls; tone down bright, harsh colors; and eliminate excess noise.	To reduce sensory input; to decrease hyperactivity.
Assign patient to private room.	To provide him with a quiet area to reduce environmental and interpersonal stimulation.
Reduce the number of contacts the patient has with people; assign the same staff members to him; discourage visitations from other patients, relatives, and personnel; and limit the patient's participation with groups.	To decrease irritability; to decrease impulsive interaction; to prevent attempts at dominating others; to protect the patient from retaliation from others; and to promote physical distance, which helps to lessen misidentification of "approach" behavior as "attack" behavior.
Monitor food intake.	To maintain nutritional needs and to plan and provide necessary adjustments in dietary intake.
Provide a high-caloric, high-vitamin diet with supplemental feedings.	To combat exhaustion and weight loss due to high energy output.
Provide finger foods such as sandwiches, cookies, fruit, milkshakes.	To provide foods that can be eaten as the patient moves about because he is "too busy" to sit down and eat.
Increase fluid intake.	To prevent dehydration and constipation and to assist in elimination of medication to prevent toxicity.
Initiate weight chart.	To monitor possible weight loss.
Supervise personal hygiene: assist with collection of necessary toilet articles; adjust temperature of shower or bath water; assist and instruct patient with bathing, oral hygiene, shaving, dressing; observe condition of skin and general state of the body for injury or misuse; and control the patient's use of toiletries, cosmetics, and jewelry.	To maintain physical well-being; to combat disorganization and distractibility; to provide for safety—needed because of the patient's poor judgment; to insure cleanliness, neatness, and appropriateness, to prevent patient from being an object of ridicule; and to promote positive self-image.
Encourage the patient to wear his own clothes.	To maintain identity and contact with reality.
Maintain patient's wardrobe—keep clothing in good repair; advise and provide changes of attire according to season, activity, and time of day; remove from pockets accumulated junk or items that belong to others.	To encourage appropriateness of appearance and to maintain identity and to set realistic limits.
Monitor physiological functioning: observe for signs and symptoms of physical distress; encourage patient to verbalize discomforts; investigate, record, and report somatic complaints.	To maintain a state of physiological homeostasis and guard against illness and to intervene and prevent the development of any pathophysiological condition.
Exercise vigilance in administration of medication: if the patient refuses the medication, don't argue, but distract his attention while offering the medication; if the patient seeks to postpone taking medication, go on to the next patient in line and then return using positive suggestions, "It's now time to take your medication"; if patient	To maintain effective therapeutic drug regime or to prevent possible misuse of drugs by the patient or others.

TABLE 22–6. CONTINUED

Intervention	Rationale
is hoarding, closely observe for swallowing, increase fluids, inspect his mouth, change to liquid or parenteral administration.	
Promote rest and sleep by observing usual sleep patterns; reducing stimuli prior to bed time; using somatic comfort measures like hot tubs, warm milk, back rubs; administering prescribed medication; and prescribing and planning for daily rest period.	To prevent fatigue, exhaustion, and circulatory collapse.
Provide a regular supervised, noncompetitive, solitary or small-group activity such as swimming, gymnastics, walking, running, housekeeping, raking grass, finger painting, or writing.	To direct excessive amount of energy into appropriate channels; to increase sedentary activity to prevent fatigue and lessen hyperactive behavior; and to allow for expression of angry feelings.
Select projects or activities that can be completed in a short time.	To provide opportunities for the patient to experience success and counteract feelings of inferiority and inadequacy, and to assist the patient to develop self-control.
Listen quietly and attentively to the patient.	To act as a sounding board for his excitement.
Attempt to interrupt flow of conversation and refocus.	To redirect attention toward "real" concerns.
Schedule short, frequent interaction sessions.	To make maximum use of the patient's short attention span.
Give short, simple, direct explanations for procedures and activities.	To maintain focus on reality.
Observe for changes in mood and behavior such as increasing irritability and increased physical or verbal activity.	To assess the need for specific intervention and to prevent hyperactive crisis.
Define firm, consistent limits for the patient.	To establish external control and to aid in the prevention of hyperactive crisis.
Guard against becoming maneuvered by the patient's excitement, impetuosity, grandiosity, and hyperactivity.	To prevent loss of personal control and therapeutic effectiveness.

COMPULSIVE BEHAVIOR

Compulsive behavior is stereotyped behavior. It is peculiar, repetitive behavior. The individual is usually intellectually cognizant that his behavior is exaggerated, impulsive, inappropriate, unreasonable, and undesirable. Nevertheless, he is unable to stop and feels compelled to carry out the ritualistic, repetitive act. With this type of behavior the individual disguises his overwhelming anxiety. Each repetitive act is significant for the individual, and its form of expression is directly related to the particular problem producing the underlying anxiety.

The majority of ritualistic acts are in effect "makeup" behaviors. The individual is attempting to atone for past or present guilt feelings either by restitution or undoing.

Compulsive behavior is essentially an avoidance and protective operation. Its use acts as a substitute for establishing constructive and satisfying relationships. It also may act as a means of escaping from the responsibility of expressing and sharing feelings. Dynamically, the specific behavior symbolizes the commission of some act that would violate the individual's value or belief system and serves as a means of restitution for the original prohibited act. Anxiety is a key factor, since the individual experiences heightened levels of anxiety before and after the performed act. The performance of the act itself only temporarily reduces and relieves tension.

Engagement in compulsive behavior produces a rigid and constricted life-style with resultant daily routines. In turn, this peculiar stylized pattern of living is perceived by the individual as reassurance that he is in control. This means that he functions under the assumption that he can predict and thereby prevent undesirable effects from disrupting his sense of equilibrium. However, this view is erroneous, since the individual becomes so involved with controlling maneuvers that his daily living experience deteriorates into chaos.

The nurse's approach should include kind, patient acceptance and understanding. The attitudes the nurse needs to implement in this approach are integrity, personal worth, open-mindedness, and involvement.

Specific nursing interventions found to be effective in dealing with the clinical problem of compulsive behavior are included in Table 22–7.

TABLE 22–7. COMPULSIVE BEHAVIOR—INTERVENTION AND RATIONALE

Intervention	Rationale
Modify environment, schedules, and routines.	To convey acceptance; to permit the patient time to carry out his ritualistic behavior without interruption; and to reduce his anxiety.
Plan, discuss, and implement with the patient an individualized schedule of daily activities.	To accommodate his need for repetitive acts and to demonstrate support for the patient.
Expect patient to adhere to planned schedule that includes time for ritualistic behavior as well as consistent limits on the behavior.	To convey acceptance and understanding by not subjecting the individual to ridicule or criticism and to meet needs through alternative means.
Anticipate needs by offering self through frequent, planned contact; listening to and encouraging verbalization; administering medication *on time*; and giving information, instructions, or items for daily living before he has to ask.	To increase feelings of security; reduce anxiety; and demonstrate personal worth and integrity.

TABLE 22–7. CONTINUED

Intervention	Rationale
Plan and participate in diversional activity with the patient.	To prevent preoccupation with self and to substitute more appropriate means for reducing anxiety.
Choose recreational and occupational therapy according to old interests and successful accomplishments.	To insure success and positive feedback that increase his self-image.
Introduce patient to small-group activity.	To release tension; to provide new interests; and to meet the needs for affection, recognition, and belonging.
Seek out and spend time with patient.	Provide the patient with therapeutic support that allays feelings of guilt and anxiety.
Listen patiently and attentively to verbalization of feelings.	To convey acceptance and interest.
Focus communication on problem areas.	To assist the patient with identification and to develop awareness of anxiety and conflict.
Explore current conflict in relationship to ritualistic behavior.	To facilitate comparison and to encourage decision-making.
Support decisions made and assist the patient to implement new behaviors.	To interrupt the use of ritualistic behavior; to promote psychological comfort; and to provide necessary reassurance to lessen anxiety.
Observe for signs of mounting anxiety and intervene before the patient resorts to ritualistic behaviors.	To prevent the need for the behavior pattern and to assist the patient to learn to deal with anxiety.

ADDICTIVE BEHAVIOR

Addictive behavior is flight from pain, an escape from responsibilities, and a search for pleasure. It is the manifestation of altered physiological and psychological processes that result in dependency on substances that permit the individual to escape, avoid, distort, obliterate, or escalate his thoughts, feelings, or actions. Substances used to produce major physiological and psychological alterations include alcohol, hallucinogenic agents, narcotics, sedatives, stimulants, and volatile chemicals. The type of substance abused, its availability, and the dynamics leading to addiction differ with each user.

Addictive behavior is one of the most prevalent, disruptive phenomena invading all strata of society. There are many forms of addiction, from the most common and socially acceptable addiction to caffeine as illustrated by the "universal coffee break" to the more bizarre, socially unacceptable, and often destructive misuse and abuse of hallucinogenic agents. The results are unmistakable, whether one is young or old, rich or poor, male or female. Prolonged abuse eventuates in both the physical and mental deterioration of the individual; causes serious disruption and often produces seemingly irreconcilable conflicts within family units; and directly or indirectly negatively affects society at large.

Addictive behavior is used by the individual as a means of changing his present reality. It is used as a prop for hope and happiness. It involves the seeking after a state of well-being in which all problems, needs, wants, and desires disappear, are magically resolved, or are relegated to a position of secondary importance. As a means to an end, addictive behavior is a substitute for problem solving and confrontation with reality. The individual uses his addiction much like the circus clown uses his "paint pots," that is, to mask his real self from the real world. The mask enables the abuser to be or not to be! It allows him to present to the world an outward show of bravado or confidence that he does not feel or that does not exist. It permits him to display outgoing or assertive behavior that covers his inner timidity or fearfulness. It enables him to deny, rationalize, and project his ideas or actions in an effort to conceal and protect himself from assuming responsibility for self and involvement with others. It lets him manifest exaggerated feeling states to relieve the discomfort of perceived boredom, routine, or loneliness. The drug abuser is firmly convinced that the drug route is the only avenue open to him in his fight for survival.

Reluctance, opposition, open conflict, and defiance of all authority are predominant behavioral characteristics of the drug abuser. This individual plays games, is a master in the art of manipulation, and uses others to achieve his own ends. The addicted individual is a person whose tolerance for stress is minimal, whose ego strengths are few, and whose ability to cope is almost nonexistent. The predominantly aggressive tactics used by the drug abuser, namely: subtle innuendoes; abusive, insulting language; loud, demanding, threatening verbalizations; or intimidating gestures, are essentially distancing maneuvers that segregate him from society and prevent the development of close, warm, human ties.

A firm, consistent, matter-of-fact, nonpunitive, and realistic approach is esssential for individuals who manifest addictive behavior. The significant attitudes that must be cultivated by the nurse in implementing this approach are integrity, personal worth, and openmindedness.

Specific nursing interventions found to be effective in dealing with the clinical problem of addictive behavior are included in Table 22–8. The interventions are divided according to the three essential phases of the treatment process: detoxification, rehabilitation, and follow-up.

TABLE 22–8. NURSING INTERVENTION IN ADDICTIVE BEHAVIOR

Intervention	Rationale
Detoxification	
Assign the same staff on a prolonged basis and initiate a therapeutic nurse–patient relationship.	To provide consistency, reduce fear, and allow for development of trust.
Remain with patient and exercise close observation.	To monitor changes in patient status; to collect data for reassessing and updating of the care plan; to offer reassurance; to provide additional emotional support; and to limit access to abused drug.
Minimize environmental stimuli.	To prevent triggering inappropriate perceptual responses to environment.
Take vital signs frequently and accurately.	To establish a data base and to prevent complications.
Monitor intake and output.	To maintain hydration and to observe for retention.
Note response to questions and directions.	To determine alterations in levels of consciousness and to identify the presence of psychopathological symptomatology.
Note changes in behavior.	To initiate preventive measures, thereby safeguarding the patient from experiencing the acute discomfort frequently associated with withdrawal, such as alcoholic hallucinosis, delerium tremens, or panic.
Check and relay laboratory findings to physician.	To keep physician informed of serum electrolyte status.
Document and report changes in patient status immediately.	To prevent crisis.
Check personal belongings of patient.	To ensure that patient or others have not secreted a supply of abused drug.
Restrict or limit visitors.	To prevent or reduce potential hazard of obtaining abused drugs from outside source.
Rehabilitation	
Continue therapeutic relationship initiated during detoxification.	To continue identification of problems, needs, and concerns; to set realistic goals and explore alternatives to addictive patterns of behavior.
Involve the patient in developing and adjusting an ongoing plan of care.	To foster the patient's sense of responsibility and accountability in the management of his own treatment; to acknowledge the patient's right to have input into his own care.
Structure activities of daily living.	To provide consistency and to limit the amount of unplanned "free" time.
Set and maintain limits.	To provide consistency, maintain structure, and minimize manipulative behavior.
Provide a variety of group experiences relating to work opportunities, drug abuse education, social interaction, gripes and unmet needs, discharge planning and community placement.	To increase interpersonal contact; to share, compare, and verify interpersonal experiences; to develop group communication skills and socialization; to assist the patient to begin

(*continued*)

TABLE 22–8. CONTINUED

Intervention	Rationale
Rehabilitation	
Hyperactive behavior (*continued*)	movement toward independent functioning; to provide another avenue for continued growth and responsibility; and to support and reinforce abstinence behavior.
Insist on active participation in total treatment plan.	To motivate the patient; to present reality; to reduce potential manipulative behavior; and assess commitment to treatment process.
Include family members, relatives, or friends in the treatment plan.	To provide support to patient and family; to enlist cooperation of significant others.
Implement a mechanism for checking patient's whereabouts at all times.	To maintain supervision and observational processes and to provide additional data for evaluating the effectiveness of care.
Follow-up	
Maintain therapeutic relationship with original staff.	To provide continuity of care.
Plan with patient a detailed schedule for outpatient clinic visits, individual counseling, group sessions, home visits, family counseling.	To provide structure, consistency, and support in assisting the patient and his family to meet the demands of adjustment outside the hospital environment; to monitor physical change; to foster and sustain continuous movement toward independent functioning; and to reduce possibility of potential relapse.
Refer patient to existing community support groups such as Alcoholics Anonymous or Narcotics Anonymous.	To help the patient adopt a supportive social network.

SUSPICIOUS BEHAVIOR

Suspicious behavior is forceful, aggressive confrontation with others. Such behavior is manifested through a consistent, persistent tendency to doubt and to mistrust the sincerity, motivation, reliability, or honesty of others. In his relationship with others, the suspicious individual makes no allowance for human error. Suspicious behavior is compensatory behavior used to disguise, project, or deny feelings of insecurity, interpersonal inadequacy, and distortions of personal identity.

This individual harbors deep-seated dependency needs and manifests morbid resentment. His primary area of difficulty is found in the manner in which he attempts to satisfy and gratify these needs as well as the manner in which he responds to authority. The behavior manifested is determined by the excessive and exaggerated use of projection as a defensive operation. The respondent behavior is often not acceptable, resulting in the individual's social isolation. This isolation, in turn, contributes to and reinforces his sense of powerlessness and alienation, thus perpetuating his self-defeating behavior.

Suspicious behavior is indicative of cognitive rigidity. This means that the thoughts are fixed and that the individual is preoccupied with his search for supporting evidence that will confirm his expectations. In this process, the individual carefully scrutinizes each bit of new information with exacting thoroughness. He then, according to his prejudicial bent, extrapolates and discards that which is not pertinent to his area of suspicion. He retains only those pieces that have relevance for the maintenance of his original belief system.

In addition to cognitive rigidity, the suspicious individual also demonstrates a highly refined and penetrating ability as an observer. This ability produces a keen sensitivity and receptivity to the prevailing environmental overtones and the specific attitudes of those with whom he comes in contact.

The suspicious individual lives and functions from a highly subjective frame of reference. From this framework of subjectivity, facts, accurately perceived, are endowed with special interpretative significance. This means that in his interaction with others, the suspicious individual does not disagree with others regarding specific facts but rather insists on his own subjective meaning for these facts. As a result, he feels isolated, lonely, fearful, anxious, and hostile. Examples of suspicious behavior include expressions of dissatisfaction; subtle sabotage; dissemination of evil tidings or pessimistic warnings; portrayal of pretentious, dramatic self-sacrifice; spreading harmful tales about others; inciting violence; demonstrating resistance to any form of compliance, including that which may be for his own welfare, such as medication.

For the psychotic patient, suspicious behavior is manifested by an internal response in the form of hallucinatory and delusional symptomatology. The hallucinatory experiences may be auditory, visual, gustatory, tactile, or olfactory. The delusional systems exhibited are those involving persecution, grandiosity, or specific ideas of reference. Each of the experiences lends itself to the creation of additional suspicion and mistrust of other people and the environment. This increase in suspicion intensifies the patient's already overwhelming feelings of insecurity.

For those patients who display suspicious behavior, a kind, helpful, nonthreatening, and somewhat detached approach by the nurse is most effective in creating a responsive therapeutic milieu. Prevailing nurse attitudes for the implementation of this approach are those of personal worth, hopefulness, and integrity.

In planning interventive strategies a note of caution for the nurse—it is essential that interventive techniques not disturb or contradict the existing delusional or hallucinatory system until such time as the patient manifests a readiness to engage in reality orientation. Premature intervention will drive the patient to withdraw further and jeopardize the nurse–patient relationship.

Specific nursing interventions found to be effective in dealing with the clinical problem of suspicious behavior are included in Table 22–9.

TABLE 22–9. SUSPICIOUS BEHAVIOR—INTERVENTION AND RATIONALE

Intervention	Rationale
Be frank, open, and honest.	To counteract the patient's mistrust.
Demonstrate dependability by keeping promises, being on time for appointments, and alerting the patient well in advance of schedule changes.	To establish trust and integrity.
Clarify and restate role; repeat with patience and understanding.	To prevent misinterpretations; to decrease fear of involvement; to establish trust; and to define the helping relationship.
Listen for expressions of fear, anxiety, and mistrust in communication.	To identify and help the patient recognize problems.
Reflect and explore feelings.	To identify and clarify the relationship between feeling and behavior.
Discuss, implement, and evaluate with the patient alternatives for suspicious behavior.	To produce behavioral change and to demonstrate to the patient a satisfactory method of adaptation through the use of problem solving.
Minimize contact with a variety of staff.	To protect the patient from feeling threatened by too much interpersonal contact.
Eliminate unnecessary physical contact—do not touch the patient.	To avoid misinterpretation of action as an attack on the patient.
Assign to solitary, noncompetitive activity such as messenger or escort service, picture puzzles, weaving, drawing, photography, and typing.	To minimize feelings of insecurity or inferiority.
Allow patient the freedom to select activities within the scope of available choices.	To decrease mistrust and to foster a potential sense of accomplishment.
Reward completion of meaningful tasks with merited praise.	To increase self-esteem and to promote a more realistic view of self.
Be alert and observe for potential problem areas in eating, sleeping, and the taking of medications.	To plan intervention before the problem becomes unmanageable.

EVALUATION

A list of projected outcomes for each of the behaviors described in this chapter is found in Table 22–10. The evaluation criteria are based on the primary nursing care goal: to bring about change in behavior resulting in more healthy functioning. This listing is general in scope

TABLE 22–10. EVALUATION CRITERIA—BEHAVIORAL DISRUPTIONS

Behavioral Disruptions	Evaluation Criteria
Negativistic behavior	Develops responsible behavior: Initiates self-care activities. Sets realistic goals. Verbalizes positive feelings about self. Engages in realistic self-appraisal. Accepts success. Displays hopeful attitude. Meets deadlines. Complies with demands of social living.
Regressive behavior	Progresses to highest level of functioning: Expresses concern for others. Demonstrates interest in people and activities. Forms and maintains relationships. Communicates spontaneously. Participates independently in activities of daily living. Free from hallucinations and delusions. Uses learned coping strategies to reduce and manage anxiety, fear, and feelings of insecurity. Verbalizes positive statements about self.
Aggressive behavior	Ceases aggressive responses: Uses assertive communication skills. Displays respect for personal integrity of self and others. Selects constructive means for dealing with anger, guilt, or frustration. Remains calm when threatened. Uses problem-solving skills to resolve conflict. Exerts self-control.
Manipulative behavior	Ceases to exploit others: Verbalizes self-worth. Accepts responsibility for self. Delays satisfaction of wants. Sets limits on self. Adapts to rules and regulations. Makes reasonable requests.
Self-destructive behavior	Relinquishes self-punishment: Verbalizes hope for future. Makes positive references about self. Mood congruent with verbalizations and actions. Establishes relationship with others. Engages in productive activities. Accepts compliments and praise. Uses learned coping strategies to deal with feelings of anger, guilt, hostility, or anxiety. Assumes responsibility for self-care.
Hyperactive behavior	Exercises control over self and environment: Decreases motor activity. Completes tasks. Performs activities of daily living. Attends to physiological needs. Recognizes signs of mounting tension.

(*continued*)

TABLE 22–10. CONTINUED

Behavioral Disruptions	Evaluation Criteria
Hyperactive behavior (*continued*)	Seeks to reduce environmental stimuli. Demonstrates ability to concentrate. Directs excess energy into appropriate channels.
Compulsive behavior	Ceases ritualistic behavior: Recognizes signs of mounting anxiety. Employs learned coping strategies to reduce anxiety. Participates in diversional activities. Takes positive action on identified concerns. Makes logical, rational decisions. Recognizes and uses personal strengths. Refrains from focusing on somatic complaints. Exhibits flexibility in carrying out daily routines.
Addictive behavior	Ceases substance abuse: Demonstrates improved self-esteem. Assumes responsibility for behavior. Ceases to place blame on others. Sets realistic goals for self. Initiates actions toward meeting goals. Copes with stress. Resumes social roles. Develops interpersonal ties and external supports. Restructures social and environmental parameters of living.
Suspicious behavior	Develops trust: Makes allowance for human error. Initiates interpersonal approaches. Decreases feelings of insecurity and felt inadequacy. Expresses personal regard and respect for others. Ceases to hallucinate or express delusional thinking. Participates in group activities. Seeks to validate perceptions with significant others. Expresses a realistic view of self.

and is intended to serve only as an example. It is important for the reader to note that outcome criteria are derived from the identification of the optimal expectations to be achieved with each patient.

SUMMARY

In this chapter we have presented nine of the most commonly encountered clinical problems involving disruptive behavior patterns. The major nursing care goal is restoration of equilibrium through behavioral change. The goal is easily stated, but somewhat more difficult to achieve. Achievement rests almost exclusively with the attitudes of the nurse and in the consistent and persistent application of the change measures rather than on the specific strategies selected and employed. Behavioral change is a slow process in which there are neither short-cuts nor assurances that any single strategy is more effective than another.

The problem behaviors described in this chapter place an exacting and demanding burden on the nursing care provider and probably tax her professionalism more than any of the other physical or psychological problems she is likely to encounter. Dealing with patients with behavioral disturbances requires the practice of patience and the maintenance of a delicate balance between the humanness of the care provider and the humanness of the patient. Undoubtedly, it is of vital importance to the total care and treatment process for the nurse to be clear that the negativism projected by these patients is not to be interpreted as a personal affront or as an effort to cast aspersion upon the nurse's character or professional integrity.

SUGGESTED READINGS

Anders, R. L. When a Patient Becomes Violent. *American Journal of Nursing,* Vol. 77, No. 7 (July, 1977), 1144–1148.

Battin, M. P. *Ethical Issues in Suicide.* Englewood Cliffs, N. J.: Prentice-Hall, 1982.

Billings, C. V. Emotional First Aid. *American Journal of Nursing,* Vol. 80, No. 11 (November, 1980), 2006–2009.

Blythe, M. M., & Pearlmutter, D. R. The Suicide Watch: A Re-examination of Maximum Observation. *Perspectives in Psychiatric Care,* Vol. 21, No. 3 (July–September, 1983), 90–93.

Boettcher, E. G. Preventing Violent Behavior: An Integrated Theoretical Model for Nursing. *Perspectives in Psychiatric Care,* Vol. 21, No. 2 (April–June, 1983), 54–58.

Briggs, P. F. Specializing in Psychiatry: Therapeutic or Custodial? *Nursing Outlook,* Vol. 22, No. 10 (October, 1974), 632–635.

Brigman, C., Dickey, C., & Zeeger, L. J. The Agitated Aggressive Patient. *American Journal of Nursing,* Vol. 83, No. 10 (October, 1983), 1409–1412.

Burns, D. D. The Perfectionist's Script for Self Defeat. *Psychology Today,* Vol. 14, No. 6 (November, 1980), 34–52.

Busteed, E. L., & Johnstone, C. The Development of Suicide Precautions for an Inpatient Psychiatric Unit. *Journal of Psychosocial Nursing and Mental Health Services,* Vol. 21, No. 5 (May, 1983), 15–19.

Cavers, A. & Williams, R. The Budget Plan (Behavior Modification of Long-Term Patients). *Perspectives in Psychiatric Care,* Vol. 9, No. 1 (January, 1971), 13–16.

Cavers, A. & Williams, R. Dealing with Rage. *Nursing '75,* Vol. 5, No. 10 (October, 1975), 25–29.

Cedog, M. Mr. Rope. *Nursing '78,* Vol. 8, No. 8 (August, 1978), 88.

Cotton, P. G., et al. Dealing With Suicide on a Psychiatric Inpatient Unit. *Hospital and Community Psychiatry,* Vol. 34, No.1 (January, 1983), 55.

Davister, K. E. The Demanding Patient. *Nursing Life,* Vol. 5, No. 1 (January/February, 1985), 41.

Doenges, M., & Morehouse, M. *Nurses' Pocket Guide: Nursing Diagnoses with Inverventions.* Philadelphia: F. A. Davis, 1985.

Finley, B. Counseling the Alcoholic Client. *Journal of Psychiatric Nursing and Mental Health Services,* Vol. 19, No. 5 (May, 1981), 32–34.

Fitzpatrick J. J. Suicidology and Suicide Prevention: Historical Perspectives from the Nursing Literature. *Journal of Psychosocial Nursing and Mental Health Services,* Vol. 21, No. 5 (May, 1983), 20–28.

Fultz, J. M., Jr., et al. When a Narcotic Addict Is Hospitalized. *American Journal of Nursing,* Vol. 80, No. 3 (March, 1980), 478–481.

Gilead, M. P., & Mulaik, J. S. Adolescent Suicide: A Response to Developmental Crisis. *Perspectives in Psychiatric Care,* Vol. 21, No. 3 (July-September, 1983), 94–101.

Glasser, W. *Reality Therapy.* New York: Harper & Row, 1975.

Glazer, G. The "Good" Patient. *Nursing and Health Care,* Vol. 2, No. 3 (March, 1981), 144–147, 164.

Goldstein, S. Impulse Control. *Journal of Psychiatric Nursing and Mental Health Services,* Vol. 14, No. 7 (July, 1976), 36–40.

Hatton, C. L., & Valente, S. M. *Suicide Assessment and Intervention.* (2nd ed.) Norwalk, Conn.: Appleton-Century-Crofts, 1984.

Hickey, B. A. Transitional Relatedness and Engaging the Regressed Borderline Client. *Journal of Psychosocial Nursing and Mental Health Services,* Vol. 21, No. 1 (January, 1983), 26–30.

Hirst, S. P. Understanding the Difficult Patient. *Nursing Managament,* Vol. 14, No. 2 (February, 1983), 68–70.

Huberty, D. J., & Malmquist J. D. Adolscent Chemical Dependency. *Perspectives in Psychiatric Care,* Vol. 16, No. 1 (January/February, 1978), 20–27.

Iyer, P. W. The Battered Wife. *Nursing '80,* Vol. 10, No. 7 (July, 1980), 52–55.

Jurgensen, K. Limit Setting for Hospitalized Adolescent Psychiatric Patients. *Perspectives in Psychiatric Care,* Vol. 9, No. 4 (1971), 173–182.

Karshmer, J. F. The Application of Social Learning Theory to Aggression. *Perspectives in Psychiatric Care,* Vol. 16, Nos. 5–6 (September/December, 1978), 223-227.

Kurose, K., et al. A Standard Care Plan for Alcoholism. *American Journal of Nursing,* Vol. 81, No. 6 (June, 1981), 1001–1006.

Lanza, M. L. The Reactions of Nursing Staff to Physical Assault by a Patient. *Hospital and Community Psychiatry,* Vol. 34, No. 1 (January, 1983), 44–47.

LeBow, M. D. *Behavior Modification.* Englewood Cliffs, N. J.: Prentice-Hall, 1973.

Loughlin, Sister N. Suicide: A Case for Investigation. *Journal of Psychiatric Nursing and Mental Health Services,* Vol. 18, No. 2 (February, 1980), 8–12.

Luna, M. L. The Patient Who Complains. *Nursing '84,* Vol. 14, No. 11 (November, 1984), 46–49.

Marks, V. L. Health Teaching for Recovering Alcoholic Patients. *American Journal of Nursing,* Vol. 80, No. 11 (November, 1980), 2058–2061.

Matiak-Mozingo, L. Ron Taught Us To Expect the Unexpected. *Nursing '79,* Vol. 9, No. 5 (May, 1979), 50–53.

McFarland, G. K., & Wasli, E. L. *Nursing Diagnoses and Processes in Psychiatric Mental Health Nursing.* Philadelphia: Lippincott, 1986.

McMorrow, M. E. The Manipulative Patient. *American Journal of Nursing,* Vol. 81, No. 6 (June, 1981), 1188–1190.

Neville, D. & Barnes, S. Suicidal Phone Call. *Journal of Psychosocial Nursing and Mental Health Services,* Vol. 23, No. 8 (August, 1985), 14–18.

Palermo, K. R. To Punish Herself, Laura Mutilated Her Body. *Nursing '79,* Vol. 9, No. 6 (June, 1979), 44–48.

Post, J. M., & Oteri, E. M. Sign-Out Rounds. *Journal of Psychosocial Nursing and Mental Health Services,* Vol. 21, No. 9 (September, 1983), 11–17.

Reubin, R. Spotting and Stopping the Suicide Patient. *Nursing '79,* Vol. 9, No. 4 (April, 1979), 82–85.

Richardson, J. I. The Manipulative Patient Spells Trouble. *Nursing '81,* Vol. 11, No. 1 (January, 1981), 49–53.

Righthand, P. How to Deal With Rude, Demanding, Unreasonable People. *Nursing Life,* Vol. 3, No. 5 (September/October, 1983), 28–32.

Rosenbaum, M. S. Depression: What To Do, What To Say. *Nursing '80,* Vol. 10, No. 8 (August, 1980), 64–66.

Royalty, D. C. "Try To Help Her Keep Her Clothes On." That Was the Staff's Only Goal. *Nursing '76,* Vol. 6, No. 4 (April, 1976), 38–40.

Scheideman, J. Remotivation: Involvement Without Labels. *Journal of Psychiatric Nursing and Mental Health Services,* Vol. 14, No. 7 (July, 1976), 41–42.

Schloemer, N. F., & Skidmore, J. W. Opiate Withdrawal with Clonidine. *Journal of Psychosocial Nursing and Mental Health Services,* Vol. 21, No. 10 (October, 1983), 8–14.

Siegel, E. Scapegoating: Manifestation and Intervention. *Journal of Psychiatric Nursing and Mental Health Services,* Vol. 19, No. 4 (April, 1981), 11–15.

Smith, T. M. The Dynamics in Time-Limited Relationship Therapy with Methadone Maintained Patients. *Perspectives in Psychiatric Care,* Vol. 16, No. 1 (January/February, 1978), 28–33.

Southwell, M. Counseling the Young Prison Prostitute. *Journal of Psychiatric Nursing and Mental Health Services,* Vol. 19, No. 5 (May, 1981), 25–26.

Stevenson, R. C. K. Dealing with Drug Abusers. *R.N.,* Vol. 48, No. 4 (April, 1985), 37–39.

Summer, A. Billy Was Totally Unresponsive. *American Journal of Nursing,* Vol. 79, No. 7 (July 1979), 1262–1263.

Tripp-Reimer, T., Brink, P. J., & Saunders, J. M. Cultural Assessment: Content and Process. *Nursing Outlook,* Vol. 32, No. 2 (March/April, 1984), 78–82.

Tupin, J. P. The Violent Patient: A Strategy for Management and Diagnosis. *Hospital and Community Psychiatry,* Vol. 34, No. 1 (January, 1983), 37–40.

Tuskan, J. J., Jr., & Thase, M. E. Suicides in Jails and Prisons. *Journal of Psychosocial Nursing and Mental Health Services,* Vol. 21, No. 5 (May, 1983), 29–33.

White, J. Working with a Dependent Client in Therapy: A Clinical Paper.

Journal of Psychiatric Nursing and Mental Health Services, Vol. 18, No. 1 (January, 1980), 21–25.

Whitley, M. P. Seduction and the Hospitalized Person. *Journal of Nursing Education*, Vol. 17, No. 6 (June, 1978), 34–39.

Wiley, L. (Ed.). Coping with a Seductive Patient. *Nursing '78*, Vol. 8, No. 7 (July, 1978), 40–45.

Wiley, L. (Ed.) The Value of Life. *Nursing '79*, Vol. 9, No. 7 (July, 1979), 30–37.

23

NURSING INTERVENTION FOR PATIENTS EXPERIENCING ALTERATIONS IN OR INTERRUPTIONS OF PATTERNS IN LIVING

LEARNING OBJECTIVES

1. Identify two major problems that lead to an alteration in or interruption of living patterns.
2. Distinguish between each of the identified problems.
3. Discuss specific concepts and principles underlying nursing intervention for clients experiencing alterations in or interruptions of patterns in living.
4. Identify specific nursing interventions for stress and crisis.
5. State the rationale on which intervention is based.

INTRODUCTION

Each person thinks, feels, and behaves according to a set of internal and external constraints that give direction, meaning, and purpose to his life. The actions and reactions precipitated by these constraints form his pattern of living. This pattern of living, in turn, governs his interaction between self and self, self and others, and between self and his environment. A **pattern of living** is a mode of operation that permits the person to grow, develop, change, and adapt. A pattern of living reflects the flow of a person's life as the person maintains his equilibrium and healthy functioning. It includes those coping mechanisms that serve to assist him in his adjustment and accommodation to life.

This chapter is concerned with alterations in and interruptions of a person's pattern of living. We identify two major areas of altered or interrupted life experience that may require nursing intervention: stress and crisis. Because NANDA's taxonomy does not reflect these actual or potential problems in living, we have chosen to state a diagnostic classification that might reflect these phenomena. An appropriate diagnostic statement might read: *Patterns in living, alterations in or interruptions of related to ineffective coping as evidenced by stress.*

> The primary nursing care goal for a client with an altered or interrupted pattern of living is restoration of equilibrium and promotion of tranquility.

The specific long- and short-term behavioral objectives evolve from the data base and resulting patient profile. Thus, the interventions detailed within this chapter are directed toward the primary nursing care goal rather than the specificity required by the uniqueness presented within each patient's care situation.

The concepts and principles underlying our discussion in this chapter are listed below. These have value and application in guiding the formulation of nursing intervention on behalf of and in partnership with a person experiencing alterations in or interruption of his usual pattern of living.

1. A pattern of living promotes homeostasis and maintains equilibrium.
2. Stressors are universal phenomena.
3. All behavior has meaning.

4. Reduction in the level of stress increases potential and receptivity for learning new or alternative methods of coping and influences adjustments in the pattern of living.
5. Unmanageable stress creates instability and increases potential for breakdown.
6. Each person responds to stressors from within his own perceptual framework and value system.
7. Stressors cannot be eliminated, but their impact can be reduced.
8. Ineffective coping intensifies stress response.
9. An extreme and prolonged state of stress can cause death.
10. Positive as well as negative changes contribute to system breakdown.
11. Effects of change accumulate over time.
12. Overstimulation or understimulation can increase a person's stress level.
13. Crisis is time-limited.
14. Stress and crisis decrease productivity and increase inefficiency of functioning.
15. Resistance resources enhance stress management and crisis resolution.
16. Health promotion enhances the quality of life.
17. Reduction of stress and resolution of crisis depend on client motivation for change.
18. Early recognition and intervention prevent the development of pathopsychophysiology.
19. Excessive stress or crisis lower resistance to disease.
20. Individuals experiencing an alteration in or interruption of their patterns of living exhibit the same need for relief.
21. An individual experiencing a crisis is more emotionally accessible to help than at any other time.
22. Crisis may stimulate new learning and personal growth.
23. Intervention requires mobilization of untapped resources.
24. Intervention requires the use of a reality-based, problem-solving approach.

STRESS

Stress can menace the quality of life. Stress occurs when a demand is made on a person's system that requires adaptations calling forth the use of coping devices. Since life consists of encountering a series of stressors, sometimes one, sometimes many, an individual is constantly experiencing readjustment. The outcome or response to the stressor and the management of the stress evoked depends on at least three factors: the meaning the stressor has for the individual; the degree of flexibility the person can exhibit in identifying options; and the variety of coping devices available. In addition, outcome is also significantly influenced by the manner in which the individual perceives his relationship to his world. If the individual views himself as being in control, he will be more likely to handle his stress effectively.

Usually a person is able to manage his level of stress. For example, an individual knows that traffic at rush hour is heavy; therefore, in order to avoid frustration and the fear of being late for a scheduled appointment, he can plan ahead and leave earlier. This problem-solving action reduces what otherwise might be an occasion leading to stress overload. However, management of stress levels is not always so simplistic or easy to handle. Suppose, given the same situation, the person who planned ahead encounters an accident that ties up traffic more than usual, causing him to be late. As a consequence, he misses his appointment, necessitating rescheduling. The rescheduling requires that he take an additional day off without pay. Now he has lost two days from work, which adversely affects his financial resources. He is unable to make his car payment, must pay a late fee, and receives a caustic letter from his creditor. As a result of this one incident, a chain of additional stressors has emerged. They have increased his level of anxiety, generated feelings of anger and frustration, and produced a sense of guilt for being late, missing work, and not being able to meet his financial responsibility. This illustration demonstrates the fact that stress can be cumulative and that it can vary in degree and kind.

Stress produces change that can be either positive or negative. It can be positive from the standpoint that stress can serve to motivate and to challenge the individual to grow and develop. For example, a person identifies that a college education is needed to fulfill his life goal. Entering an educational setting increases the demands placed on self and is therefore a potential stressor. However, the goal of education is valued, and sacrifices are acknowledged. The individual encounters the stress, produced by this challenge to his intellectual capacities and determines that the expenditure of energy in coping is worth the effort. The outcome is that the individual experiences satisfaction and grows as a result of achieving the desired goal.

Stress can be negative in that it can create a demand upon the system that exceeds available coping resources. To illustrate, a person desires a college education, but his preadmission testing shows that he has marginal skills in reading comprehension, mathematical ability, and abstract thinking. His scores indicate that his potential for successful completion is marginal. Despite recommendations from a counselor to enroll with a light load, he insists on carrying an excess load. He is attracted to several organizations on campus and becomes very involved in the social life of the college. Of the six courses attempted, he withdraws from two, fails two, and earns a C grade in the remaining two. He is placed on probation and treats this event with indifference, blaming the faculty for his prior performance. Additional courses attempted earn more Ds than Cs. His behavior and social interaction becomes increasingly more aggressive, as evidenced by verbal abuse in class and acting out in the student center. His behavior and academic standing warrant dismissal. Thus, when demands exceed resources, breakdown occurs.

When normal coping and adaptive strategies are ineffective, the individual experiences alterations in cognitive, affective, behavioral, social, and physiological functioning. If stress is prolonged, maladaptive responses may be evidenced, which in turn, if not interrupted, can lead to complete breakdown and eventual death.

Tension management requires involvement and commitment and a desire to change, plus a readiness and willingness to participate in that change. There is no single magical formula that can be applied across the board, like a panacea, to reduce the adverse effects of stress. What will be effective for one person may not be the answer for another. However, in designing creative interventive strategies for tension management, the nurse should focus her attention on assisting the client to:

1. Develop self-awareness and self-understanding.
2. Improve or expand intellectual capabilities and functioning.
3. Develop healthy attitudes.
4. Manage emotional responses.
5. Restore or repair body processes and physiological responses.
6. Improve and expand interpersonal relationships.
7. Cultivate a spiritual self.
8. Manage job and job-related activities.
9. Modify the environment.
10. Pursue a healthy life-style.

To create and maintain a therapeutic atmosphere conducive to the establishment of a satisfying pattern of living, the nurse should approach the client in a calm, assured, concerned, and nonthreatening manner. The attitudes the nurse needs to cultivate in dealing with clients experiencing stress are those of personal worth, hopefulness, and advocacy.

Specific interventions found to be effective for clients experiencing stress are included in Table 23–1.

TABLE 23–1. STRESS—INTERVENTION AND RATIONALE

Intervention	Rationale
Assess level of stress.	To identify the extent of alterations in cognitive, affective, and behavioral functioning.
Isolate specific stressors.	To increase the client's perceptual awareness and to clarify the problem.
Identify usual coping mechanism.	To determine pattern of functioning.
Assess outcome of coping mechanisms used.	To determine effectiveness of coping.
Determine client's attitude toward stressor and resultant state of tension.	To establish readiness of client to engage in change.
List client resources.	To identify strengths and potential supports.
Reduce, modify, or eradicate stressors when possible.	To promote immediate relief and comfort; to enhance rapport and trust.
Formulate a detailed plan of action with time frames.	To clearly define the goal for intervention.
Allow client to express his perceptions.	To release pent-up emotions; to reduce emotional charge; to clear mind for sensible actions; and to facilitate problem-solving concentration.
Listen carefully.	To demonstrate respect; to increase client's level of confidence; and to demonstrate sympathy and understanding.
Permit client to escape or retreat from the tension as needed.	To reduce tension and regain equilibrium.
Assist the client to develop diversional outlets.	To provide safe, pleasurable forms of release from mounting tension.
Encourage the client to act, taking one step at a time and one day at a time.	To initiate a starting point for action; to provide opportunity for positive feedback; and to allow the client to experience self-control and satisfaction of accomplishment.
Assist the client to acknowledge and accept the universal presence of stressors.	To establish a frame of reality.
Facilitate the appropriate discharge of anger and frustration.	To prevent displacement of anger on self or others; to reduce potential risks and promote safety and security for client.
Promote client's self-acceptance.	To allow client to recognize that there is no perfect self.
Promote client's acceptance of others.	To decrease the potential for negative response to interpersonal stressors; to promote interpersonal harmony; and to create a network of social support.
Encourage the client "to do" for others.	To create a feeling of strength and satisfaction; to counteract moodiness; and to share generous impulses.
Assess progress of client's ability to manage tension.	To evaluate and revise creative strategies that promote continuation of a healthy pattern of living.

CRISIS

Crisis is a state of disequilibrium, a reaction to a jeopardized ego or life-threatening event that produces a temporary loss or interruption of ego functioning, resulting in a person's inability to act constructively. Crisis is always viewed as an emergency situation that demands immediate relief, even though crisis is known to be time-limited.

The outcome of crisis is affected by the availability of coping mechanisms and the person's ability to use these coping mechanisms appropriately. If a person can marshal or be assisted to marshal all available resources, positive adjustment and accommodation can occur. The end result is restoration of equilibrium. When a person has successfully lived through a crisis, there is evidence to indicate that the person has developed increased ego strength and may have added to his cognitive functioning by learning new skills. Furthermore, in mastering the crisis and in being once again in charge of his life, the person often expresses a sense of satisfaction with self.

If, on the other hand, the individual evidences a lack of appropriate coping mechanisms or is unable to employ those he has, the outcome is negative and results in a maladaptive response. The individual will continue to experience disequilibrium, disharmony, and dissonance. This outcome leaves the person in a position of increased vulnerability for potential breakdown and the development of an identifiable mental disorder.

In dealing with crisis, the nurse must establish a therapeutic, interactive–interventive environment that is action-oriented. In crisis there is immediacy of need that must be addressed. The rapid establishment of rapport and trust with the client is a critical factor. The approach most crucial for the nurse to adapt is one that demonstrates concern, conveys decisiveness and intentionality, and fosters quiet assurance. Cultivation of the attitudes of personal integrity, personal worth, open-mindedness, and advocacy are required for facilitation of the approach and the implementation of the appropriate strategies.

Specific interventions for clients in crisis are detailed in Table 23–2.

TABLE 23–2. CRISIS—INTERVENTION AND RATIONALE

Intervention	Rationale
Reach out to the client.	To establish contact; to gain rapport and trust; and to facilitate direct action.
Speak clearly in a quiet, well-modulated tone.	To promote a feeling of comfort and to decrease distortions.
Use clear, simple words and phrases.	To decrease misinterpretation and to prevent confusion.

(*continued*)

TABLE 23–2. CONTINUED

Intervention	Rationale
Obtain description of situation or event surrounding the problem.	To collect background data needed for assessment.
Identify client's perception of the problem.	To determine meaning and extent of the problem for the client.
Formulate with the client a clear definition of the problem.	To facilitate mutual understanding and give direction to further action.
Determine areas of client strength.	To determine the availability and kind of resistance resources.
Discuss with client past coping mechanisms and their effectiveness.	To provide data for the construction of creative strategies unique to the needs of the client.
Establish interactive–interventive goals with the client.	To prevent excessive dependence; to reinforce the client's involvement; and to strengthen client's ego functioning within a reality orientation.
Formulate a plan of action with the client, using the problem-solving and decision-making strategies.	To move the client toward successful resolution of the crisis event.
Support the client as he mobilizes and translates the plan into action.	To allow the client to experience mastery and growth and regain control in the reestablishment of equilibrium.
Advocate on behalf of the client as needed.	To remove obstacles; to allow for dependency; and to decrease the potential for additional stress.
Facilitate closure.	To resolve the crisis and to prepare for termination through restoration of independent and interdependent functioning.
Plan with the client for follow-up.	To evaluate with client the outcome of the interventive processes to reinforce cognitions and skills; to insure that the client has regained control and reestablished equilibrium.

EVALUATION

A list of projected outcomes for each of the altered or interrupted patterns in living described in this chapter is found in Table 23–3. The evaluation criteria are based on the primary nursing care goal: restoration of equilibrium and promotion of tranquility. This listing is general in scope and is intended to serve only as an example. It is important for the reader to note that outcome criteria are derived from the identification of the optimal expectations to be achieved with each patient.

TABLE 23–3. EVALUATION CRITERIA—ALTERATIONS IN OR INTERRUPTIONS OF PATTERNS IN LIVING

Alteration/Interruption	Evaluation Criteria
Stress	Manages stress effectively: Clarifies goals and values. Makes firm commitments. Takes active control of time management. Works toward achieving goal(s). Plans tasks. Reflects confidence in making decisions. Seeks out supportive relationships. Invests self and acts on plans.
Crisis	Resolves crisis: Demonstrates decreased anxiety or depression. Ceases to be helpless. Learns new coping strategies. Employs learned coping strategies. Functions at same or better level prior to onset of crisis. Expresses satisfaction with problem resolution.

SUMMARY

Stress and crisis are two major problems that alter or interrupt an individual's usual pattern of living. These disruptions that bring disorganization and chaos can either facilitate the health and well-being of the person or contribute to the development of maladaptive chronicity or complete breakdown. The outcome of an encounter with an event, perceived by an individual as a stressor, depends on the availability of resistance resources and supports along with the person's ability to utilize these in the management of tension. Therapeutic intervention can only occur with the full cooperation and coparticipation of the client. Interactive–interventive strategies in stress and crisis are reality-based and address the immediacy of need presented by the client.

SUGGESTED READINGS

Adams, J. Renewal: A Prescription For Coping Failure. *Nursing Forum*, Vol. 28, No. 3 (1984), 28–30.

Antonovsky, A. *Health, Stress, and Coping*. San Francisco: Jossey-Base, 1981.

Bahr, Sr. R. Management of Common Stressors in the Later Years. *Responding to Stress: Community Mental Health in the 80s*. New York: National League for Nursing, Pub. No. 52-1870, 1981, 18–23.

Beard, M. T. Life Events, Method of Coping, and Interpersonal Trust: Implications for Nursing Actions. *Issues in Mental Health Nursing*, Vol. 4, No. 1 (January–March, 1982), 25–50.

Benson, H. Your Innate Asset for Combating Stress. *Nursing Digest*, Vol. 3, No. 3 (May/June, 1975), 38–41.

Blainey, C. G. Six Steps to Personal Fulfillment in Nursing. *Nursing Management*, Vol. 16, No. 2 (1985), 37–38.

Dixon, S. L. *Working with People in Crisis*. St. Louis: C. V. Mosby, 1979.

Donnelly, G. F. *RN's Survival Sourcebook: Coping with Stress*. Oradell, N.J.: Medical Economics Books, 1983.

Ewing, C. P. *Crisis Intervention as Psychotherapy*. New York: Oxford University Press, 1978.

Everstine, D. S., & Everstine, L. *People in Crisis: Strategic Therapeutic Interventions*. New York: Brunner/Mazel, Inc., 1983.

Farquahr, J. W. *The American Way of Life Need Not Be Hazardous To Your Health*. Stanford, Calif.: Stanford Alumnae Association, 1978.

Garland, L. R. M., & Bush, C. T. *Coping Behaviors and Nursing*. Reston, Va.: Reston Publishing, 1982.

Gaston, S. K. Death and Midlife Crisis. *Journal of Psychiatric Nursing and Mental Health Services*, Vol. 18, No. 1 (January, 1980), 31–35.

George, G. Exercise and Coping with Stress. *Topics in Clinical Nursing*, Vol. 4, No. 2 (July, 1982), 13–19.

Guzzetta, C. E. Relationship Between Stress and Learning. *Advances in Nursing Science*, Vol. 1, No. 4 (July, 1979), 35–49.

Hamburger, L. K., & Lohr, J. M. *Stress and Stress Management Research and Applications*. New York: Springer, 1984.

Hoover, R. M., & Parnell, P. K. An Inpatient Educational Group on Stress and Coping. *Journal of Psychosocial Nursing and Mental Health Services*, Vol. 22, No. 6 (June, 1984), 17–22.

Johnson-Saylor, M. T., Pohl, J., & Lowe-Wickson, B. An Assessment Form for Determining Patient's Health Status and Coping Responses. *Topics in Clinical Nursing*, Vol. 4, No. 2 (July, 1982), 22–32.

Kogan, H. N., & Betrus P. A. Self-Management: A Nursing Mode of Therapeutic Influence. *Advances in Nursing Science*, Vol. 6, No. 4 (July, 1984), 55–73.

Knowles, R. D. Control Your Thoughts. *American Journal of Nursing*, Vol. 81, No. 2 (February, 1981), 353.

Lancaster, B. J., & Brekovsky, D. An Ecological Framework for Crisis Intervention. *Journal of Psychiatric Nursing and Mental Health Services*, Vol. 16, No. 3 (March, 1978), 17–23.

McGee, R. F. Hope: A Factor Influencing Crisis Resolution. *Advances in Nursing Science*, Vol. 6, No. 4 (July, 1984), 34–44.

McGuigan, F. J., et al, (Eds.). *Stress and Tension Control*. New York: Plenum Press, 1980.

Meissner, J. E. Measuring Patient Stress with the Hospital Stress Rating Scale. *Nursing '80*, Vol. 10, No. 8 (August, 1980), 70–71.

Mengel, A. The Concept of Coping. *Topics in Clinical Nursing*, Vol. 4, No. 2 (July, 1982), 1–3.

Miller, C. M. Crisis Intervention and Health Counseling: An Overview. *School Health Review* (September, 1970), 16–17.

Mitchell, C. E. Identifying the Hazard—Key to Crisis Intervention. *American Journal of Nursing*, Vol. 77, No. 7 (July, 1977), 1194–1196.

Otte, E. *Retirement Rehearsal Guidebook*. Indianapolis, Ind.: Pictorial, 1974.

Richter, J. M. Crisis of Mate Loss in the Elderly. *Advances in Nursing Science*, Vol. 6, No. 4 (July, 1984), 45–54.

Savitz, J. Diagnosing and Counseling Bored and Confused Patients. *Responding to Stress: Community Mental Health in the 80s*. New York: National League for Nursing, Pub. No. 52-1870, 1981, 65–75.

Schubin, S. Rx for Stress—Your Stress. *Nursing '79*, Vol. 9, No. 1 (January, 1979), 52–55.

Scully, R. Stress in the Nurse. *American Journal of Nursing*, Vol. 80, No. 5 (May, 1980), 911–914.

Shaffer, M. *Life After Stress*. New York: Plenum Press, 1982.

Sifneos, P. E. *Short-Term Psychotherapy and Emotional Crisis*. Cambridge, Mass.: Harvard University Press, 1972.

Sredly, D., Klenke, C., & Rojkind, M. Offering the Rape Victim Real Help. *Nursing '79*, Vol. 9, No. 7 (July, 1979), 38–43.

Stubbs, D. C. Family Crisis Intervention: A Study. *Journal Of Psychiatric Nursing and Mental Health Services*, Vol. 16, No. 1 (January, 1978), 36–44.

Zeimer, M. M. Coping Behavior: A Response to Stress. *Topics in Clinical Nursing*, Vol. 4, No. 2 (July, 1982), 4–12.

24

NURSING INTERVENTION FOR PATIENTS EXPERIENCING ADJUNCTIVE THERAPY

LEARNING OBJECTIVES

On completion of this chapter the reader should be able to:

1. Define **adjunctive therapy**.
2. Discuss the nurse's role in carrying out adjunctive therapy.
3. State the purpose and expected therapeutic results of psychotropic chemotherapy, activity therapy, electroconvulsive therapy, and physical constraint.
4. Identify the patient's pattern of response to adjunctive therapy.
5. Identify actual, potential, or possible nursing care concerns for the patient involved in adjunctive therapy.
6. Discuss the rationale upon which interventions are based.

INTRODUCTION

In this chapter we address four frequently used adjunctive therapies: psychotropic chemotherapy, activity therapy, electroconvulsive therapy (ECT), and physical constraint, any or all of which may be included as part of a patient's total treatment program. We define **adjunctive therapy** as a treatment modality in which physical manipulation of the patient's internal or external environment produces both a physical response and a social and psychological change in the patient's perception of self and others.

The major principle underlying the use of somatic intervention is that the body and mind operate as an integrated whole that cannot be separated. Therefore, from this premise adjunctive therapy is prescribed and undertaken as a viable treatment strategy to strengthen the integration of psychomotor, cognitive, and affective expressions of the client's thoughts and feelings. Involvement of the client in adjunctive therapy is useful in altering negative perceptions, thus decreasing resistance to change and increasing socially acceptable behavior. To achieve therapeutic effectiveness these adjunctive therapies need the patient's full cooperation and participation; therefore, *the primary nursing care goal is to secure, promote, and maintain the patient's collaborative assistance.*

The concepts and principles underlying our discussion in this chapter are listed below. These have value and application in guiding the formulation of nursing interventions on behalf of and in conjunction with an individual for whom adjunctive therapy has been prescribed.

1. The psyche and soma are inseparable.
2. The rights of clients must be protected when they are subjected to adjunctive therapy.
3. Collaboration between nurse and client fosters client's compliance.
4. Belief systems and values of the client influence the client's positive or negative perception of adjunctive therapy.
5. Goal-directed activity promotes self-esteem.
6. Adjunctive therapy facilitates the development of socially acceptable behavior.
7. Successful adaptation can be achieved through the use of adjunctive therapy.
8. Adjunctive therapy mandates attention to biophysical and psychosocial needs of the client.
9. The attitudes of staff directly influence the client's response to adjunctive therapy.

PSYCHOTROPIC CHEMOTHERAPY

Psychotropic chemotherapy is an adjunctive treatment that produces a direct relief of symptoms, thereby enabling the patient to make maximum use of the total treatment regime. Specifically, it is used to bring about changes in an individual's disrupted thinking, distorted feelings, and disturbed behavior. Those chemical agents that fall within this classification include: the antipsychotic, antianxiety, antimanic, antidepressant, and anticholinergic/antiparkinsonism drugs. These psychotropic agents are employed in the treatment of mental and emotional disturbances and are directly responsible for interrupting psychotic symptomatology, decreasing disruptive psychomotor activity, increasing perception, alleviating anxiety, decreasing depression, and controlling adverse extrapyramidal effects. These drugs enable the client to feel more comfortable. They also allow for the introduction of needed psychotherapeutic interventions, that is to say, they foster within the client a state of readiness and amenability to therapy.

For information regarding specific drugs, the reader is referred to current pharmacology textbooks, handbooks, pharmaceutical literature, and journal articles. Information contained in this segment of the chapter is designed to provide the practitioner with current baseline data regarding specific, commonly used psychotropic drugs. It also includes nursing interventions that might be useful in enhancing the therapeutic effectiveness of this treatment modality. This section is intended to increase the knowledge and skill of the nurse in the administration and monitoring of drugs and in the assessment of the patient's response behavior.

Antipsychotic Agents

The drugs within this category are commonly referred to as **major tranquilizers**, **ataractic** or **neuroleptic** agents. They were first introduced as a part of the treatment regime in psychiatric care in the mid-1950s, and their impact on patient care has been phenomenal. For the first time, nurses were able to engage in nursing activity directed toward meeting the patient's psychological needs as opposed to merely providing custodial care.

The term **tranquilizer** is somewhat misleading in that it tends to convey the idea that the chief use of the drug is confined to the production of a state of calmness or reduced anxiety. *However, the primary therapeutic effect of antipsychotic drugs is found to lie in their ability to reduce, modify, or influence major psychotic manifestations.* These manifestations include hallucinations, delusions, illogical thought processes, and perceptual distortions as well as exaggerated psychomotor activity. These drugs act within the subcortical structure of the brain, resulting in suppression of cortical functioning. The most recent theory indicates that therapeutic effectiveness is achieved by decreasing neurotransmitter activity within the cerebral cortex.

Severe adverse reactions have been noted. Many of these are common. In fact, they occur so frequently that the nurse can almost anticipate their presence. Therefore, the nurse needs to be vigilant in observing the client for early signs and symptoms. When therapy is initially begun, the nurse will most likely observe and hear the patient complain about drowsiness, dizziness, dryness of the mouth, constipation, blurriness of vision, or urinary retention. Other observations and comments frequently made by patients are related to weight gain, impotence in males, and menstrual irregularities in females.

More serious but less frequently noted adverse reactions include dermatological conditions, tachycardia, photosensitivity, orthostatic hypotension, pseudoparkinsonism, jaundice, dystonia, and akathisia. Two of the most severe and serious adverse reactions are agranulocytosis and tardive dyskinesia. Agranulocytosis is a potentially fatal blood dyscrasia whose prodromal signs are similar to those observed with influenza. Early recognition is essential and is facilitated through monitoring of laboratory findings. Immediate discontinuation of the drug is mandatory if agranulocytosis is found to be present. Tardive dyskinesia is a syndrome involving gross motor movements of the entire muscular system. Characteristically, the client displays hyperkinetic activity of the mouth, such as sucking and smacking of the lips and protrusion of the tongue along with side-to-side movements of the chin. Facial grimaces, tics, and spastic distortions are also evidenced. This condition usually appears in patients after long-term therapy and is irreversible.

Table 24–1 lists five of the more common antipsychotic drugs (Thorazine, Mellaril, Prolixin, Haldol, and Navane). It includes both the generic and trade names, the daily therapeutic range, how the drug is supplied, contraindications, and pertinent remarks.

Antianxiety Agents

The drugs within this category are commonly known as **minor tranquilizers**. Today these drugs are prescribed with far greater frequency than almost all other medications currently on the market. Their discovery was fostered when it became evident that the major tranquilizers produced little or no effect on the overwhelming anxiety experienced by patients. The first antianxiety drug to be marketed was Meprobamate. It was introduced in the middle 1950s.

The primary effectiveness of antianxiety agents lies in their ability to control emotional responses to stress and anxiety. They modify

TABLE 24–1. DESCRIPTION OF SELECTED COMMONLY USED ANTIPSYCHOTIC DRUGS

Drug Trade (Generic)	Therapeutic Range (mg)	Contraindications	Remarks
Thorazine (Chlorpromazine)	50–1500. Supplied as: tablets, spansules, ampules, concentrate, suppositories, and syrup.	Sensitivity. Comatose and unconscious patients. Bone marrow depression. Convulsive disorders. Glaucoma. Prostatic hyperthrophy.	Cautious and close observation is mandatory for clients with a history of respiratory dstress, impaired liver and kidney function, and cardiovascular disease. Potentiates action of narcotics, alcohol, and barbiturates. Known to produce contact dermatitis in both client and nurse. Avoid contact of liquid preparations with skin, eyes, or clothing. Wear rubber gloves when preparing liquid forms. Protect liquid preparation from light. Discard yellowed solutions (indicates chemical change). Dilute liquid concentrates with juice and inform patient. I.V. administration may produce extravasation of tissue. I.M. administration causes postural hypotension. Instruct patient to lie down for I.M. administration. If hypotension is severe, place patient in Trendelenburg's position. Volume expansion may be required. Vasopressors may be needed; norepinephrine is frequently used. Epinephrine should not be given because it can produce a further lowering of the blood pressure. Give injection deeply and slowly into the upper, outer quadrant of buttocks; alternate sites. If tissue irritation is observed or patient verbalizes discomfort, consult with physician regarding dilution of medication with saline or 2% procaine. Do not administer more than 2 cc at a time in

(continued)

TABLE 24–1. CONTINUED

Drug Trade (Generic)	Therapeutic Range (mg)	Contraindications	Remarks
Thorazine (Chlorpromazine) (*continued*)			one site. After administration instruct patient to remain in a recumbent position for at least 1/2 hour after injection. Caution patient to rise slowly. Initially, monitor blood pressure before and after administration for at least 1 to 2 weeks and periodically thereafter. In children, drug may produce excessive sedation and interfere with cognitive behavior and learning.
Mellaril (Thioridazine)	100–800. Supplied as: tablets, concentrate, and suspension.	Sensitivity. Comatose and unconscious patients. Extremes in hypertension or hypotension. Others—same as those listed for Thorazine.	Low incidence of extrapyramidal effects. Little or no antiemetic effect. Is often a substitute when patients manifest sensitivity to other phenothiazines. Drowsiness is a common complaint during initial therapy. Effect can be managed by administering a single dose 1 to 2 hours before bedtime. Observe patient closely for increased pigmentation of the retina. Known to inhibit ejaculation. Effects in children are similar to those encountered with Thorazine.
Prolixin (Fluphenazine Hydrochloride)	2.5–20. Supplied as: tablets, elixir, and ampules.	Liver damage. Patients receiving large doses of hypnotics. Others—same as those listed for Thorazine.	May produce anaphylactic shock. High incidence of reversible extrapyramidal side effects. Patients may be prone to upper respiratory infections referred to as "silent pneumonias."
(Fluphenazine Enanthate)	12.5–100. q̄ 2 wk Supplied as: ampules.		Observe for fluctuations in blood pressure. Long-term therapy may result in renal complications. Parenteral preparations with an extended duration of action are usually ordered for

TABLE 24–1. CONTINUED

Drug Trade (Generic)	Therapeutic Range (mg)	Contraindications	Remarks
(Fluphenazine Enanthate) (*continued*)			patients who are unwilling or unable to take drugs orally. Detailed documentation is needed to identify patterns of individual response when an extended-action preparation is used.
Haldol (Haloperidol)	1–30. Supplied as: tablets, concentrate, and ampules.	Hypersensitivity. Parkinson's disease. Depression. Patient on lithium.	Concentrate is colorless, odorless, and tasteless. Highly potent. High incidence of extrapyramidal side effects. No photosensitivity. Eliminated slowly and tends to have cumulative effect. Cautious use with elderly individuals who are lethargic and dehydrated because of reduced pulmonary ventilation and hemoconcentration; may result in death. Decreases effects of anticoagulant therapy due to increased breakdown in the liver. High incidence of extrapyramidal effects in children. Produces minimal sedation and orthostatic hypotension.
Navane (Thiothixene)	6–60 Supplied as: capsules, concentrate, and ampules.	Circulatory collapse. Hypersensitivity. Others—same as those listed for Thorazine.	Less likely to produce serious side effects. A more potent inhibitor of postural reflexes and motor coordination than Thorazine. Observe patient closely for increased pigmentation of the retina. Not recommended in children under 12.

the intensity of the anxiety and produce a physiological reduction in muscular tension. These agents are drugs of choice in the treatment of anxiety and in somatoform and some affective disorders. They are also frequently employed as adjunctive treatment in any pathophysiological condition in which anxiety and tension play a key role. For example, they have been known to be beneficial in such conditions as low back pain, osteoarthritis, angina pectoris, torticollis, chronic alcoholism, alcohol withdrawal delirium, selected convulsive disorders, nocturnal enuresis in children, and as a premedication for surgery or electric cardioversion.

Drugs of this category fall within three major classifications and each classification has its own unique action. However, it does appear that these drugs have in common their ability to depress neurotransmission. As a result of this decreased transmitter activity, there is a reduction in the impact of stimulus reception and response.

Theoretically, antianxiety drugs are considered relatively safe when prescribed in small doses. That is, when comparing the adverse reactions of antipsychotic drugs to those manifested by the antianxiety agents, the disabling side effects of the minor tranquilizers are fewer and less severe. However, this does not mean that adverse reactions do not occur and cannot be deleterious to the client. The major adverse reactions produced by these drugs include drowsiness, fatigue, dizziness, ataxia, blurred vision, slurred speech, tremor, and hypotension. In addition, it has been noted that paradoxical reactions have occurred, even though their incidence is rare. These reactions include excitement, hostility, rage, confusion, and depersonalization. Because psychological and physical dependency occur with long-term use or abuse, withdrawal reactions are common. These reactions appear as increased restlessness, heightened levels of anxiety, muscular weakness, and convulsions. Overdosage may lead to coma and death.

Table 24–2 lists four of the more common antianxiety agents. These are Vistaril, Valium, Equanil, and Librium. The table provides

TABLE 24–2. DESCRIPTION OF COMMONLY USED ANTIANXIETY DRUGS

Drug Trade (Generic)	Therapeutic Range (mg)	Contraindications	Remarks
Vistaril (Hydroxyzine)	25–100. Supplied as: capsules, suspension.	Pregnancy. Hypersensitivity.	Potentiates effects of CNS depressants such as narcotics or barbiturates. Patient should be warned about possibility of impaired coordination that may hazardously affect driving or the operation of machinery.
(Hydroxyzine Hydrochloride)	Ampules.	Any parenteral route except intramuscular.	May produce marked discomfort, induration, and even gangrene at I.M. injection sites.
Valium (Diazepam)	2–40. 2–20. Supplied as: tablets, ampules.	Hypersensitivity. Children under 6 months. Narrow angle glaucoma.	Irritating to tissue; may produce desquamation at intramuscular injection site. Should be avoided in first trimester of pregnancy

TABLE 24–2. CONTINUED

Drug Trade (Generic)	Therapeutic Range (mg)	Contraindications	Remarks
Valium (Diazepam) (*continued*)			because of the possibility of congenital malformations. Crosses placental barrier and is found in milk of nursing mothers. Cumulative effects occur with repeated use. If administered intravenously should be injected slowly, taking at least 1 minute for each 5 mg of drug given. Should not be mixed with other injectables or added to I.V. fluids. Store protected from light. May potentiate antihypertensive effects of diuretics and antihypertensive drugs.
Equanil (Meprobamate)	400–1800. Supplied as: tablets, ampules.	Grand mal epilepsy. Chronic alcoholism. Pregnancy. Concomitant use of MAO inhibitors. Suicidal tendencies.	Seizures may be precipitated in patients with epilepsy. I.V. injection may cause thrombosis or hemolysis. Hypnotic doses at bedtime tend to increase sleep motor activity; padded side rails necessary. Periodic blood cell counts and liver function tests required for patients on prolonged therapy.
Librium (Chlordiazepoxide)	15–300. Supplied as: capsules, tablets, and ampules.	Hypersensitivity. Same as for Valium. History of convulsive disorder. Psychoses. Suicidal tendencies.	Long duration of action and cumulative effect. Less potent than Valium, produces less drowsiness. Excreted slowly, action may persist 3 or more hours; has less anticonvulsant activity. I.V. administration requires slow injection. When reconstituting injectables, make sure solution is clear. Discard opalescent or hazy solutions. Parenteral administration requires the patient to remain recumbent for at least 3 hours after injection.

the following information: the generic and trade names, the daily therapeutic range, how the drug is supplied, contraindications, and specific remarks pertinent to each drug.

Antimanic Agent

Lithium is the only agent currently falling within this category. The generic term for this drug group is **lithium salts**. The most frequently used lithium salt is **lithium carbonate**. Trade names include Lithane, Lithonate, and Eskalith.

Lithane was first introduced in 1970 in the management of manic and hypomanic episodes in patients with major affective disorders. It is used effectively in the treatment of acute episodes, although it may also be employed prophylactically where the patient experiences recurrent mood swings. Lithane acts by blocking the release of norepinephrine and stimulating its uptake at the neural synapse. There is additional evidence indicating that Lithane alters sodium ion transport in both nerve and muscle cells. The effectiveness of this drug is evidenced by decreased motor activity, a reduction in cognitive dissonance, and a decrease in elation, along with stabilization of mood at a more normal level. It is known to decrease the intensity of the feelings rather than the frequency of mood changes.

Lithane is supplied in capsule and tablet form. It is considered a toxic drug whose therapeutic range is extremely narrow. Dosage is highly individualized and ranges from 300 to 1800 milligrams. The dosage regulation is based on the severity of presenting symptoms, the individual's renal lithium clearance, serum lithium determinations made at onset of therapy, and observation of clinical response, particularly the appearance of toxic symptomatology.

Since such a narrow range exists between therapeutic and toxic doses, serum lithium levels are monitored daily or biweekly when initial therapy is begun and monthly thereafter for as long as the patient is on a maintenance dose. The normal serum blood level ranges from 0.9 to 1.5 mEq/L. The maximum therapeutic serum drug concentration during therapy is 2mEq/L. The range of concentration between 1.5 and 2 mEq/L is potentially toxic. This necessitates extremely close observation of the patient, and some authorities advocate withholding administration of the drug for a 24-hour period and then resumption of therapy with a lowered dosage.

Routine side effects indicative of minor lithium toxicity include fine hand tremors, transient nausea, fatigue, thirst, polyuria, diarrhea, and muscle weakness. These symptoms usually occur with onset of therapy and generally subside during the first few weeks of treatment. Where side effects persist, a temporary reduction in dosage is recommended. Discontinuation of the drug will result in cessation of symptoms.

The onset of lithium toxicity is gradual and may result in major toxic effects. These effects include the presence of coarse tremors, vomiting, diarrhea, general sluggishness, lassitude, and drowsiness, followed by confusion, slurred speech, and ataxia. Extreme toxicity produces impaired levels of consciousness, muscular hypertonicity, coma, and death. Not only must the patient be observed for the development of these clinical signs, but also the dietary intake of sodium must be closely supervised in order to prevent onset of toxicity. It has been noted that lithium ions substitute for sodium ions when sodium ion levels are reduced. With such reduction, there is an increase in reabsorption of lithium ions in the distal renal tubules. This action elevates the serum level concentration. Therefore, patients must be instructed to maintain sodium chloride intake at normal level (5 gm/day) and to maintain a fluid intake of approximately 3 L/day. In addition, supplementary salt may be required to replace sodium depletion that occurs when the patient experiences increased diaphoresis during prolonged periods of elevated environmental temperatures or sustained periods of strenuous physical activity.

The use of this agent is contraindicated in at least eight major conditions. These include significant renal disorders; congestive heart failure; sodium restricted diets; organic brain disorders; severe debilitation; epilepsy; pregnancy; and fluid and electrolyte imbalance. Furthermore, close observation and careful evaluation are strongly recommended for patients with existing thyroid disorders or cardiovascular disease and for any patient who has a history of an endocrine or metabolic disorder such as diabetes mellitus.

Antidepressant Agents

The drugs in this category are subdivided into two main classes, the tricyclic agents and the monoamine oxidase (MAO) inhibitors. They are commonly referred to as **psychic energizers** because of their effectiveness in the treatment of affective disorders. Both classes of antidepressant agents are believed to act by overcoming a deficiency of monoamines within the brain. Specifically, the tricyclic agents are thought to produce their mood-elevating effect by increasing the amount of free norepinephrine available for transmission and by prolonging the activity of the transmitters. MAO inhibitors are thought to be effective because they interfere with the breakdown of catecholamines, such as norepinephrine and dopamine, in nerve cells. They interfere with the function of the monoamine enzyme, thereby increasing the amount of amine stores within the brain. Generally, the tricyclic antidepressants are considered safer and more effective in the treatment of depressive disorders. However, MAO inhibitors are frequently the drugs of choice in the case of a patient who does not appear to respond to tricyclic therapy.

Adverse reactions, common to both classes of antidepressants, are orthostatic hypotension, dryness of the mouth, blurred vision, constipation, tachycardia, urinary retention, anorexia, and leukopenia. Although the literature reports that the therapeutic doses of the tricyclic compounds seldom produce the severe toxicity sometimes associated with the MAO inhibitors, the tricyclics are capable of producing a wide variety of discomforting and potentially injurious side effects. Some of the most frequently observed reactions reported are disorientation, hallucinations, increased anxiety, insomnia, palpitations, tremor of the extremities, parotid swelling, paralytic ileus, changes in libido, jaundice, agranulocytosis, photosensitivity, edema of face and tongue, and tinnitus.

The most dangerous toxic effect of the MAO inhibitors is **hypertensive crisis**. This reaction is caused by interaction between drugs and foods containing large amounts of tyramine, a pressor amine that is normally inactivated by MAO. When the individual ingests this pressor amine, there is a corresponding increase in the norepinephrine levels in the body, producing severe vasoconstriction resulting in hypertensive crisis. Other adverse reactions noted include dizziness, confusion, edema, impotence, and hepatitis.

Table 24–3 contains five of the most widely used antidepressant agents. Elavil, Tofranil, and Sinequan are tricyclic compounds, while Marplan and Nardil belong to the MAO inhibitor class. The generic and trade names, the daily therapeutic range, how the drug is supplied, contraindications, and specific remarks are provided for each of these drugs.

TABLE 24–3. DESCRIPTION OF COMMONLY USED ANTIDEPRESSANT DRUGS

Drug Trade (Generic)	Therapeutic Range (mg)	Contraindications	Remarks
Elavil (Amitriptyline)	75–300. Supplied as: tablets, ampules.	Hypersensitivity. Concomitant administration of MAO inhibitors.	Has greater sedative properties than Tofranil. Hyperpyretic crisis, severe convulsions, and death have been known to occur in patients receiving both classes of antidepressant drugs. When one class is replaced with another, a time lag is essential—that is, a minimum of 14 days is required when changing from a tricyclic compound to an MAO inhibitor.

TABLE 24–3. CONTINUED

Drug Trade (Generic)	Therapeutic Range (mg)	Contraindications	Remarks
Elavil (Amitriptyline) (*continued*)			Antidepressant effect may be noted in 3 to 4 days; however, in some patients, as much as 30 days elapse before effectiveness becomes apparent. Close observation for changes in thoughts, feelings, and behavior is mandatory to prevent suicidal attempts. May turn urine a blue-green color.
Tofranil (Imipramine)	50–300. Supplied as: capsules, tablets, and ampules.	Hypersensitivity. Concomitant use of MAO inhibitors. Patients initially recovering from an acute M.I.	Same drug interaction occurs as is noted with Elavil. Therapeutic effectiveness varies from patient to patient; time span observed has been from 2 to 8 weeks. Monitor vital signs during initial therapy. Periodic evaluation of blood cell counts, liver function, and cardiac status is required in prolonged therapy. Ambulatory outpatients should be cautioned in regard to using dangerous machinery or operating motor vehicles. Alcohol ingestion potentiates effects. White crystals sometimes form inside ampules. These are not indicative of chemical change and can be redissolved by immersing the ampule in warm water for about 1 minute.
Sinequan (Doxepin)	75–300. Supplied as: capsules, concentrate.	Hypersensitivity. Glaucoma. Urinary retention. Children under 12. Concomitant administration of MAO inhibitors.	Well tolerated by the elderly. Dilute concentrate with orange juice. Controversial opinions exist regarding its effectiveness in controlling anxiety. Same conditions regarding close observation, alcohol ingestion, use of machinery, and drug interaction prevail.

(*continued*)

TABLE 24–3. CONTINUED

Drug Trade (Generic)	Therapeutic Range (mg)	Contraindications	Remarks
Marplan (Isocarboxazid)	10–30. Supplied as: tablets.	Hypersensitivity. Impairment of liver or renal function. Congestive heart failure. Pheochromocytoma. Patients on sympathomimetic drugs such as Dopamine or epinephrine. Concurrent administration of other MAO inhibitors.	Elective surgery requiring a general anaesthetic is not recommended while patient is on Marplan. Spontaneous death has been reported after a single dose of Demerol. Tends to have cumulative effects. Hypertensive crises may be caused by food and drug interactions. Restricted foods for patients taking any MAO inhibitor include cheese—Cheddar, Gruyere, Camembert; any aged product; alcoholic beverages—beer, sherry, or red wines, such as Chianti; organ meats, such as chicken livers; any pickled products; fruits, such as raisins, bananas, avocados, canned figs; broad beans; chocolate; soy sauce; yeast products, such as yogurt; excessive caffeine, such as coffee, tea, colas. Nonprescription drug products, such as patent cold remedies; antiallergic compounds; weight-reducing remedies; or nasal sprays, along with any other medication that may contain sympathomimetic drugs, may also precipitate hypertensive crisis. These foods and drug products cannot be taken for at least 2 to 3 weeks after discontinuation of the MAO inhibitors. Blood pressure should be monitored regularly.
Nardil (Phenelzine)	15–75. Supplied as: tablets.	Hypersensitivity. Other—same as for Marplan.	Lower incidence of hypertensive crisis as compared to other drugs in this class. Store between 59° and 86°F. Restrictions regarding food and nonprescription drugs apply.

Anticholinergic/Antiparkinsonism Agents

This drug classification is included in the discussion of psychotropic chemotherapy primarily because of its use in the control of drug-induced extrapyramidal reactions, such as rigidity, akinesia, tremor and akathisia, caused by the antipsychotic drugs. These agents cross the blood-brain barrier and act by blocking acetylcholine at certain cerebral synaptic sites. The objective of treatment is to provide maximum relief of uncomfortable symptoms and to promote the patient's functional capacity.

Adverse reactions seen with this group are related chiefly to their anticholinergic action. When initial therapy is begun, most likely the patient will manifest evidence of a dry mouth, dizziness, blurred vision, nausea, and increased nervousness. Other problematic conditions that may appear with more prolonged therapy include constipation, tachycardia, urinary hesitancy or retention, anhidrosis, drowsiness, weakness, vomiting, or headache. In addition, the literature indicates that there is evidence of increased central nervous system stimulation, which is usually manifested by increased restlessness and agitation, disorientation, memory loss, confusion, delirium, or visual hallucinations.

Table 24–4 contains three anticholinergic agents in current use: Cogentin, Artane, and Akineton. The table provides the reader with information identifying the trade and generic names, the therapeutic range, the form in which the drug is supplied, contraindications, and pertinent remarks regarding each one.

TABLE 24–4. DESCRIPTION OF COMMONLY USED ANTICHOLINERGIC/ANTIPARKINSONISM DRUGS

Drug Trade (Generic)	Therapeutic Range (mg)	Contraindications	Remarks
Cogentin (Benztropine Mesylate)	0.5–6. Supplied as: tablets, ampules.	Pregnancy. Glaucoma. Prostatic hypertrophy.	Has a cumulative effect. Adverse reactions are more likely to develop in debilitated, aged, or alcoholic patients. Anhidrosis (suppression of perspiration) especially in hot weather or with increased physical exertion requires dosage adjustments or discontinuation because of the body's inability to regulate temperature that may precipitate fatal hyperthermia. Administer drugs during or after meals to reduce gastric irritation.

(continued)

TABLE 24–4. CONTINUED

Drug Trade (Generic)	Therapeutic Range (mg)	Contraindications	Remarks
Cogentin (Benztropine Mesylate (*continued*)			Monitor pulse and blood pressure. Measure intake and output.
Artane (Trihexypheni-dyl)	2–15. Supplied as: elixir, tablets. and spansules.	Same as for Cogentin.	Increases intraocular pressure. All precautionary implications identified with Cogentin also apply to Artane.
Akineton (Biperiden)	2–20. Supplied as: tablets, ampules.	Same as for Cogentin.	Side effects noted have been minimal to date.

The nurse should be aware that drug therapy is not to be considered a panacea for the patient's problems. Neither should it be a replacement for good clinical practice nor a routine procedure carried on without sound clinical judgment. Therefore, the nurse's approach to the patient undergoing chemotherapy should be one that is knowledgeable, firm, confident, and actively observant. To achieve this approach the nurse must cultivate the attitudes of involvement, hopefulness, open-mindedness, and advocacy.

Specific interventions designed to assist patients undergoing psychotropic chemotherapy are listed in Table 24-5.

TABLE 24–5. PSYCHOTROPIC CHEMOTHERAPY—INTERVENTION AND RATIONALE

Intervention	Rationale
Be aware of the specific drugs prescribed for the patient.	To make accurate assessment of the effectiveness of chemotherapy.
Be familiar with the purpose for which the specific drug is prescribed.	To give meaning and purpose for the interpretations of the clinical observation.
Be alert to the action, desired effects, usual dosage, side effects, contraindications, precautions, and nursing implications related to the prescribed drug.	To exercise vigilance on behalf of the patient in order to protect him and to maintain his physical comfort and well-being. Older or debilitated patients require lower dosage ranges.
Instruct the patient and his family members about the drug therapy program, including the name of the drug, usual side effects, danger signals, and comfort measures.	To secure the patient's and the family's cooperation through education to decrease anxiety for all.
Elicit and explore with the patient his thoughts and feelings regarding taking the prescribed medications.	To identify his value system, to determine his level of understanding, to provide support, and to alleviate fear and anxiety.

TABLE 24–5. CONTINUED

Intervention	Rationale
Answer the patient's drug-related questions openly and honestly.	To establish trust, to provide the patient with correct information, and to clarify misinterpretations.
Administer the prescribed medication to the right patient, in the right dose, at the right time, and use the right route of administration.	To protect the patient's right to quality treatment and care.
Keep phenothiazines separate from other medications; do not mix in same syringe.	To prevent formation of a precipitate.
Administer tricyclic antidepressants no later than 5:00 P.M.	To prevent insomnia.
Plan to observe the patient and evaluate the clinical effectiveness of the patient's drug program.	To determine the patient's response to drug therapy and to provide a data base for making recommendations for change in the nursing care and treatment plan.
Encourage the patient to promptly report untoward reactions.	To provide protection and implement appropriate nursing intervention.

STUMBLING BLOCKS AND STEPPING STONES

There is an abundance of reference material on psychotropic drugs and chemotherapy readily available to the nurse. This material supplies information on effects, side effects, untoward reactions and contraindications. But information related to necessary precautions and specific nursing interventions is limited. Therefore, we identify some of the more common problems or stumbling blocks encountered and provide some suggestions, or stepping stones, for effective intervention. These are listed in Table 24–6.

TABLE 24–6. COMMON STUMBLING BLOCKS AND STEPPING STONES ASSOCIATED WITH CHEMOTHERAPY

Stumbling Blocks: What if . . .	Stepping Stones: Try this . . .
1. The patient complains of dizziness?	Change the patient's position slowly.
	Lower the patient's head down between his knees.
	Instruct patient to remain in a recumbent position 1/2 to 1 hour after parenteral administration.
	Check and record blood pressure in lying, sitting, and standing position.
	Have the patient sit down periodically.

(*continued*)

TABLE 24–6. CONTINUED

Stumbling Blocks: What if . . .	Stepping Stones: Try this . . .
	Instruct the patient to walk close to the walls in corridors.
	Note frequency and duration of the complaint.
2. The patient complains of a dry mouth?	Have the patient take frequent *small* sips of water.
	Suggest sucking ice chips or hard *sour* candies.
	Suggest chewing gum.
	Have the patient rinse his mouth frequently.
	Lubricate the patient's lips.
3. The patient complains of blurred vision?	Provide adequate lighting.
	Provide large-print books and newspapers.
	Have the patient read with a light over his right shoulder.
	Recommend an opthalmological consultation and periodic eye examination.
4. The patient has slurred speech?	Listen carefully and patiently.
	Encourage the patient to speak slowly.
	Ask him to repeat when necessary.
5. The patient has an unsteady gait?	Instruct the patient to walk slowly.
	Encourage him to wear sturdy, supportive shoes.
	Show him how to use his arms for balance and support.
	Have him use railings and walls for support.
	Provide a cane or walker if necessary.
	Remind and encourage him to walk erectly.
	Assist and supervise ambulation.
6. The patient gains weight?	Keep a weight record.
	Reduce his caloric intake.
	Discourage or restrict his eating "junk foods."
	Discourage or restrict his eating between meals.
	Insure, adequate, regular exercise.
7. The patient complains of drowsiness?	Discourage staying in bed all day.
	Plan schedules so that major activities occur immediately after drug administration.
	Include time for rest periods in the patient's schedule.
8. The patient has edema?	Check intake and output.
	Restrict fluid intake.
	Instruct the patient to elevate his legs periodically.
	Elastic stockings to prevent venous pooling.

TABLE 24–6. CONTINUED

Stumbling Blocks: What if . . .	Stepping Stones: Try this . . .
9. The patient experiences photosensitivity?	Provide patient with protective clothing to cover exposed skin areas. Encourage him to wear a wide-brimmed hat outdoors. Advise him to keep out of direct rays of sun. Apply sun screening lotion to his exposed areas. Plan for and encourage indoor activities.
10. The patient complains of sore throat, runny nose, or cold?	Check vital signs. Observe and report the condition of his throat. Report symptoms to physician. Initiate laboratory request to check for agranulocytosis.
11. The patient experiences drooling, twitching of facial muscles, swelling and protrusion of tongue?	Alert physician immediately. Withhold drug. Observe patient closely while waiting for physician's intervention. Force fluids. Maintain patent airway. Administer oxygen.
12. The patient experiences anorexia, nausea, or other gastrointestinal symptoms?	Restrict food high in fats and carbohydrates. Give medication with skim milk. Plan for small, frequent feedings. Observe closely for jaundice.
13. The patient complains of feeling cold?	Provide proper clothing. Check temperature periodically. Regulate temperature of bath water. Advise patient to be cautious in handling hot coffee, tea, water; to avoid direct contact with radiators, hot water bottles, or heating pads.
14. The patient complains of constipation?	Increase roughage, bulk, and fluid intake. Check frequency and consistency of stool. Encourage the patient to increase physical exercise.
15. The patient experiences itching or redness of skin?	Report symptoms to physician. Suggest baking soda or cornstarch baths. Discourage use of colognes, shaving lotions, perfumed soaps. Encourage use of hypoallergenic soaps and toiletries.

(*continued*)

TABLE 24–6. CONTINUED

Stumbling Blocks: What if . . .	Stepping Stones: Try this . . .
16. The patient's drug therapy includes a monoamine oxidase inhibitor such as Nardil, Marplan, or Niamid?	Instruct the patient regarding diet. Eliminate the following foods: chicken livers, aged or natural cheeses, pickled herrings, yeast extract, broad beans, etcetera. Limit intake of coffee, tea, or cola beverages. Eliminate beer and wine. Observe for hypertensive crisis. Caution the patient to avoid taking any medication not prescribed by his physician, including over-the-counter drugs such as aspirin, Dristan, cough syrups, and weight reduction pills.
17. The patient's chemotherapy includes lithium carbonate?	Observe the patient for signs of excessive voiding or extreme thirst. Encourage high fluid intake. Provide a high caloric diet. Report symptoms to physician. Monitor lithium levels in blood.
18. The patient is not swallowing medication?	Check patient's mouth, especially under tongue. Give additional fluids to facilitate swallowing. Discuss the patient's reasons or fears for not swallowing; assist patient to deal with concerns and resolve, if possible. Consult with physician regarding possible change in route of administration.
19. The patient is going home on medications?	Emphasize the importance of taking medications as scheduled. Provide the patient with written instructions including a list of drugs, time each is taken, and special precautions required with each. Remind the patient to immediately report any changes in his physical or emotional states and any headache, palpitations, tremulousness, crying, or lethargy. Remind the patient to continue special dietary modifications. Remind the patient to avoid driving a car, using hazardous equipment or machinery, engaging in strenuous exercises, and drinking alcoholic beverages. Inform the family of special instructions given to the patient. Set up next appointment to reevaluate the patient's response to drug therapy and to reinforce and clarify instructions.

ACTIVITY THERAPY

Activity therapy is a necessary and vital treatment that provides the individual with opportunities for personal, interpersonal and intrapersonal interaction and growth. Activity therapy is a broad term that encompasses occupational, recreational, educational, industrial, manual arts, and exercise therapy. Within residential facilities activity therapy is used in conjunction with chemotherapy and psychotherapy. This type of therapy expands an individual's social, recreational, physical, occupational, and leisure-time skills. It brings out talents and lets the individual feel proud of his achievements. There are suitable activities for everyone.

Activity therapy is used to promote recovery through the release of excess energy and the prevention of regression; provide a vehicle for self-expression; provide practice of social skills in a protected, accepting environment; help to acquire new knowledge; help to develop new technical and creative skills; correct physical and psychological impairment; help to achieve self-actualization; and help develop a sense of responsibility. Activity therapy is not merely used to occupy the patient's time. It is as important as any other part of the treatment program. The nurse's approach should be firm, patient, persistent, observant, and helpful. To achieve this approach and to convey to the patient the importance activity therapy plays in his total treatment program, the nurse must demonstrate the attitudes of personal worth, involvement, and advocacy.

Specific interventions designed to assist patients who are participating in activity therapy are listed in Table 24–7.

TABLE 24–7. ACTIVITY THERAPY—INTERVENTION AND RATIONALE

Intervention	Rationale
Acquire knowledge about kinds of activities available.	To select the appropriate activity for the patient.
Assess the patient's emotional and physical needs.	To plan nursing intervention and to demonstrate personal interest in the patient.
Assess strengths and weaknesses through interviewing and determine former interests, areas of success, and possible areas for developing new interests.	To devise an individualized plan that supports the patient, decreases his level of anxiety, reduces stress, and promotes the possibility of successful involvement.
Collaborate with colleagues, multidisciplinary team members.	To share information, provide consistency, and to secure cooperation in devising an effective therapeutic plan.
Plan activity schedule and allow for free time.	To prevent exhaustion and to demonstrate the concept of a balance between work, rest, and play.

(continued)

TABLE 24–7. CONTINUED

Intervention	Rationale
Discuss activity schedule with the patient.	To provide information to the patient and create an opportunity for patient input, to maintain a bond of trust, and to involve the patient in the decision-making process.
Elicit the patient's thoughts and feelings regarding his schedule.	To demonstrate acceptance and understanding and to facilitate the clarification of misinterpretations.
Encourage the patient to make choices in terms of activities offered.	To assist him to take responsibility for involvement in his own therapeutic regimen.
Provide the patient with a copy of his schedule.	To decrease confusion and guard against manipulation and resistance.
Indicate firm expectation of adherence to schedule.	To demonstrate care and concern for the patient and to foster his sense of responsibility.
Accompany the patient to activity therapies.	To provide security and support, to alleviate anxiety and fear, and to convey interest and concern.
Stay with the patient for the first few sessions.	To assist the patient in adjusting to a new environment and to observe his initial response to activities and people.
Plan and schedule progress conferences with the therapists involved.	To promote collaborative effort on behalf of the patient and to maintain the highest level of effectiveness for the treatment regime.
Plan for additional visits and make periodic observations of patient's involvement and responses during activity programs.	To gather information for assessing the patient's progress and to demonstrate sustained interest and concern in his progress.
Discuss progress with the patient.	To provide feedback, to give merited praise, and to elicit patient's self-evaluation of progress.
Revise schedule based on progress reports and patient's input.	To adjust activity therapy to the changing needs of patient.

ELECTROCONVULSIVE THERAPY

Electroconvulsive therapy is a form of shock therapy used to interrupt a patient's current maladaptive pattern of thinking, feeling, and behaving. It is an adjunctive somatic treatment that is most commonly utilized for those patients experiencing severe depression, excitation, or agitation, or for those who are actively suicidal. In essence the procedure is undertaken to produce emotional regression of the patient in time, thereby bringing about modification of the patient's affective response and behavior. This effect is produced when an electrical current is applied to the brain through electrodes placed on the temporal areas of the skull, producing an artificially induced grand mal seizure. Its exact mechanism of action is unknown, but it is believed that the electrical charge induces a biochemical response.

The treatment is considered effective if the patient begins to evidence a feeling of well-being, ceases to be preoccupied with morbid ideation, or is free from agitation. The outcome of this form of treatment permits the individual to be more accessible to others. This accessibility is observed when the patient demonstrates a readiness to socialize and to engage in intensive psychotherapy.

The treatment necessitates the use of specific drugs, each of which is employed to meet a particular need of the treatment process. Prior to treatment the patient is given an agent that dries secretions. This is done to prevent aspiration during treatment. The drug of choice is usually atropine sulfate. The second drug used is a short-acting barbiturate, administered intravenously, which induces anaesthesia. This allows the patient to sleep through the procedure and therefore have no recall or feel no panic related to the convulsive experience or the feeling of suffocation. The drug most frequently employed for this purpose is brevital sodium. The third and final drug utilized is anectine chloride. This drug is a curare derivative and produces complete muscle relaxation, which prevents injury during the seizure. It is also administered intravenously. At the point where this drug takes effect, the patient ceases to breathe, and the current is administered. Since there is no known antidote for this drug, it is imperative that the nurse make absolutely no mistake in preparing the dosage required. A mistake in dosage can be lethal.

In electroconvulsive therapy, nursing intervention is divided into three areas of concern: preparation of the patient prior to the procedure; care of the patient during the procedure; and care of the patient immediately after the procedure. A quiet, firm, confident, nonthreatening approach contributes to the development of a therapeutic atmosphere. The attitudes needed by the nurse to successfully implement such an approach are those of involvement, hopefulness, and advocacy.

Specific interventions designed to assist patients undergoing electroconvulsive therapy are listed in Table 24–8.

TABLE 24–8. ELECTROCONVULSIVE THERAPY—INTERVENTION AND RATIONALE

Intervention	Rationale
Preparation	
Explain the treatment to the patient in simple, clear, concise terms.	To provide information, to prevent misinterpretation, and to alleviate the patient's anxiety and fear.
Prepare the patient for and carry out pretreatment workup: assist with the physical examination;	To assist in the gathering of clinical data, to safeguard the patient, to protect the patient's

(*continued*)

TABLE 24–8. CONTINUED

Intervention	Rationale
Preparation	
check and verify completion of x-rays, EKG, and EEG; secure written consent of the patient or guardian.	rights, and to provide legal protection for the treatment team and the hospital.
Schedule the treatment and inform the patient of the time, place, and frequency.	To implement the therapeutic prescription and to decrease the possibility of additional anxiety.
Procure, set up, and maintain treatment supplies and equipment: oxygen, carbon dioxide, resuscitator, airway, tracheotomy tray, emergency medication tray, I.V. standard and parenteral fluids, treatment machine, saline solution or electrode jelly, electrodes, headband, mouth gag, tourniquet, syringes, needles, atropine sulfate, Brevital, and Anectine.	To prepare the treatment area for the safe and efficient administration of therapy.
Keep the patient NPO for at least 4 hours prior to treament.	To prevent aspiration during therapy.
Administer prescribed dose of atropine sulfate.	To decrease secretions.
Assist the patient to remove all metal objects such as hairpins, watch, rings, medals or other jewelry, glasses, dentures or other prosthetic devices.	To promote safety and prevent injury.
Remind the patient to void.	To prevent possibility of a ruptured bladder; to prevent incontinence and save the patient from social embarrassment.
Stay with the patient; listen to and closely observe for expressions of anxiety, fear, and resistive or manipulative behavior.	To promote psychological comfort through the alleviation of fear and anxiety; to enhance therapeutic effectiveness of treatment.
Encourage the patient to identify and discuss his feelings about the therapy.	To provide support, to give assurance, to promote comfort, and to convey the nurse's acceptance and understanding.
Administration	
Accompany the patient to the treatment room.	To provide security, support, and reassurance.
Proceed with implementation of procedure: instruct the patient to lie supine, assisting if necessary; remove shoes; loosen restrictive clothing; recheck for metal objects or dentures; assist in the administration of the Brevital and Anectine; apply conductor to temple area; secure headband in place; insert airway; hyperextend neck; hold jaw in place; assume position needed to apply soft restraint to extremities; advise physician of the patient's and team's readiness.	To prepare the patient for the administration of the treatment and to decrease the patient's level of anxiety.
Observe the patient for grand mal seizures, changes in color, and restoration of spontaneous inhalation.	To observe patient's response to treatment and to be ready to institute emergency measures if necessary.

TABLE 24–8. CONTINUED

Intervention	Rationale
Administration	
Cleanse temple areas.	To prevent irritation to skin.
Turn patient on side.	To promote patent airway and prevent aspiration.
Check for patency of airway.	To ensure maintenance of respiration.
Raise side rails.	To protect the patient.
Remove the patient to recovery room.	To allow time for anaesthetic to wear off; to provide continuous monitoring of patient's condition.
Recovery	
Check pulse and respiration periodically and observe for changes in their rate and in the color of the patient.	To assess physiological functioning and to provide data for emergency intervention.
Allow patient to sleep until effect of anaesthetic has worn off.	To allow for individual differences in reaction time based on individual physiological response or amount of drug given.
Reorient the patient to reality as his level of consciousness increases.	To promote patient's feeling of security, to minimize disorientation and confusion, and to provide reassurance.
Ease the patient to a sitting position on the side of his bed.	To allow for reestablishment of equilibrium.
Assist the patient with personal appearance by dressing or rearranging clothing, combing hair, and returning personal effects.	To convey personal interest, to minimize anxiety, and to promote psychological comfort.
Serve meal and assist, if needed.	To meet nutritional needs.
Listen to the patient for expressions of physical complaints such as headache, pain, muscle soreness, dizziness, memory deficits, or misinterpretations of treatment or procedure.	To gather information for future interventions, to provide reassurance, and to convey interest, acceptance, and concern.
Complete treatment record form.	To provide information regarding patient's response to treatment.
Encourage the patient to participate in his regularly scheduled activities.	To deemphasize preoccupation with ECT and to emphasize the patient's need for involvement in his total treatment program.

PHYSICAL CONSTRAINT

Physical constraint is a protective, adjunctive treatment procedure requiring the application of external control measures that are time-limited. These measures are employed when the client experiences a loss of self-control that distort his perceptions and judgments to the point where he is at risk to himself or others. Physical constraint provides for containment or immobilization. It is used to create a therapeutic situation in which the client is held safe and secure until such time as restoration of equilibrium can be achieved. The application of physical constraints is intended to assist the client to maintain dignity and to minimize, in so far as possible, loss of self-esteem due to uncontrollable behavior.

Seclusion and mechanical restraints are two common forms of physical constraint frequently encountered in clinical practice. **Seclusion** is the deliberate therapeutic separation and isolation of a client from his usual, daily living environment. Seclusion can be partial or complete. **Partial seclusion** involves the withdrawal of the client to a designated quiet area that is private, free from dissonant stimuli, and conducive to rest and relaxation. **Complete seclusion** requires that the client be placed in a locked room devoid of stimuli and containing the minimum of a mattress and bedding on the floor or the maximum of a bed, mattress, and bedding. Seclusion offers time out to the client, an opportunity to promote a feeling of security and to develop a sense of comfort and peace with self and with the environment. **Restraints** are immobilizing mechanical devices that minimize the risk of self-injury or harm to others and assist the client to regain self-control.

It should be noted that both the use of seclusion and the application of restraint are subject to legal ramifications. Specifically, both require a written physician's order and are further governed by state law, hospital policy, and ethical considerations such as informed consent.

Currently, there are no standards for practice or clear-cut guidelines to suggest when one mechanism of physical constraint is more appropriate than another. In our clinical practice, we have found that seclusion is therapeutically effective for those clients whose:

1. Hyperactivity is increased or exaggerated by environmental stimuli
2. Self-control is so marginal that they are unable to respond appropriately to redirection or verbal limit setting
3. Anger is externalized in argumentative behavior with other patients or staff
4. Level of insecurity or fear results in severe agitation
5. Dissatisfaction with self or life's circumstances results in the agitation of others
6. Behavior demonstrates pronounced, exaggerated responses to environmental stimuli that indicate an imminent loss of control

Leather restraints are employed only when the client exhibits behavior that places him at risk to himself or jeopardizes the immediate safety of others. They are used only when all other avenues of therapeutic strategies have failed to produce a restoration of equilibrium.

Most often, when the decision has been reached to use physical constraint with a client, the client is already experiencing a loss of control. In this situation the nurse is confronted with a person who may be angry, severely agitated, destructive, violent, fearful, or in panic. The implementation of physical constraint must be executed in an efficient and humanistic manner to safeguard the rights of the patient and to protect the nurse from harm. The approach should be one that is calm, organized, and supportive. The attitudes that facilitate the adoption of this approach are those of advocacy, hopefulness, personal worth, and integrity.

The nursing interventions designed to assist clients experiencing physical constraint may be found in Table 24–9. The reader should note that the interventions detailed below are general in nature and form an overall guide, the specifics of which should be found within the policies and procedures of each clinical facility.

TABLE 24–9. PHYSICAL CONSTRAINT—INTERVENTION AND RATIONALE

Intervention	Rationale
Identify the number of personnel needed.	To insure safety and protection for client and staff.
Organize nursing team.	To promote efficiency.
Assign specific duties to team members.	To clarify roles and promote efficiency of action.
Prepare the environment; for example: clear the area of patients, gather supplies or equipment, remove hazardous objects.	To prevent chaos and promote the dignified execution of the procedure.
Inform the client of intent to seclude or restrain.	To elicit cooperation, if possible; to alert the client of the need to alter his plan of care.
Tell the client clearly and concisely what is to take place.	To orient the client to the experience of physical constraint and to potentially reduce fear and anxiety.
Initiate procedure.	To implement the plan.
Closely monitor client's response; observe behavior, and check vital signs.	To determine effect of procedure on client.
Implement schedule for meeting biological needs such as feeding, toileting, bathing, exercise, and medication.	To provide safety and comfort for the client; to preserve biological integrity.
Schedule periodic, brief contacts with client.	To prevent feelings of abandonment, to offer support and reassurance, and to promote physical and psychological comfort and safety.
Monitor and document observations and interactions.	To assess client progress and to determine readiness for reintegration into the living community.
Wean client gradually as ability to control self increases.	To promote a smooth transition from isolation to resocialization.

EVALUATION

A list of projected outcomes for the adjunctive therapies presented in this chapter is found in Table 24–10. The evaluation criteria are based on the primary nursing care goal: to secure, promote, and maintain the patient's collaborative assistance. This listing is general in scope and is intended to serve only as an example. It is important for the reader to note that outcome criteria are derived from the identification of the optimal expectations to be achieved with each patient.

TABLE 24–10. EVALUATION CRITERIA—ADJUNCTIVE THERAPY

Adjunctive Therapy	Evaluation Criteria
Psychotropic chemotherapy	Experiences relief of symptoms: Verbalizes feelings of increased comfort. Initiates self-care activities. Demonstrates alertness. Controls impulsivity. Seeks information about prescribed medications. Assumes responsibility for self-medication. Resumes daily activities. Communicates effectively with others. Socializes.
Activity therapy	Learns adaptive social and coping skills: Works collaboratively. Expresses interest, satisfaction, and enjoyment. Completes tasks or projects. Exhibits pride in accomplishment. Demonstrates a balance between work, rest, and play. Manages anxiety. Tolerates frustration. Exhibits patience.
Electroconvulsive therapy	Evidences interruption of maladaptive thoughts, feelings, and behavior: Expresses a feeling of well-being. Ceases to be preoccupied with morbid ideation. Free from agitation. Accessible to others. Demonstrates a willingness to socialize. Resumes pursuit of usual interests and daily activities.
Physical constraint	Restoration of self-control and equilibrium: Ceases aberrant behavior. Verbalizations indicate congruency between thoughts and feelings. Decreases hyperactivity. Initiates problem-solving to deal with anger, fear, or insecurity. Follows directions.

SUMMARY

In this chapter we have discussed adjunctive therapy, focusing on the use of chemotherapy, activity therapy, electroconvulsive therapy, and physical constraint. Each is a viable adjunctive treatment modality. Probably the nurse will be most closely involved with chemotherapy and activity therapy, since these are universally used both in and outside the hospital. The therapeutic effectiveness to be derived from each of these modalities depends to a large extent on the nurse's attitude and behavior. It is absolutely essential that the nurse be involved, not only to observe the patient's response, but also to encourage, support, and teach the patient. The nurse's involvement in adjunctive therapy also demands collaborative efforts: first, collaborative effort with other health professionals to insure that the outcome of the treatment is meeting therapeutic expectations on behalf of the patient; second, collaborative effort with the patient to secure compliance with the prescribed treatment regime and to ascertain from the patient's standpoint the effectiveness of the particular adjunctive therapy in meeting individualized needs.

SUGGESTED READINGS

Allen, M. D. Drug Therapy in the Elderly. *American Journal of Nursing*, Vol. 80, No. 8 (August, 1980), 1474–1475.

Amdur, M. A., & Cohen, M. Medication Groups for Psychiatric Patients. *American Journal of Nursing*, Vol. 81, No. 2 (February, 1981), 343–345.

Baradell, J. G. Humanistic Care of the Patient in Seclusion. *Journal of Psychosocial Nursing and Mental Health Services*. Vol. 23, No. 2 (February, 1985), 9–14.

Beard, M. T., Enelow, C. T., & Owens, J. G. Activity Therapy as a Reconstructive Plan on the Social Competence of Chronic Hospitalized Patients. *Journal of Psychiatric Nursing and Mental Health Services*, Vol. 16, No. 2 (February, 1978), 33–41.

Berstein, J. G. *Handbook of Drug Therapy in Psychiatry*. Littleton, Mass.: John Wright, PSG, Inc., 1983.

Breggin, P. R. *Electro-Shock: Its Brain-Disabling Effects*. New York: Springer, 1979.

Chamberlain, A. Providing Motivation. *American Journal of Nursing*, Vol. 78, No. 1 (January, 1978), 80.

Cochran, C. C. A Change of Mind About ECT. *American Journal of Nursing*, Vol. 84, No. 8 (August, 1984), 1004–1005.

Cole, J. O. (Ed.). *Psychopharmacology Update*. Livington, Mass.: D.C. Heath and Company, 1980.

Conference on Creative Arts Therapy. *The Use of Creative Arts in Therapy: Art Therapy, Dance Therapy, Music Therapy, Psychodrama*. Washington, D.C.: American Psychiatric Press, 1980.

Cook, J. D. The Therapeutic Use of Music: A Literature Review. *Nursing Forum*, Vol. 20, No. 3 (1981), 252–266.

DeGennaro, M. D., et al. Antidepressant Therapy. *American Journal of Nursing*, Vol. 81, No. 7 (July, 1981), 1304–1310.

Durel, S. H., & Munjas, B. A. Client Perception of Role In Psychotropic Drug Management. *Issues in Mental Health Nursing*, Vol. 4, No. 1 (January-March, 1982), 65–76.

Gerlock, A., & Solomons, H. C. Factors Associated with the Seclusion of Psychaitric Patients. *Perspectives in Psychiatric Care*, Vol. 21, No. 2 (April–June, 1983), 46–53.

Gever, L. N. Anticholinergics. *Nursing 84*, Vol. 14, No. 9 (September, 1984), 64.

Gordon, M. Assessing Activity Tolerance. *American Journal of Nursing*, Vol. 76, No. 1 (January, 1976), 72–75.

Harris, E. Antidepressants: Old Drugs, New Uses. *American Journal of Nursing*, Vol. 81, No. 7 (July, 1981), 1308–1309.

Harris, E. Antipsychotic Medications. *American Journal of Nursing*, Vol. 81, No. 7 (July, 1981), 1316–1323.

Harris, E. Extrapyramidal Side Effects of Antipsychotic Medications. *American Journal of Nursing*, Vol. 81, No. 7 (July, 1981), 1324–1328.

Harris, E. Lithium. *American Journal of Nursing*, Vol. 81, No. 7 (July, 1981), 1310–1315.

Harris, E. Sedatives-Hypnotic Drugs. *American Journal of Nursing*, Vol. 81, No. 7 (July, 1981), 1329–1334.

Hinds, P. S. Music: A Milieu Factor with Implications for the Nurse-Therapist. *Journal of Psychiatric Nursing and Mental Health Services*, Vol. 18, No. 6 (June, 1980), 28–33.

Hoepfel-Harris, J. A. Improving Compliance with an Exercise Program. *American Journal of Nursing*, Vol. 80, No. 3 (March, 1980), 449–450.

Hunn, S. et al. Nursing Care of Patients on Lithium. *Perspectives in Psychiatric Care*, Vol. 18, No. 5 (September/October, 1980), 214–220.

Jefferson, J. W., & Griest, J. H. *Lithium Encyclopedia for Clinical Practice*. Washington, D.C.: American Psychiatric Press, 1983.

Kelley, S. J. The Use of Art Therapy With Sexually Abused Children. *Journal of Psychosocial Nursing and Mental Health Services*, Vol. 22, No. 12 (December, 1984), 12–18.

Klerman, G. L. Psychotherapeutics and Somatic Therapies in Affective Disorders. *Psychiatric Clinics of North America*, Vol. 6, No. 1 (March, 1983), 85–103.

Knowles, R. D. Handling Depression through Activity. *American Journal of Nursing*, Vol. 81, No. 6 (June, 1981), 1187.

Lancaster, J. Activity Groups as Therapy. *American Journal of Nursing*, Vol. 76, No. 6 (June, 1976), 947–949.

Lehmann, P. Food and Drug Interactions. In *Consumer*. Health, Education and Welfare Publication No. (FDA) 80-3070. Washington D.C.: U.S. Government Printing Office, March, 1978.

McAfee, H. A. Tardive Dyskinesia. *American Journal of Nursing*, Vol. 78, No. 3 (March, 1978), 395–397.

McCoy, S. M., & Garritson, S. H. Seclusion: The Process of Intervening. *Jour-*

nal of Psychosocial Nursing and Mental Health Services, Vol. 21, No. 8 (August, 1983), 8–15.

O'Brien J. Teaching Psychiatric In-Patients about Their Medications. *Journal of Psychiatric Nursing and Mental Health Services*, Vol. 17, No. 10 (October, 1979), 30–32.

Overcoping with Valium. In *Consumer*. Health, Education and Welfare Publication No. (FDA) 80-3100. Washington D.C.: U.S. Government Printing Office, January, 1980.

Pilette, W. L. Caffeine: Psychiatric Grounds for Concern. *Journal of Psychosocial Nursing and Mental Health Services*, Vol. 21, No. 8 (August, 1983), 19–24.

Rodman M. J., & Smith, D. W. *Pharmacology and Drug Therapy in Nursing*. Philadelphia: Lippincott, 1968.

Roper, J. M., et al. Restraint and Seclusion: A Standard and Standard Care Plan. *Journal of Psychosocial Nursing and Mental Health Services*, Vol. 23, No. 6 (June, 1985), 18–23.

Sackheim, H. A. The Case for ECT. *Psychology Today*, Vol. 19, No. 6 (June, 1985), 36–40.

Schmidt, R. M., & Margolin, S. *Harper's Handbook of Therapeutic Pharmacology*. Philadelphia: Harper & Row, 1981.

Schoolar, J. C., & Claghorn, J. L. (Eds.). *The Kinetics of Psychiatric Drugs*. New York: Brunner-Mazel, 1979.

Singerman, B. et al. An Evening Diversional Activity Program for Psychiatric Patients. *Journal of Psychiatric Nursing and Mental Health Sevices*, Vol. 18, No. 12 (December, 1980), 28–31.

Smith, J. E. Improving Drug Knowledge in Psychiatric Patients. *Journal of Psychiatric Nursing and Mental Health Services*, Vol. 19, No. 4 (April, 1981), 16–18.

Thomas, S. P. The Uses and Abuses of Electric Convulsive Shock Therapy. *Journal of Psychiatric Nursing and Mental Health Services*, Vol. 18, No. 11 (November, 1978). 17–23.

Whiteside, S. E. Patient Education: Effectiveness of Medication Programs for Psychiatric Patients. *Journal of Psychosocial Nursing and Mental Health Services*, Vol. 21, No. 10 (October, 1983), 16–21.

VII

PROFESSIONAL PRACTICE

Nursing Process Exemplified

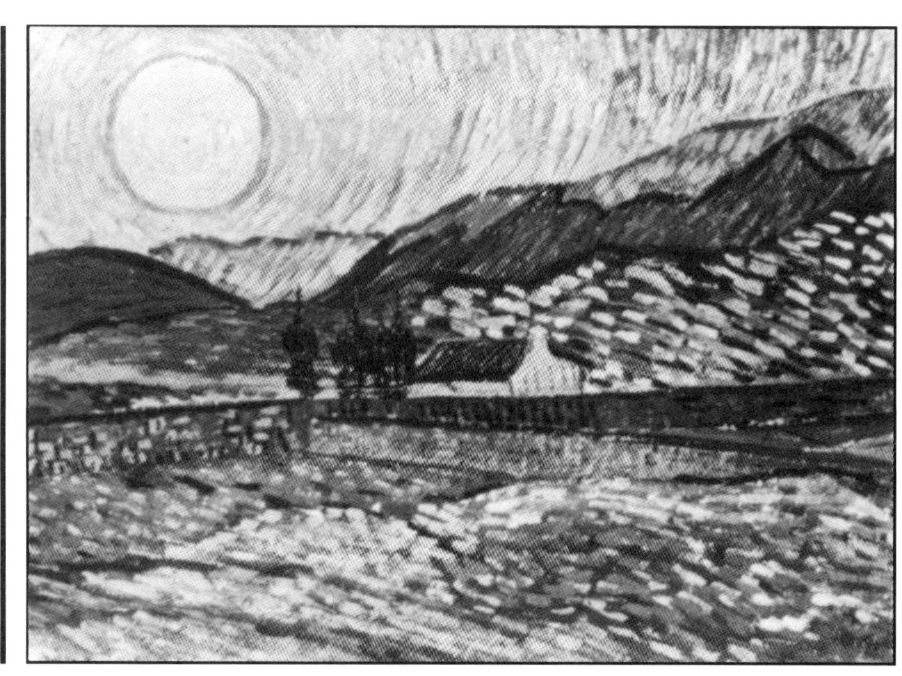

25

A CASE PRESENTATION: MRS. SHEILA FRANKLIN

LEARNING OBJECTIVES

On completion of this chapter the reader should be able to:

1. Identify relevant social data.
2. Describe the relationship of social data to the formation of dysfunction.
3. Identify specific symptomatology from the social data base.
4. Describe the psychosocial dynamics as they relate to the developmental process, the effects of stress and crisis, and the sequence of pathology.

INTRODUCTION

Students tend to feel overwhelmed when they are confronted with the task of reading a patient's history, deciding which portions are relevant, and from this developing a nursing care plan. Another task they seem to find difficult is the completion of a thoughtful, organized assessment. Although current nursing practice emphasizes the importance of assessment, students and inexperienced practitioners sometimes feel baffled about how to do an assessment. A third major task students and beginning practitioners must cope with is forming therapeutic relationships by establishing and maintaining communication with assigned patients.

In the previous chapters we have presented basic theories, concepts, and processes along with definitive interventions necessary for the beginning practice of psychiatric–mental health nursing. Knowledge and understanding of the prior content should enable the reader to move from a level of abstract conceptualization to a level of practical application. To facilitate this progress and to enhance the reader's movement toward developing needed competency, we have included the following patient profile, the history of Mrs. Sheila Franklin, who was diagnosed as having schizophrenia, paranoid type.

It is our belief that an in-depth analysis and synthesis of this case material will operationalize for the reader the cognitive assessment process that the nurse employs as she attempts to extrapolate assessment data from which the remainder of the nursing process flows. In addition, this learning tool fulfills several other functions. First, it illustrates the psychodynamics involved in interpersonal interaction. Second, it demonstrates the development of psychopathology within the patient's living experiences, and third, it points out characteristic symptomatology associated with the identified clinical condition illustrated.

The knowledge acquired and assimilated through the use of case material leads to understanding and to the development of effective nursing care. It is only with understanding that the nurse moves into a position of being able to apply psychological principles, theories, and concepts learned to actual patient care.

FAMILY CONSTELLATION AND BACKGROUND

The case history to be considered is that of Mrs. Sheila Franklin, a 30-year-old, widowed, Caucasian female. She is the mother of an 8-year-old daughter, Debby. Mrs. Franklin's immediate family consists of her father, William J. Mitchell, her mother, Mary Rose, and two siblings, Evelyn James and Thomas. William Mitchell, age 56, is a professional golfer and amateur musician. He presents himself as a quiet, rather retiring individual. He married at the age of 21 and appears content to allow his wife complete management of family life. He has never been known to countermand any of her directives. Mary Rose is 52. She was raised as a strict Methodist, attends church regularly, and requires that all her family members participate as well. She is exacting and controlling, more aggressive than assertive. Mary Rose makes all the rules in the family and sees to it that they are enforced. Whenever it is necessary for William to be away from home for a tournament, she makes lists for him—what he is to wear and when; what he can eat; how much he should pay; where he is to stay; the time he should get up; and the time he should go to bed. And, too, she requires that he return the lists checked off. Furthermore, William must call home twice a day to report. To all this, William meekly complies and in response to inquiries or humorous comments from friends merely states very matter-of-factly that, "Mary Rose knows best."

Evelyn James, age 32, is the oldest sibling. She is married and resides in Arizona with her husband John and their three children: Jimmy, Jane, and Susan. Their ages respectively are 10, 9, and 7. It is known that Evelyn had a "nervous breakdown" after the birth of her first child, from which she has apparently recovered.

Thomas, a senior at State College, is 20 and unmarried. He lives at home and has a part-time job in a delicatessen. He aspires to be an architect. Thomas feels there is a "closeness" between Sheila and himself that he does not share with their sister Evelyn.

Family history reveals the familiar pattern found in histories of schizophrenic patients—domineering mother, passive father.

DEVELOPMENTAL HISTORY

As a child, Mrs. Franklin was quiet and obedient—"a good little girl"—who never got into trouble like her sister Evelyn. Sheila seldom needed discipline and was content to sit on the floor and play with her dolls or to spend hours sitting silently listening to her father practice on the piano. When her brother Thomas was born, she took charge of him whenever her mother permitted and incorporated his care into her fantasy play with her doll family. Sheila and Evelyn shared the same room, attended the same schools, but were never very close. They did not participate in the same activities or cultivate similar interests.

Her teachers considered her a good student except they wished she would "talk a little more and look out the window less." During her high school years she liked to read and never complained about her school work. She made friends easily but established no close relationships. She was considered a "loner." In her junior year she began having occasional dates with Paul Franklin, a college student whom Sheila had known all her life. She refused to join in school social activities because she "needed the time to 'bone up' on math and sciences" since she planned to enter nursing school after graduation.

"Good" behavior during early childhood is used to gain approval from adults. Playing alone, talking little, and gazing out of the window might be considered early manifestations of autistic behavior. The pattern of withdrawal appears to become more pronounced during high school years, as does the pattern of isolation from social involvement. Both are evidenced through poor interpersonal relationships. Relationships formed are superficial and lack warmth. Sheila uses rationalization regarding studies to camouflage avoidance and noninvolvement behavior. Healthy aspects of personality are displayed through attempts to establish identity, acknowledge love object of opposite sex, and engage in future planning to establish place and role in society.

Sheila was accepted into a school of nursing. After 6 months, she contracted infectious mononucleosis. During convalescence she decided that she was no longer interested in nursing and that she would leave school to get her trousseau ready for her forthcoming marriage with Paul Franklin. She made plans, placed orders for clothes and household articles, and was very much involved in the total preparation for the wedding. However, she failed to keep appointments for fittings and alterations; she scheduled two appointments for the same time and as a result, her mother and fiancé completed most of the transactions she started. The night before the wedding, she paced her room for 2 hours, packed and unpacked her suitcase three times and finally insisted on telling her parents all the factors that indicated to her that she was definitely ready for marriage.

Increased levels of anxiety interfere with the completion of projects begun and give rise to feelings of insecurity and self-doubt as evidenced by indecisiveness and vacillation.

In the first 2 months of her marriage, she seemed to enjoy taking care of the apartment, shopping, and learning to cook the things her husband liked. She and her husband visited her parents on occasion, but she was reluctant to invite anyone in or to go out. She stated that she felt uncomfortable at the home of her in-laws; she felt sure they thought she was not good enough for Paul. She began to complain of being tired and used this complaint to reject Paul's sexual advances. As the months passed she slept later than usual and found it more difficult to care for the apartment and herself. She took to wearing her pajamas and housecoat all day. This change in behavior concerned her husband, and he insisted that she have a physical examination, which revealed that she was about 3 months pregnant. Upon learning of the pregnancy, Paul immediately assumed many of the usual household routines that she had previously neglected.

Apathy is clearly demonstrated by a loss of interest in her surroundings and lack of attention to her physical appearance. These two behaviors also indicate early signs of regressive behavior. Social noninvolvement is again manifested. Her behavior with respect to limiting contact with others and her expression of discomfort about her in-laws illustrate projection, isolation, and mistrust.

Before the baby was born, her husband left on a business trip and was killed in an airplane accident. Mrs. Franklin accepted the news of her husband's death calmly and displayed no observable signs of grief during or after the funeral service. Her mother urged Sheila to close the apartment and return to the family home, at least until the baby was born. Sheila willingly complied. Shortly after returning to her parents' home, Sheila again complained of tiredness, took less and less interest in her surroundings, and spent increasingly longer periods in her room. Frequently Mrs. Franklin missed appointments at the prenatal clinic, saying either that she forgot or "there was no need to go." Her mother said that during this period she never cried, just sat in the rocker, continuously rocking back and forth, staring out of the window.

Lack of response to husband's sudden death is indicative of inappropriate affect. Emotional detachment and withdrawal are becoming more pronounced. In addition, symptoms of rationalization and denial are beginning to appear.

After the baby was born, Mrs. Franklin said that she was happy that the baby was a little girl. But she expressed fear about caring for her. She told her mother that she thought she might drop or hurt the baby in some way. One day Mrs. Franklin was observed bending over the baby's crib, gently stroking the baby's arm. Suddenly, she squeezed Debby's hand until the infant started to cry.

This behavior toward the child displays marked ambivalence toward herself and motherhood as well as feelings of inadequacy and inability to cope with the stress of additional responsibility.

After this incident she ran out of the room, left the house, and was gone for 2 hours. Her brother found her sitting on a park bench several blocks from home. As soon as she saw him, she asked if he came to tell her that Paul was home. Without waiting for him to respond, she continued, "If only he would come back. I know Mom and Dad did not want us to get married, but we did. I should be living with him—not at home with them. Why are they keeping me away from him? Debby needs a father. Oh! Why am I sitting here. I have so much to do, the baby must be hungry—it's too nice a day to work, the sun feels good . . . warm and bright but I feel cold and alone. . . ."

This segment of social history demonstrates autistic thinking and dissociation as indicated by her belief that Paul was still alive. The stream of thought begins to show looseness of association and confabulation. However, this is the first indication of it, and it is still minimal. Other symptoms displayed are those of loneliness, possible feelings of isolation, and again, mistrust.

Mrs. Franklin's parents and her obstetrician were able to convince her that she should seek psychiatric help. She was placed on an antipsychotic medication and saw a psychiatrist each week for 6 months. She made continuous progress and was discharged after this 6-month period.

Mrs. Franklin enrolled in a secretarial school, completed the course of study and obtained a job in an office, which she held for 5 years. She and Debby lived with her parents. Mrs. Franklin helped her mother, assumed some of the ordinary household expenses, and managed to devote a great deal of time to her daughter, especially on weekends. She seldom dated, said she compared all men to Paul and they just didn't measure up. She received three pay raises at the office, expressed satisfaction with the job, and never had any complaints about the work.

One day about a year ago she came home from work and suddenly announced to her family that she and Debby were moving to Arizona to live near her sister. She said she was unhappy at work: "The other girls leave me the hardest and most complicated assignments, and they blame me for the mistakes in the files. Now they don't like the color of my clothes—my blouse would be prettier if it were yellow instead of blue. I'm getting tired of their checking up on me, always asking, 'Did you do this—did you finish that job—will you type this for me.' I finally said no; I cleared out my desk and quit."

Sudden onset of suspiciousness, ideas of reference, delusional ideation, and impulsiveness may be indicative of exacerbation of psychopathology.

Evelyn James and her husband were glad to have Sheila come to Arizona and promised to help her find a job and an apartment. Meanwhile, they agreed that Sheila and Debby could live with them. Mrs. Franklin got along well with Evelyn—they made up for lost time since they hadn't seen each other for at least 4 years. Evelyn and her children had fun showing Sheila and Debby around the city. They toured various sections so that Mrs. Franklin could decide where she'd like to live. The sisters shared the work at home. Mrs. Franklin studied the daily newspaper ads and made lists of people to contact both for an apartment and for a job interview. After 6 months there was still no job nor had she found a place to live. When Mrs. James tried to discuss the situation with her, Sheila offered numerous reasons why the apartments were unsuitable. As for the job interviews, she gave multiple reasons why none of the positions were acceptable: they wanted to know too much about her personal life; one employer expected too much for the money he was willing to pay; one placement was like the job she just left—too many girls in the office, she would be the newest employee, and therefore they would soon take advantage of her.

Geographic removal produced relief of stress with a return to a relatively normal level of functioning. However, relief was only temporary. As adaptation to a new environment occurs, pressure begins to build. Sheila again demonstrates inability to assume responsibility for self as evidenced through increased passive-dependent behavior. Excuses indicate excessive use of rationalization and projection.

Mrs. James and her husband tried to be understanding and reassuring and told Sheila to keep looking until she found something more to her satisfaction. At the end of another month, Evelyn tried again to discuss the situation. Sheila began to cry, insisting she was trying but there was really very little available. If she and Debby were creating financial problems for the James' she could pay board; it wouldn't take long to transfer the money from her savings account. A few more weeks passed; this time both Mr. and Mrs. James talked with Mrs. Franklin. She listened for awhile, then in an angry tone blurted out that it was clear to her that they really did not care about her and she certainly would not stay where she was not wanted. She abruptly left the living room, helped Debby get settled into bed, and immediately started packing. The next day she bought bus tickets for herself and Debby and returned to Cleveland.

Pressure from family precipitated an increase in irrational behavior in the form of impulsiveness, hostility, and reappearance of ideas of persecution.

Her parents met them at the bus station. On the way home, she told her parents that they were no longer welcome in Arizona. Evelyn bossed Debby around and her kids made trouble, caused fights and then blamed Debby for them. Debby said, "No! Mommy! No! Aunt Evelyn was nice to me, and I liked Jimmy and Janey and Susie." Mrs. Franklin told her, "Shush," and said she certainly knew better than a little girl what was really going on. Sheila then proceeded to relate to her parents how Evelyn had grown jealous of her, interfered with her getting any of "those good jobs," and prevented her from renting "wonderful apartments." The next few days Sheila was illogical, unreasonable and argumentative. Her mother tried to convince her that she should see her former therapist or be admitted to a hospital.

Behavior at this point indicates Sheila is demonstrating increasing deterioration of her thought processes. The distortion of the situation with her sister and her inability to maintain an objective viewpoint illustrate this increase in her pathology.

Sheila refused, stating, "Everyone seems to think there is something wrong with me. No one considers that anyone else is wrong. As long as I do what you all want then everything is okay, but as soon as I say no, it's a different story. Nobody cares when I am being pushed around, but as soon as I complain then there is something wrong with me!"

Her statement is an example of denial, rationalization and projection. Unable to think logically and clearly, yet needing to defend herself, Sheila increases her use of automatic coping devices. Specifically, there is marked increase in denial—there's nothing wrong with me; rationalization—it's someone else's fault, not mine; and projection—going against others brings retaliation.

For the next 2 weeks Sheila kept to her own room except for meals. She ate little, stating she wasn't hungry. She did not talk much but did respond to questions.

There is an increase in her pattern of withdrawal and apathetic behavior. Her behavior also demonstrates negativism, loss of appetite, and mutism.

One day during lunch she told her mother that she again dreamed that someone tried to kill her and Debby. The mother became frightened after hearing this, and the family agreed to make arrangements for an emergency admission for Sheila.

Her repeated dreams of someone trying to harm her is part of a now well-developed system of persecutory delusions. The dream may indicate the possibility of suicidal and homicidal tendencies.

During the admission procedure Mrs. Franklin was obviously anxious and overtalkative. She told the doctor that she had been fighting strange incidents and plots against her for at least 7 years.

Persecutory delusions have become more pronounced and expansive.

"Everything has been so hard. It would have been different if Paul had lived. People don't pick on women when their husbands are around. Have you any idea what it is like for a mother to bring up a child alone? Debby is a good girl but sometimes she does strange things."

She makes a transition from one thought to a completely different one, indicating more pronounced looseness in association. Rationalization is also apparent.

"I did not tell anybody before because they just wouldn't believe me. John, my sister's husband, made improper advances toward me.

That's why we came back. I was afraid. What really scared me was all those men on the bus and at the bus station looking at me so funny. Even my own brother; I keep my door locked 'cause you just can't trust anyone these days, not even your own family."

Denial of normal sexual feelings resulting in projective behavior.

Mrs. Franklin was admitted to a psychiatric unit of a general hospital with an initial diagnosis of schizophrenia, paranoid type.

SUMMARY

This social history details and demonstrates the sequence of events that eventuated in psychiatric hospitalization. It is at this point in time that those nurses who function in the institutional treatment setting begin to implement a realistic, operational nursing care plan to enable Mrs. Franklin and her family to resume their usual daily living experiences.

26

APPLICATION OF THE NURSING PROCESS WITH MRS. SHEILA FRANKLIN

LEARNING OBJECTIVES

On completion of this chapter the reader should be able to:

1. Trace the development of an effective nursing care plan.
2. Extract relevant data that contributes to the assessment and the care of the patient.
3. Identify the application of theory to practice.

Nursing care for any patient begins when the patient enters the door and meets the nurse for the first time. In the initial encounter with the patient, the nurse begins the nursing process. The nursing care plan that is eventually formulated takes into account the admission procedure and the patient's response to it, the assessment interview, and the physical, sociocultural, and psychological findings as well as the continuous assessment of the patient's response to the care provided. The following is a graphic representation of the hospital experience of Mrs. Sheila Franklin and the actual step-by-step process the nurses used in planning for and implementing her care.

ADMISSION TO THE HOSPITAL

Miss Elizabeth Maris, R.N., responded to the call from the emergency room and escorted Mrs. Franklin to the ward. Mrs. Franklin acknowledged the introduction of the nurse by nodding her head but said nothing. Walking down the hall toward the elevator, the nurse observed that Mrs. Franklin avoided walking next to her, looked from side to side, and peered intently at any open doorway. As they approached the elevator, Mrs. Franklin said, "You don't expect me to get into that cage!" Miss Maris replied, "This is the elevator, but we could walk up the stairs to the next floor, if you'd rather."

Mrs. Franklin's behavior demonstrates suspiciousness. Her verbal and behavioral responses evidence an increased level of anxiety, fear, and distrust based on threats to the self-system. The nurse responds matter-of-factly, offers factual information, avoids argument with paranoid thoughts, and provides reasonable alternative to allow choice and to decrease anxiety.

On reaching the ward, Miss Maris introduced Mrs. Franklin to the head nurse. Mrs. Franklin looked at her and said, "What do you think you are going to do for me here? There's nothing wrong with me!"

The repeated use of denial indicates a lack of insight. Mistrust of the physical and personal environment is conveyed though her actions and comments.

Neither of the nurses directly referred to Mrs. Franklin's statements. Miss Maris calmly and with self-assurance said, "Come, I'll take you to your room. I'll show you where to put your things. I will wait for you until you put them away or I'll help you, if you like." After the unpacking was completed, Miss Maris sat down with Mrs. Franklin to explain the admission and other hospital routines and to answer whatever questions she might have. The nurse decided to forego the actual procedures and initial interview because she assessed that Mrs. Franklin needed time to adapt herself to her new environment.

This decision was based on the assessments the nurse had already made regarding Mrs. Franklin's level of anxiety and degree of suspiciousness.

The nurse kept her explanations short and to the point and briefly answered questions asked by the patient. In less than an hour Mrs. Franklin was ready to leave her room to see the ward and continue with the admission procedures. In the meantime Miss Maris consulted the ward social worker about the patient's history and planned to continue the assessment interview after lunch.

The following "Assessment—Psychiatric Nursing History" form was completed by Miss Maris and is shown in Figure 26–1.

ASSESSMENT - PSYCHIATRIC NURSING HISTORY FORM:

A. PERSONAL INFORMATION

Name *Sheila Franklin* Date of Admission *3/1*

Date of Birth *5/30* Date of Assessment *3/1*

Age *30* Sex *F* National Origin *English - Irish*

Marital Status: __ M ✓ W __ D __ S

Address *1243 Meadowbrook Rd.* Phone *909-1275*

Name of Nearest Relative *Wm. J. Mitchell* Relationship *Father*

Address *(same as above)* Phone *909-1275*

Religious Preference *Protestant*

Church Affiliation *St. Paul's Methodist*

Do you want your clergy to visit? Yes __ No ✓

Do you want the hospital chaplain to visit? Yes __ No ✓

Previous Hospitalizations:

Diagnosis	Date
Pregnancy	*1980*
D and C	*1966*

Medications Currently Being Used:

Drug	Dosage
None	

Do you have any known sensitivity to drugs? Yes __ No ✓

If yes, please identify. ____________

Do you have any allergies? ____________

B. SOCIAL FUNCTIONING

1. Family Constellation:

   a. Position and role in family. *2nd. of three siblings*

Figure 26–1. An Assessment–Psychiatric nursing history form

(continued)

b. Spouse: Name *Paul Franklin* Age *Deceased*

Parents: Name *Wm. J. Mitchell* Age *56*

Parents: Name *Mary Rose* Age *52*

Siblings: Name *Evelyn James* Age *32*

Name *Thomas Mitchell* Age *20*

Name ______ Age ______

Children: Name *Debby Franklin* Age *8*

Name ______ Age ______

Name ______ Age ______

c. Living arrangements: *Lives with parents, daughter and unmarried brother in parent's home.*

d. To whom do you relate the best? *Brother*

2. Occupational and Educational Status:

a. Occupation *Secretary*

b. Place of employment *Unemployed.*

c. Date of last employment *Approx. one year ago*

d. If unemployed, source of income *Social security - Survivor benefits*

e. Education *High school plus six months secretarial course*

3. Recreational Activities:

a. Interest? *Did not respond.*

b. Hobbies? *??*

c. Membership in clubs or organizations? *??*

C. BIOPHYSIOLOGICAL FUNCTIONING

1. Vital Signs: T *98.8* P *86* R *20* BP *124/72*

a. Signs and symptoms indicating possible deficit: *None*

b. Nursing intervention required: *None at present.*

2. Sensory Functions:
   a. Any hearing difficulty? Yes ____ No ✓
      1. Describe: ____________
      2. Hearing aid: Yes ____ No ✓
      3. Provision for batteries ____________
   b. Any Visual difficulty? Yes ____ No ✓
      1. Describe: ____________
      2. Wear glasses: For reading ______ All day ______
      3. Has glass eye: Yes ____ No ✓
   c. Any other prosthetic devices? Yes ____ No ✓
      1. Describe: ____________
      2. Nursing intervention required: ____________
   d. Any decreased ability or inability to detect changes in skin temperature? Yes ____ No ✓
   e. Any numbness, tingling, dizziness, blurred vision? Yes ____ No ✓
   f. Other: ____________
3. Motor Functions:
   a. Physical limitations and disabilities? Yes ____ No ✓
   b. Seizures? Yes ____ No ✓
4. Personal Hygiene:
   a. Bathing: Time: A.M. ____ (P.M) 10 Type: Shower ____ Tub ✓
   b. Care of teeth:
      1. Dentures: Yes ____ No ✓
      2. Usual cleaning time: Morning and Night
   c. Care of skin:
      1. Condition: Oily ____ Dry ✓ Moist ____
2. Color: Pale ____ Flushed ✓ Jaundiced ____ Cyanotic ____ Normal ____
3. Skin is: Broken ____ Bruised ____ Edematous ____ Intact ✓
4. Abnormalities: Rash ____ Lesion ____ Other ____ None ✓
   a. Describe location and extent: —
   b. Nursing intervention required: —
5. Do you use anything on your skin at home: No

(continued)

d. Care of hair:

1. Length: Average ✓ Long ___ Short ___

2. Appearance Clean ___ Well Groomed ___ Unkempt ✓ Stringy ___

3. Condition: Dry ___ Oily ___ Shiney ___ Dull ✓

4. How often do you wash your hair: *weekly*

Self ✓ Beauty shop ___ Barber shop ___

e. Care of nails (hands and feet):

1. Condition: Hard ___ Soft ___ Long ___ Short ✓ Average ___

2. Uses: File ___ Emery boards ___ Buffer ___ Scissors___ Clipper ___Polish___

Evidence of nail biting

f. Feminine hygiene:

1. Menstrual cycle:

a. Frequency of period? *q 28 da.* Number of days: *5*

b. Amount of discharge: Sm ____ Mod ✓ Heavy ___

c. Type of absorbent protection used? Napkin ✓ Tampons ___

d. Date of last menstrual period *2/27/–*

2. Birth control measures: Yes ___ No ✓

a. Contraceptives: Oral ___ I.U.D. ___

b. Rhythm: Yes ___ No ___

c. Other: Yes ___ No ___ Describe ______________________________

3. Douching: Yes ___ No ✓

a. Solution __________________ Equipment used _________________

4. Hair removal: Yes ✓ No ___

a. Uses: Depilatory cream ___ Razor ✓

b. Type of razor: Electric ___ Safety ___

5. Cosmetics used: None ___ Powder ✓ Perfume ___ Lipstick ✓

Deodorant ✓ Cremes ___ Lotions ___ Hairspray ___

g. Masculine hygiene:

1. Shaving: Razor: Electric ___ Safety ___

2. Cosmetics: Shaving creme ___ Skin conditioner ___ Cologne ___

After shave lotion ___ Hairspray ___

3. Athletic support: Yes ___ No ___

5. Elimination (usual pattern):

   a. Bowel: Frequency _daily_ Time _a.m._

      Laxative (Specify) _No_ Colostomy: Yes ___ NO ✓

   b. Bladder: Frequency _2-3 times_ Time _"I don't know"_

      Nocturnal Voiding: Yes ___ No ✓

   c. Any changes noted since illness? Yes ___ No ___

      Describe ___

6. Sleep and Comfort Pattern:

   a. Usual bedtime _11:30 p.m._ Number of hours sleep _9-10 hrs._

      1. Uninterrupted: Yes ___ No ✓

      2. Up during night: ~~Time~~ _yes_ Frequency _could not specify. "Sometimes I sleep, sometimes I don't, my thoughts keep me awake."_

   b. Accustomed to a single room: Yes ✓ No ___

   c. Nap: Yes ___ No ✓

   d. Comfort Measures:

      1. Pillow: Yes ✓ No ___ Number _2_

      2. Blanket: Yes ✓ No ___ Number _1_

      3. Night Light: Yes ✓ No ___

      4. Window: Open ___ Closed ✓ _Sleeps with room door locked._

      5. Bedtime Snack: Yes ✓ No ___ Specify _anything_

      6. Sleeping pills: Yes ___ No ✓ Drug ___ Dosage ___

7. Nutritional Pattern:

   a. Height _5'6"_ Weight _130 lbs._

   b. Food habits:

	Meal Pattern	Time	Usual Food
B		8^{30} - 9^{30}	Juice and coffee
L	Skips lunch		
D	"When I feel like eating"		anything
S		Before bed	anything

   c. Food likes: _"I'm not fussy"_

   d. Food dislikes: _"My mother cooks what I like"_

   e. Food allergies: _None_

   f. Religious restrictions: _None_

(continued)

g. Fluid habits: Beverage Temperature

B Black coffee and water — hot

L

D Black coffee — milk — hot / cold

S Fruit juice — pop — cold

h. Beverage Dislikes: tea — diet pop

i. Any difficulties with food or fluid intake? Yes ___ No ✓

Appetite___Chewing___Swallowing___Nausea___Vomiting___Distention___Other___

j. What do you usually do for a stomach upset at home? "I don't have any, there's nothing wrong with me." Mother reports that Sheila chews Rolaids constantly.

D. MENTAL-EMOTIONAL-BEHAVIORAL FUNCTIONING:

1. Appearance on admission:

a. Facial expressions:

Angry	✓	Worn	___	Smiling	___	Questioning	✓
Blank	___	Cheerful	___	Tearful	___	Bewildered	___
Happy	___	Frowning	✓	Disinterested	___	Interested	___
Sad	___	Haggard	___	Dissatisfied	___	Surprised	___

b. Eyes:

Open	✓	Sparkling	___	Staring	___
Closed	___	Darting	✓	Fixed	___

c. Complexion: Healthy ___Sallow___Pasty___Ruddy___Other slightly flushed

d. Grooming and dress:

1. C[illegible]hing: Clean___ Pressed___ Wrinkled ✓ Ragged___ Soiled___ Burned___
2. Shoes: Shining___ Scuffed___ Worn ✓
3. Stockings: Yes ___ No ✓
4. Socks: Yes ___ No ✓

e. Body Language:

1. Posture: Erect ✓ Sagging ___ Slouched ___ Stiff ___
2. Movement: Normal ___ Slow ___ Fast ✓ Relaxed ___ Coordinated ___

   Hyperactive ___

	Head	Face	Torso	Extremities
Trembling	___	___	___	___
Twitching	___	___	___	___
Spastic	___	___	___	___
Rocking	___	___	___	___
Immobile	___	___	___	___
Rigid	✓	___	✓	✓
Tics	___	___	___	___

2. Behavior:

Shy	___	Confused	___	Demanding	___	Suspicious	✓
Bold	___	Agitated	___	Confident	___	Ritualistic	___
Aloof	✓	Critical	✓	Apathetic	___	Distrustful	✓
Bossy	___	Oriented	✓	Irritable	✓	Uninhibited	___
Alert	✓	Restless	✓	Impulsive	___	Disoriented	___
Labile	___	Euphoric	___	Seductive	___	Apprehensive	✓
Fearful	✓	Sarcastic	✓	Impatient	✓	Antagonistic	___
Playful	___	Withdrawn	✓	Attentive	___	Distractible	___

3. Communication:

a. Tone: Soft ___ Loud ✓ Average ___ Clipped ___ Whispering ___

b. Speech difficulties: Language barrier ___ Lisping ___ Stuttering ___ Other___

c. Flow of speech:

Talkative	✓	Relevant	___	Irrelevant	___
Mute	___	Repetitious	✓	Monosyllabic	✓
Average	___	Mumbling	___	Gregarious, Initiating	___
Guarded	✓	Continuous	___	Quiet, Noninitiating	___
Hesitant	___				

Talkative but when questioned about specifics resorted to monosyllabic responses.

4. Perception and Thinking:

a. Intellectual functioning:

1. Impaired memory: Yes ___ No ✓ Recent ___ Remote ___
2. Impaired judgment: Yes ✓ No ___ *suspicious*
3. Brief attention span: Yes ✓ No ___
4. Lacks ability to concentrate: Yes ✓ No ___ *appears preoccupied*
5. Misinterprets: Yes ✓ No ___

(continued)

6. Logical: Yes ___ No ✓
7. Ability to abstract: Yes ___ No ✓
8. Concrete: Yes ✓ No ___ see admission note.

b. Perception:
1. Impaired: Yes ✓ No ___ perceived elevator as "cage"
2. Types of impairment:
a. Illusions: Yes ✓ No ___
b. Hallucinations: Visual ___ Auditory ___ Tactile ___ Gustatory ___ Olfactory ___
c. Other: Describe: Denied - Seemed guarded in response to question about hearing voices
d. Thought progressions: Normal ___ Abnormal ✓ Blocking ___ Flight of Ideas ___ Incoherence ___ Circumstantiality ✓ Retardation ___
e. Thought content:
1. Delusions: Somatic ___ Ideas of reference ✓ Grandeur ___ Persecutory ✓ Self-accusatory ___ "People take advantage of me"
2. Obsessions: Yes ___ No ___ Describe none stated
3. Phobias: Yes ___ No ___ Describe none discerned

5. Ego Assessment:
a. Defense mechanisms used:

Denial	✓	Conversion	___	Compensation	___
Undoing	___	Suppression	___	Substitution	___
Repression	___	Sublimation	___	Identification	___
Regression	___	Introjection	___	Rationalization	✓
Projection	✓	Displacement	___	Reaction formation	___

b. Self-evaluation:
1. How do you see yourself?

Polite	✓	Friendly	✓	Easygoing	___
Loving	___	Likable	___	Trustworthy	___
Honest	✓	Reliable	✓	Independent	✓
Unkind	___	Cautious	___	Considerate	___
Selfish	___	Dependent	___	Short tempered	___

2. What is your usual mood? Has it changed? "Sometimes I feel sad. I miss my husband."

3. What kinds of things make you feel better/worse? "When people blame me for things that happen."

4. Is there any time of day in which you think more clearly, do things better, or feel best? "At night." Wasn't able to give any reason or further explanation.

5. What are some of the things you think and worry about? "My little girl - Debby."

6. Does time go quickly or slowly for you? "Don't know."

7. Do you find it easy to talk to other people? "What do you want to know for?" (Before I could respond, answered yes.)

8. What kind of person do you find most interesting? "Haven't thought about it - someone like my Paul."

9. What do you expect of yourself? "To work and to be a good mother."

   Of family? "Leave me alone!" (Sounds angry)

   Of friends? "To be friends."

   Of people in general? "Not to fuck me around - to live and let live."

10. What were the circumstances which led up to your coming to the hospital? "My parents think I need to be here."

11. Have you ever felt a desire or tried to injure yourself in any way? No verbal response - shook head no. Moved back in chair - appeared angry.

12. Have you noticed any changes in your sexual interest/functioning? No verbal response - shook head no.

(continued)

13. What would you like the nursing staff to help you with while you are in the hospital? "I don't know."

14. What did you find most helpful/least helpful when you were hospitalized before? "They had good food."

15. What do you expect to happen to you after your experience in the hospital?
"I don't know—work I suppose and care for Debby 'til she grows up."

E. VISTORS:

1. Are your friends and family able to visit you? Yes ✓ No ___

2. Do you want any limitations of visitors? Yes ✓ No ___
"I don't want to see my parents. They put me here—now they can stay away!"

NURSING SUMMARY:

1. What does the patient "want" or need? Wants: to be left alone
Needs: a. decrease in suspiciousness
b. develop positive relationships
c. develop trust.
d. develop realistic sense of responsibility.
e. increase self-esteem.

2. Is attainment within the realm of the patient's capabilities and potential?
Yes. Previous past experiences indicates potential.

3. What prevents the individual from reaching identified goals? Poor self-concept; feelings of inadequacy; guilt re- husband's death; suspiciousness; anxiety; inability to focus on reality; illogical and unreasonable sequencing of thoughts.

4. What changes in behavior could result in more productive living patterns through health teaching? Better dietary habits; priority setting and use of time; organization; learning to cope with feelings of anger, anxiety, guilt and loneliness.

5. What role does the family play in the individual's pattern of living? Parents are very much interested in her welfare but contribute to her dependency. Brother is supportive and encouraging.

6. To what extent can the family be involved in the individual's care? To a large extent, expressed interest and willingness to help.

7. What resources are available to the individual and family upon returning to the community? Mental Health Clinic, Family Service, Job Counseling, Social groups and Church groups.

INITIAL NURSING CARE PLAN

After completing the interview, Miss Maris made her initial nursing diagnoses and wrote a preliminary care plan based on the available data. She then scheduled a total conference with the ward staff (physician, psychologist, social worker, occupational and recreational therapists, the nursing assistants assigned to her team, the head nurse, and herself) and Mrs. Franklin for 10:00 A.M. the next day. The purpose for the conference was to formulate a total treatment program for Mrs. Franklin. The outcome of the ward conference provides the nurse with the necessary information to design a nursing care plan in conjunction with the interdisciplinary team.

In developing the initial nursing care plan, Miss Maris identified three major nursing care goals:

1. To assist Mrs. Franklin in achieving successful adaptation to the hospital environment.
2. To prepare Mrs. Franklin for involvement in the total treatment plan.
3. To obtain needed information through observation and interaction with Mrs. Franklin in order to facilitate the ongoing development of her nursing care plan.

The initial nursing care plan devised by Miss Maris is shown in Table 26–1.

TABLE 26–1. INITIAL NURSING CARE PLAN

Name: Sheila Franklin | Nurse: Miss Maris | Date: 3/1/19__

Nursing Diagnosis	Goals/Objectives	Nursing Intervention	Rationale	Results of Intervention
1. Behavioral disruption due to inadequate self-concept and lowered self-esteem as evidenced by suspicious behavior; for example: a. Sits facing the door. b. Looks over her shoulder as she walks down the hall. c. Distressed because she cannot lock her room door.	1. By the end of the first week of hospitalization, Mrs. Franklin will achieve successful adaptation to the hospital environment as evidenced by: a. Expressing a sense of safety and security. b. Establishing rapport with staff.	1. Approach in a calm, self-assured manner. 2. Take time to explain scheduled procedures. Tell her: a. Laboratory technician will take blood samples at 8 A.M. b. She will go to x-ray and EKG at 8:30 A.M. c. Breakfast will be served when she returns to ward. 3. Answer call bell promptly.	People displaying symptoms of suspicion, distrust, and fear are often threatened by interpersonal relationships; therefore, a friendly but reserved approach is more likely to succeed.	Patient responded to information with: "I hope they are on time—I hate to wait."
2. Behavioral disruption due to feeling of inadequacy as evidenced by regressive behavior; for example: a. Wishes to stay in her room. b. Refuses to meet other patients.	2. By the end of the first week of hospitalization, Mrs. Franklin will be involved in her total treatment plan through: a. An increasing number of contacts with staff and patients. b. Exploring with the nurse relevant current and past experiences.	4. Make positive approaches several times during evening. a. Invite Mrs. F. to: 1) Watch T.V. 2) Meet other patients. 3) Have a snack. b. Attempt to find out: 1) What she usually does with her free time. 2) Interests or hobbies, past and present.	Opportunities for satisfying relationships and feelings of security are increased when the individual is able to see others as truthful, dependable, and capable. Trust and confidence are enhanced by a demonstration of concern and interest.	Refused to come out of her room and said, "Maybe tomorrow." Responded to all questions briefly and factually.

(*continued*)

TABLE 26–1. CONTINUED

Name: Sheila Franklin | Nurse: Miss Maris | Date: 3/1/19__

Nursing Diagnosis	Goals/Objectives	Nursing Intervention	Rationale	Results of Intervention
		3) Offer assistance at bedtime: a. Check on need for toilet articles. b. Remind not to drink fluids after midnight.		
3. Feeling disturbance related to threat to self-concept and unmet needs as evidenced by anxiety; for example: a. Talks rapidly in a loud tone of voice. b. Repeats herself. c. Asks nurses to repeat, says, "I didn't hear." d. Possible refusal of h.s. medication because she is afraid to sleep with door unlocked.	3. Within the first 48 hours of hospitalization, Mrs. Franklin will feel comfortable on the unit as evidenced by: a. Readiness to complete orientation to the unit. b. Speaking at a moderate rate and tone. c. Listening attentively to direction.	5. Speak a. Clearly. b. Slowly. c. Briefly. d. In a quiet tone. 6. Ask for and answer questions in a friendly, unhurried manner. 7. Has Dalmane 30 mg. reordered for h.s. a. Withhold h.s. medication until night nurse is on duty. b. Introduce night nurse. c. Have night nurse (Miss Jeffrey) explain: 1) Night rounds. 2) Cleaning details. 3) Possible unexpected sounds.	Anxiety occurs when one is confronted with a situation that threatens one's self-image. A moderate degree of anxiety produces a decrease in perception. Therefore, clear, brief, repeated communications are needed to lessen level of anxiety and increase sense of trust.	Accepted the sedatives after being reassured that rounds were really made.

MORNING REPORT: 3/2/19___

Miss Jeffrey, the night nurse, reported that Mrs. Franklin had agreed to take the sedative ordered after being assured that the door to her room could be kept closed. Mrs. Franklin was awake twice during the night. The first time was at 2 A.M.; as the nurse entered the room, Mrs. Franklin said, "I'm still awake." But before the nurse could respond, Mrs. Franklin was already asleep again. The second time occurred about 4:30 A.M. This time when the nurse entered her room, Mrs. Franklin wanted to know if it was time to get up.

Miss Jeffrey related that Miss Valor, the evening nurse assigned to Mrs. Franklin, had reported that Mrs. Franklin had refused to go to the lounge but that she did agree to meet Mrs. Jones, a patient in the room next to hers, and that Mrs. Franklin stayed to talk with Mrs. Jones for a few minutes. Miss Valor spent about half an hour talking with Mrs. Franklin and learned that she liked to read romantic, adventure, and historical novels. She also discovered that Mrs. Franklin did some painting when she was in school but had not had much time for it since her little girl was born. She does sew for herself and Debby: "simple things—nothing too complicated."

After the scheduled interdisciplinary team conference, Miss Maris and the head nurse conducted the nursing care conference to plan specific nursing interventions related to the identified objectives. The nursing care plan they developed (Table 26–2) reflects the philosophy and treatment plan of the interdisciplinary team.

TABLE 26–2. REVISED NURSING CARE PLAN

Name: Sheila Franklin **Nurse: Miss Maris** **Date: 3/2/19___**

Nursing Diagnosis	Goals/Objectives	Nursing Intervention	Rationale	Results of Intervention
1. Behavioral disruption due to inadequate self-concept as evidenced by suspicious behavior; for example: a. Sits facing door. b. Looks over her shoulder as she walks down the hall. c. Distressed because she cannot lock her room door. d. Avoids contact with staff.	1. By the end of the first week of hospitalization, Mrs. Franklin will achieve successful adaptation to the hospital environment as evidenced by: a. Expressing a sense of safety and security. b. Establishing rapport with primary care nursing staff.	1. Show acceptance by being: a. Scrupulously honest. 1) Respond with correct, accurate information to questions. 2) Explain routines and procedures clearly. 3) Keep promises.		
		b. Consistent, friendly, and persistent. 1) Initiate approaches. 2) Assign particular staff members: a. Days—Miss Maris, R.N. b. Evenings—Miss Valor, R.N. c. Nights—Miss Jeffrey, R.N.	Attitudes and actions indicating that an individual is worthy of attention or concern contribute to a feeling of being cared about.	Requested clarification of schedule from Miss Maris on two occasions. Appears more comfortable with staff; will respond to overtures.
2. Behavioral disruption due to feelings of inadequacy as	2. By the end of the first week of hospitalization, Mrs. Franklin will be	2. Plan schedule with patient and adhere to it:	Familiar routines and persons contribute to a sense of security and	Reluctant to leave room. Will interact with nursing staff, if

evidenced by regressive behavior; for example: a. Wishes to stay in her room. b. Refuses to meet other patients.	involved in her total treatment plan through: a. An increasing number of contacts with staff and patients. b. Exploring with primary nurse(s) relevant current and past experiences. c. Participation in planned scheduled activities.	a. Rising—7:30 A.M. 1) Wash and dress before breakfast. 2) Give positive recognition when Mrs. F. complies with policy regarding clothes. b. Bath—10 P.M. Prefers tub bath. c. Meals 1) Inform about dinner hours: 7:30–9:00; 11:30–1:00; 4:30–6:00. 2) Observe eating habits; amount, selection, and frequency. 3) Encourage to sit with Mrs. Jones in dining room. (Be sure chair faces door.) 4) Evening snack—8:30 P.M. d. Medications 1) Stelazine 10 mgm. b.i.d. 9 A.M.–9 P.M.	provide a reality orientation for the patient. Commitment to a schedule is a base for developing a successful identity and decreases the fear of the unknown, thereby promoting security. Modification of hospital routines assists in individualizing care and demonstrates to the patient the staff's concern.	approached. Skips lunch. Refuses evening snack. Agreed to sit at the same table with Mrs. Jones. Responds but does not initiate conversation. Asked questions of Miss Jeffrey regarding Stelazine and its side effects.

(*continued*)

TABLE 26–2. CONTINUED

Name: Sheila Franklin | **Nurse: Miss Maris** | **Date: 3/2/19__**

Nursing Diagnosis	Goals/Objectives	Nursing Intervention	Rationale	Results of Intervention
		2) Dalmane 30 mgm. at 11 P.M. prn. —Observe and record response to medications. —Discuss medication with Mrs. F.		
		e. Counseling session: 1:00–1:30 daily with Miss Maris.	Consistent approach by one nurse to develop a relationship increases the likelihood of significant trust being developed.	Agreed to attend sessions. Reported to designated place on time; left after 15 minutes; does not assume initiative in conversation.
		f. Occupational therapy: 10:00–11:30 daily. 1) Miss Maris to escort and introduce patient first time. 2) Supply therapist with additional needed information. 3) Confer with therapist on regular basis for a mutual exchange regarding progress.	Collaboration with other disciplines provides for consistency and continuity of care.	Looking at blouse patterns, Mrs. F. said she might make herself a blouse. Therapist reported that patient sat and looked at patterns but couldn't make a decision.

	g. Visitors—2:00–4:00; 7:00–9:00 P.M. daily		
	1) Inform parents of Sheila's request that they not visit.	To demonstrate advocacy and respect for patient's decision.	Mother very upset and verbalized that she felt hurt and would worry if she didn't see that Sheila was okay.
	2) Discuss with parents: Relationship of request to symptomatology; their feelings in response to request;	To provide an opportunity for maintaining family support system. To allow parents an opportunity to ventilate their concerns about Sheila.	Father agreed to the request, said he would not come until Sheila asked to see him. Mother said she would come the following day and see if Sheila would see her.
	Suggest that they come at the usual time and speak to Miss Maris; time limitation of 1/2 hour.	To offer reassurance. To prevent the patient from feeling overwhelmed.	Sheila agreed to see mother.
	3) Observe interaction between patient and visitors:	To add to data base.	Mother visited for 1/2 hour. Mrs. Franklin had very little to say. Mother did most of the talking.
	Observe for signs of mounting anxiety;	To help patient clarify thoughts and feelings.	Frequently observed lying on bed.
	Communication patterns; Visitor interaction and reaction.	To promote comfort, security, and safety of patients and visitors.	
	4) Explore with patient initial request to restrict parental visit.	To provide appropriate information.	

(continued)

TABLE 26–2. CONTINUED

Name: Sheila Franklin | Nurse: Miss Maris | Date: 3/2/19__

Nursing Diagnosis	Goals/Objectives	Nursing Intervention	Rationale	Results of Intervention
		5) Talk with visitors and acquaint them with regulations of ward. 6) Answer questions for visitors. h. Recreational therapy: 7:00–8:30 on ward. i. Rest periods or free time: 1:30–2:00 P.M. 4:00–4:30 P.M. 6:30–7:00 and 9:00–10:00 P.M. j. Retiring—after the 11 P.M. news.		
		3. Approach and invite Mrs. F. to leave her room during free periods. a. Stay with her for a few minutes each time she refuses. b. Recognize it may take time before she is willing to leave her room. c. Try positive suggestions:	To experience satisfying relationships with others, the individual must be able to feel that he will not be harmed by the relationship.	Says she stays in her room because she needs quiet to read. However, she is unable to discuss her book.

		1) I'd like—. 2) I need—. 3) I'd appreciate—.		
3. Feeling disturbance related to feelings of inadequacy and poor self-concept as evidenced by hostility; for example: a. Responds in an abrupt, critical, and sarcastic manner to members of interdisciplinary team. b. Uses delaying tactics to avoid participating in scheduled activities.	3. Within 2 weeks, Mrs. Franklin will recognize situations evoking hostility and identify appropriate means for dealing with them as evidenced by: a. Talks with Miss Maris about incidents on unit or past life experiences. b. Identifies feeling of hospitality and labels it. c. Explores behavior resulting from feeling and evaluates effectiveness. d. Suggests possible alternative means for dealing with the problem.	4. Become aware of, anticipate, and observe negative feelings and behavior. a. Observe for signs of mounting hostility: 1) Listen to complaints without making excuses or becoming angry. 2) Keep calm.	Hostility is usually a negative response that occurs when one's sense of independence is threatened, particularly in relationships with authority figures.	Refused to discuss hostile feelings during counseling session.
		b. Help Mrs. F. to identify specific cues to hostility: 1) Allow and encourage Mrs. F. to discuss the situation: What happened and when did it occur? What provoked the behavior? Who was involved? 2) How did Mrs. F. express her feelings? 3) What might she do next time?	Discussion of hostility-producing situations allows the individual to identify feelings and behavior without fear of judgment or retaliation. It also provides an opportunity for learning alternate methods of responding that will increase feelings of satisfaction.	

EVALUATION OF CARE

On March 8 at the end of the first week of hospitalization, the nursing care plan was reviewed, evaluated, and revised. Mrs. Franklin is not completely adhering to the planned schedule. She goes to the dining room for breakfast and dinner, skips lunch, and refuses the evening snack. She usually wakes up once during the night. The first 2 days Mrs. Franklin received Stelazine she complained of feeling sleepy and noted some dryness of the mouth. Mrs. Franklin attends occupational therapy but is still looking at the pattern book and is unable to decide what she is going to make. The recreational therapy sessions in the evenings were refused with such excuses as: "I would rather read"; "I cannot dance"; "I do not like to play games." Mrs. Franklin is not as abrupt with the nursing staff, but she did tell at least two patients who approached her and asked her to join them in a card game to "mind their own business." The staff agreed to give priority to:

I. Focusing the interactive–interventive process on:
  1. Mrs. Franklin's inability to relate with other people as evidenced by her noninvolvement in ward activities and
  2. Identifying those factors that seem to prevent Mrs. Franklin from assuming the necessary responsibility for committing herself to decision-making

II. Introducing those solitary activities that have been identified as successful experiences in the past

Mrs. Franklin was asked to join the nursing staff conference to discuss these treatment goals and the way in which they could be implemented. The following revision of the nursing care plan was developed and a time was set for evaluation of progress (Table 26–3).

TABLE 26–3. NURSING CARE PLAN III

Name: Sheila Franklin **Nurse: Miss Maris** **Date: 3/8/19__**

Nursing Diagnosis	Goals/Objectives	Nursing Intervention	Rationale	Results of Intervention
1. Behavioral disruption due to inadequate self-concept and lowered self-esteem as evidenced by suspicious behavior; for example: a. Nonparticipation; b. Social isolation; c. Poor interpersonal relationships; d. Misinterprets motives of others.	1. Within two weeks, Mrs. Franklin will demonstrate a decrease in suspicious behavior as evidenced by: a. Active involvement in solitary activities; b. Participation in counseling sessions with Miss Maris; c. Exploration of factors influencing participation.	1. Continue daily nurse–patient interaction. a. Increase time to 1 hour. b. Try two half-sessions: one in the morning, and one in the afternoon. 2. Approach patient at the beginning of each scheduled activity. a. Talk with her about the situation. b. Encourage participation by joining her in the activity.	Demonstration of continued acceptance toward patient results in lessening of suspicion and provides opportunities for testing reality.	Kept two morning sessions but made excuses for avoiding the afternoon sessions. Would agree to participate; starts an activity but loses interest after 15–20 minutes.
2. Feeling disturbance related to feelings of inadequacy and poor self-concept as evidenced by hostility; for example: a. Excessive use of rationalization; b. Abrupt and caustic comments.	2. Within 2 weeks Mrs. Franklin will experience success in accomplishments as evidenced by: a. Increased participation in activities; b. Completion of O.T. project; c. Verbalizing positive comments about self.	3. Provide meaningful tasks and assistance in: a. Occupational therapy: 1. Selecting a pattern. 2. Arranging for buying fabric. 3. Pinning and cutting the fabric. 4. Completing the task. b. On the ward:	Identifying achievements and positively acknowledging her accomplishments will foster feelings of adequacy and increase her self-confidence.	Selected two patterns and agreed to go to shopping center with nurse.

(continued)

TABLE 26–3. CONTINUED

Name: Sheila Franklin **Nurse: Miss Maris** **Date: 3/8/19___**

Nursing Diagnosis	Goals/Objectives	Nursing Intervention	Rationale	Results of Intervention
		1) To maintain typing skills, obtain a typewriter for her to use. 2) Request that Mrs. F. type ward lists, bed charts, time sheets.	Providing an opportunity to demonstrate real skills and earn appropriate recognition.	Complained she couldn't type lists because of staff's illegible writing. Became angry when Miss Maris offered to read lists to her and said, "You're just like my boss, setting impossible tasks."
		3. Ask for her assistance in maintaining the ward library: a. Arrange books on shelf. b. Dispose of outdated magazines and newspapers. c. Buy daily newspaper in hospital lobby.		Arranged *all* books upside down. Threw out all magazines.

A CRISIS SITUATION

On March 12 at 3:20 A.M., Miss Jeffrey heard a scream coming from the direction of Mrs. Franklin's room. On investigation, the nurse found Mrs. Franklin cowering in her bed. As Miss Jeffrey approached Mrs. Franklin, the nurse could hear her whimpering over and over, "No! No! Stay away from me! You're dead! Dead!" Mrs. Franklin sobbed and mumbled incoherently for approximately 15 minutes. When asked what was happening, Mrs. Franklin denied that anything was the matter. As the nurse tried to focus on the incident and her outcry, Mrs. Franklin insisted that she was all right saying, "It's nothing, just a nightmare! I'm fine." Miss Jeffrey got Mrs. Franklin a glass of warm milk and sat with her until she dropped off to sleep again. The nurse checked on her every half-hour and found that Mrs. Franklin was sleeping but was restless. When Miss Jeffrey entered Mrs. Franklin's room at 5:30 A.M., she found her lying rigidly, staring up at the ceiling, and nonresponsive to verbal communication.

The nursing staff held a short conference to plan for immediate revision of the nursing care plan and goals previously set for Mrs. Franklin's care. The changes were based on Miss Jeffrey's report and the observations Miss Maris made during her morning rounds. During the conference, the goals were revised and the nursing staff discussed their own feelings and reactions to Mrs. Franklin's apparent setback. The priorities they established at this time were identified as follows:

1. Limit the regression by encouraging Mrs. Franklin to focus outside self.
2. Meet dependency needs while encouraging and assisting in activities of daily living.
3. Convey the expectation of resuming full functioning in a short period of time.
4. Encourage her to verbalize her feelings.

A revised nursing care plan (Table 26–4) was initiated for Mrs. Franklin.

TABLE 26–4. NURSING CARE PLAN IV

Name: Sheila Franklin | **Nurse: Miss Maris** | **Date: 3/12/19___**

Nursing Diagnosis	Goals/Objectives	Nursing Intervention	Rationale	Results of Intervention
1. Behavioral disruption due to feelings of inadequacy and movement away from reality as evidenced by regressive behavior; for example: a. Immobility; b. Body rigidity; c. Staring at the ceiling; d. Muteness.	1. Within 72 hours will be able to focus on reality and gradually resume activity and responsibility as evidenced by: a. Decreased muscular rigidity; b. Mobility; c. Verbal responsiveness; d. Resumption of usual activities of daily living.	1. Assign counseling nurse to provide total care (Miss Maris). a. Approach in a matter-of-fact manner. b. Be patient and understanding. c. Demonstrate concern: "Mrs. Franklin, something happened last night. Perhaps you'll tell me . . ."	Regression is a means of relieving anxiety. Collapse of adult behavioral patterns occurs as frustration and conflict increase. Concerted effort in terms of staff attitude is required to influence the degree and time span of the regressive process.	Followed movements of nurse with eyes but did not move head.
		1) Sit quietly. 2) Allow ample time for the patient to respond. 3) "I'll spend more time with you today. Maybe later . . ." 4) "Now, I'll help you get ready for breakfast."	Direct verbal communications are used to focus on reality.	
		2. Make no demands this morning. a. Give positive instructions:	Expression of intense dependence connotes a need for recognition and attention.	Took 15 minutes to wash face and hands. No verbal response.
		1) Personal hygiene: a) "Wash and dry your face	Equilibrium is restored when dependency needs are met.	

and hands." b) "It's time to brush your teeth." c) Comb your hair." 2) Breakfast, lunch: a) "Drink your juice, Mrs. F." b) "Eat the oatmeal." c) "Shall I add cream and sugar to your coffee?"		Drank juice, ate half-serving of oatmeal, refused toast and eggs. Nodded head negatively. Refused lunch.
b. Prepare any articles needed for use such as washcloth, towels, toothbrush, meal tray, and eating utensils.		
c. Offer assistance if unable to do for self: 1) Bathe, comb hair, apply makeup. 2) Prepare meal tray. 3) Feed.		
d. Offer and encourage fruit juice several times during the day.	To prevent the possibility of dehydration.	Total fluid intake from 7:30 A.M. to 1:00 P.M. was 500 cc.

(continued)

TABLE 26–4. CONTINUED

Name: Sheila Franklin | Nurse: Miss Maris | Date: 3/12/19__

Nursing Diagnosis	Goals/Objectives	Nursing Intervention	Rationale	Results of Intervention
		3. Approach Mrs. Franklin every hour for at least 15 minutes each time during remainder of the day. a. Address her by name. b. Mention the time limits: "Mrs. F., it's 10:00 A.M. I'll be here for 15 minutes. I'll sit and talk with you now." c. Wait for response: 1) Sit quietly in silence. 2) Focus attention on patient. 3) Make short, nonanxiety-producing statements. a) "I'll be in and out to see you throughout the morning." b) "I'll bring a magazine for us to look at next time." c) "I'll be here 5 more minutes."	Continuous interest, persistence, and "thereness" of the nurse communicate a concern and willingness to help and assist the patient in maintaining a sense of personal worth.	Nonresponsive on verbal level. No eye contact.

	4. Encourage and assist Mrs. Franklin to get dressed in the afternoon.		Became rigid when approached with own clothes. Allowed self to be dressed in bathrobe; was helped out of bed.
	5. Provide solitary activities:	Simple, solitary activities reduce stress and promote comfort.	
	a. Furnish two or three current magazines focusing on previous expressed interests: 1) *Vogue.* 2) *Ladies Home Journal.* 3) *Good Housekeeping.*	Activities are an effective means of encouraging self-expression. Increasing responsibility implies a therapeutic optimism and expectation of patient participation in routine.	Would not turn pages or look at magazine.
	b. Page through the magazine and attempt to elicit Mrs. Franklin's comments on color, styles, recipes.		
	c. Secure finger paints from O.T. and introduce to Mrs. F.		Smeared finger paints over self and clothes. Permitted nurse to wash hands and face.
	d. Set up a small colorful picture puzzle of no more than 25 to 30 pieces.		Threw puzzle on floor. Refused to leave room.
	e. Offer to accompany Mrs. F. on a short walk in the hallway.		

PROGRESS REPORT

Mrs. Franklin remained mute and demanded a great deal of assistance in meeting her most basic needs. Bathing and dressing were very slow processes that required detailed instructions, encouragement, and supervision from the nurse every step of the way. Reminders to eat, to take her medications, and to go to the bathroom were constantly reiterated.

The physician decided to increase Mrs. Franklin's medication, and the Stelazine order was changed to 10 mg q.i.d. Miss Maris observed that Mrs. Franklin noted the change in medication as evidenced by her questioning glance at the nurse when she brought them to her at 1:00 and 5:00 in the afternoon. Mrs. Franklin did not make any comment when Miss Maris pointed out the change.

Since Mrs. Franklin still had not spoken after 3 days, the staff decided that Miss Maris should provide her with a notebook and suggest to her that she write in diary form her thoughts and feelings. Miss Maris tried to convey the attitude that she understood how difficult it was to talk about some things. She told Mrs. Franklin that it might even be painful. However, sometimes writing one's thoughts and feelings might make it easier to share them. Miss Maris offered to help her identify those thoughts and feelings that might be causing her present discomfort. The nurse also suggested that together they could explore these concerns and work out possible solutions.

Because of the intensive demonstration of concern displayed by the entire staff, the regressive period was interrupted after 5 days. Improvement resulted following patient's recognition that dependency needs were met. Staff did *not* reject her; she was still worthwhile and acceptable despite extreme behavior. Therefore, she *could* choose to change and improve her behavior. Gradually, Mrs. Franklin was able to resume functioning at a level comparable to that which existed prior to the crisis situation.

From this point on, the staff, Mrs. Franklin, and her family were actively involved in trying out different methods to deal more effectively with her fears, feelings of hostility, guilt, and suspiciousness. The plan provided for gradual resocialization through increasing Mrs. Franklin's contact with selected patients and other staff members both on and off the ward. Initially, competition was avoided or kept to a minimum. As the patient developed more self-confidence, she was included in daily group therapy sessions to further provide positive feedback in developing relationships with others.

THERAPEUTIC COMMUNICATION: A COUNSELING SESSION WITH MRS. FRANKLIN

An actual nurse–patient interaction between Miss Maris and Mrs. Franklin is reported here (Table 26–5) to provide an example of an effective therapeutic nurse–patient communication process. Inclusion of this sample will demonstrate the following:

1. The use of an interactive–interventive session as means of carrying out the nursing care goals.
2. The use of a counseling session as part of the total treatment process.
3. How the techniques of communication can be used effectively in the practical application of a theoretical framework.
4. The way in which the nurse and patient together identify a problem area and seek a workable solution.
5. The way in which the learning process is implemented to bring about a desired change in behavior.
6. The part evaluation plays in determining effective communication.
7. The planning for subsequent sessions based on achievements of mutually derived goals.

EVALUATION OF INTERACTION BY MISS MARIS

"As I reviewed this interaction immediately after the session, I was convinced that the total interaction clearly demonstrates that we are in the working phase of the therapeutic relationship. Mrs. Franklin's responses indicated that she felt secure and was able to verbalize her real feelings. This made me feel very good. I felt I had accomplished a major task. The areas which require additional work on my part to make the process more therapeutic are:

1. Using more reflection in order to elicit and clarify her feelings
2. Allowing Mrs. Franklin more time to express her feeling before I attempt to translate her comments into feelings
3. Broadening my use of a variety of therapeutic techniques of communication

With respect to Mrs. Franklin, I think that she needs:

1. Exposure to a variety of situations where she can experiment with testing her reactions and responses
2. Reinforcement of the learning process as a means of dealing effectively with uncomfortable situations
3. Time to deliberate and validate her feelings with others

TABLE 26–5. COUNSELING SESSION

Patient Name **Mrs. Sheila Franklin** **Date 3/20/19___**
Nurse Name **Miss Elizabeth Maris** **Number of Interactions 25th Hour**

GOALS:

1. For Patient:
   a. Continue to explore and describe manifestations of her anxiety and anger.
   b. Recognize the precipitating factors in the development of her anxiety.
   c. Identify one or more ways to cope with the expressed feelings.
2. For Nurse:
   a. Use therapeutic techniques appropriately.
   b. Allow Mrs. Franklin as much time as she needs to think and respond.
   c. Identify my own thoughts, feelings, and behavior as Mrs. Franklin talks about stressful situations with which I am familiar.

Nurse	Patient	Comments	Evaluation
"Good morning, Mrs. F."		Give recognition	
	"Good morning. I'm ready. Where do we begin today?"	Mrs. F. was eager to begin today's session. Looked bright. Greeted me with a half-smile.	I did not respond to question. Allowed Mrs. Franklin time to assume the initiative.
"You sound pleased."		Translating into feelings. First time Mrs. F. has spoken of her weight. Signs of positive feelings about self. Grimaces, shrugs shoulders, and looks disgusted.	Try at later point to validate interpretation.
	"I've actually gained 5 pounds since last week. I think I've gained this much because I'm eating better. My appetite is enormous. I even eat lunch now I am . . . but—oh well, it doesn't matter."		
"What doesn't matter?"		Exploring.	
	"If I continue to gain weight, I won't have any clothes to wear. I don't have a job. I can't afford to buy new clothes. I can't depend on my parents forever. My insurance money is almost all gone."	Expresses concern over welfare. Sounds distressed.	Confirms level of significance of distress.

"You're really worried about this?"		Verbalize the implied.	
	"Well, wouldn't you be? What do you do when you don't have any money? It's important to have money. Without it, how can I care for Debby?"	Mrs. F. avoided a direct response and focused on the nurse.	
		Gives second reason for needing money. May feel threatened by possibility of returning to work.	Allow her to pursue these factors and focus on threat later.
"What do you think you could do?"		Reflecting.	
	"Go to work, I guess. How can I go to work or even look for a job? I'm stuck in this place."	Tone of voice is harsh and angry.	
"You seem to have two areas of concern, getting a job and leaving the hospital. Let's talk about the job first."		Verbalizing the implied and asking for clarification. Focusing and setting priority. Asking her to collaborate with me to pursue one problem at a time.	
	(Mrs. F. nods head affirmatively.)	Patient quiet. I waited about 2 minutes before continuing.	
"You've worked as a secretary before."		Offering a broad opening, or general lead, from nurse's knowledge of patient's background.	
	"Yes, but not for the last year or so. I used to be a pretty good typist, and I could do shorthand, but I can't concentrate anymore."	Some elements of rationalization. Increased level of anxiety noted or evidenced by restless movements in chair, play with buttons on blouse, and looking out window.	Client displays readiness to focus on identified concerns. Some basis in fact for feelings of inadequacy; however, has helped with ward typing and does job well.

(continued)

TABLE 26–5. CONTINUED

Nurse	Patient	Comments	Evaluation
"Can't concentrate or feel uncomfortable because you're out of practice?"		Seeking clarification.	
	"It doesn't matter, does it? I'm stuck in this hospital."	Picked up nonverbal cues of discomfort. Looks angry. Sounds sarcastic..	Did not help Mrs. F. to recognize increasing anxiety. Discomfort continues to increase resulting in angry outbrust.
"You sound angry . . ."		Verbalizing implied feelings.	
	"I'm better now than I've ever been before. I know it. I feel it. . . . But I wonder if I can handle a job. I've been away so long."	Leans forward in chair. Looks directly at nurse. Reflects feeling of inadequacy.	Statement made with conviction and firmness, which is indicative of increasing self-confidence. Possible demonstration of ambivalence.
"You're afraid—"		Translating her thoughts into feelings.	
	"Yes, I'm afraid. I know that I'm strong enough physically and mentally. I worry, I'm nervous, and I used to get upset at work before. You know, working in an office with a bunch of other girls isn't conducive to good nerves. I've had people tell me—'Boy, I wouldn't have your job for anything.' But, you work with a lot of women too. Don't you run into the same kind of problems?"	Able to recognize and name the anxiety. This is the first step in the learning process. Use of rationalization. Giggled. Evidence again of increased discomfort. Tries to decrease feelings of uncomfortableness by shifting focus onto the nurse.	The next step in the learning process would be to encourage her to describe her feelings of "nervousness." Indirectly asking for agreement rather than looking at self in relation to situation.

The next step in the learning process would be to encourage her to describe her feelings of "nervousness."			
Indirectly asking for agreement rather than looking at self in relation to situation.			
"What kind of problem?"		Exploration.	I avoided being trapped into agreement.
	"Oh! You know! Someone expecting you to do more than the next guy. In my last job, I didn't mind helping out once in awhile, staying over, and doing the last-minute jobs. But a couple of the girls were young and had boyfriends. They had dates or plans, so most of the time they wouldn't stay. The other lady was married and had small children, so she had a good excuse for leaving on time. That left me to work all the extra, 'cause they figured I'm a widow. Mom is there to look after Debby, so I didn't have a good excuse."	Automatic knowing is a part of magical thinking. This account of behavior and expectations of her co-workers toward her fed into her feelings of suspiciousness and could be the basis for some of her delusions of persecution and ideas of reference.	Tried to remain objective.
"Did this happen often?"		Placing events in sequence.	This technique was used in order to begin to help her make comparisons.
	"Often enough. I kept track the last month I worked; it happened five times out of 2 weeks."		

(*continued*)

TABLE 26–5. CONTINUED

Nurse	Patient	Comments	Evaluation
"Do you recall what you were feeling when each of these situations occurred?"		Asking for description of feelings.	Asked for a description of feelings to help her complete the second step of the learning process.
	"Overworked, tired, mad! I remember one time especially. I was really feeling bad; my head hurt, I was sneezing, and my eyes burned. I thought I was catching a cold. The boss wanted three letters typed and mailed before morning. They all said, 'Sheila will do them.' I felt rotten, but I got the letters out."	Limited ability to describe. Uses broad, general terms. Mrs. F. has a pattern of handling anxiety through the development of physical symptoms. She uses illness as a rationalization to explain her behavior.	
"Then what happened?"		Offering a general lead to encourage her to continue.	
	"Then I went home and went to bed. I didn't even eat supper. I slept through 'til 10 o'clock the next morning, but I didn't care. I didn't go to work until noon that day."	Extreme fatigue and excessive sleep without feeling rested connotes high level of anxiety. Behavior demonstrates withdrawal as a coping mechanism. Manifests anxiety in retrospect.	
"You seem very uncomfortable about the situation you just described. Earlier in today's session you said, 'I'm better now than I've ever been before.' "		Making observation and encouraging comparison and evaluation.	Tried to get Mrs. F. to take a look at the way she deals with situations that produce anger. Did not have time for client to respond. Have to watch this behavior!
	"Yes, that's right! And I still think so! Before when this happened I got sick and mad. I mean really mad!"	Emphatic.	Realizes differences in degree of felt anger. Recognizes the

			influence of her feelings on her behavior. This awareness demonstrates increasing amounts of insight.
"And now?"		Encouraging evaluation.	
	"Now, I guess I'll say I get upset when I think about people using me. Before I couldn't do anything different but be mad. Now, I do get mad, but it's different."	Pauses, looking angry. Appears thoughtful. Expression changes to one of determination.	Nurse feels she could take a bow. Overjoyed with the patient's progress.
		Making comparisons and noting differences, which is the third step in the learning process.	
"Different—in what way?"		Encouraging comparison and asking for further description of perceptions.	
	"I used to feel tied up in knots when I was angry. I'd shut myself away in my room. I'd feel sick and go to bed. I still feel tight, but it's not so bad. Like the other day when Mrs. Jones came in and picked up my diary. I got mad. I felt like I wanted to push her out. Instead I said, 'That's a very personal thing, and I prefer you don't look at it.' She apologized and put it down. Then we started talking about something else."	Able to supply a specific example to illustrate comparison.	Used assertive behavior versus aggressive behavior.
			Patient's use of an alternative acceptable method of dealing with anger met with success.
		Mrs. F. sounded surprised.	
"You feel this is different?"		Encouraging evaluation.	
	"Oh yes! I told somebody what I really thought, and it worked out okay. I didn't get sick."	Stated with confidence.	Patient has recognized that she has learned a new method of coping.

(*continued*)

TABLE 26–5. CONTINUED

Nurse	Patient	Comments	Evaluation
"That really is different."		Presenting reality.	
	"It sure is—I feel that I can do something about it now."	Sounds pleased with self. Continues after slight pause. Acknowledges difference.	Recognized accomplishments and made a point of providing merited praise for use of assertive behavior outside of counseling session.
"Like what?"		Exploring. To help Mrs. F. formulate a plan of action for dealing with her discomfort and anger.	
	"Well, I don't have to let people use me."		
"Go on."		General lead.	
	"If I don't feel like doing something, I could say no or tell them I don't like what they are doing."	Hesitated briefly before responding, then let the words rush out.	
"How do you feel about saying no?"		Encouraging description of perception.	
	"I never thought about it, I guess. I've never liked to say no, but I found out it doesn't hurt."	Perplexed. Conveys a sense of insecurity but a willingness to try.	Needs continued support and reassurance. Possibly plan opportunities where she can further test out her solution. May need help with developing compromises in some situations.
"How would you apply this to the work situation you described earlier?"		Encouraging comparison and evaluation. Helping Mrs. F. to formulate a plan of action	

	"I guess now I would feel more confident. I could take a chance and say no when I don't want to work over."	Sounds more sure of self and action to be taken.	
"What would you do if your co-workers did not go along with your no?"		Presenting reality.	
	"Well, I don't know—I'll have to think about that—"	Realistic approach to unknown situation. Decision demonstrates ability to plan action rather than respond impulsively.	
"Perhaps next time we could explore this point further."		Encourage formulation of a plan of action. Setting up goal for next interaction session.	
"Mrs. Franklin, there's 5 minutes remaining in the session. As you and I talked, it became evident that you had two important areas of concern, getting a job and your continued hospitalization. In the course of our discussion you identified your feelings of nervousness and anger on the job. You explored these in detail and gave me the impression that you can better deal with these feelings now."		Summarizing. Organizing the important points of the interaction.	Demonstrates significant improvement in use of healthy behavior.
		Giving recognition, acknowledgment, and merited praise to Mrs. Franklin's accomplishment of a difficult task.	
	"I feel pretty proud of myself."		
"On Wednesday we can discuss your getting a job and feelings about leaving the hospital."			
	"See you Wednesday."		

Mrs. Franklin shows an increased ability to deal more effectively with current living situations. She displays an interest in self, concern for her appearance, and an awareness of financial responsibility, all of which indicates to me an increase in her level of independence. She is also showing signs of irritability concerning continued hospitalization, which seems to me to be a readiness to move constructively toward discharge. In the next two sessions, I will prepare for her inclusion into the family counseling sessions I am presently having with her parents and brother."

SUMMARY REPORT

After an additional 2 weeks in group therapy, Mrs. Franklin was included in the family counseling sessions with her parents and brother. She met with Miss Maris and her family a total of four times over the next 2 weeks. As a result of these meetings, Mrs. Franklin was able to scan the want ads and initiate calls to placement agencies for job interviews. The brother supported Mrs. Franklin by agreeing to provide transportation to the interviews. She joined a Parents Without Partners group that is active in her community. She attended her first meeting while still hospitalized and requested that Miss Maris accompany her. The school counselor was contacted because the grandparents expressed concern that Debby "is not doing her work, she is afraid to go to bed at night, and she cries a lot."

At the end of Mrs. Franklin's 7th week of hospitalization, the interdisciplinary team met to finalize discharge plans with her. Mrs. Franklin was discharged 1 week later. Arrangements were made through referral for her to attend weekly group therapy sessions in a nearby mental health clinic. Miss Maris was to maintain contact and to visit in the home once a month until such time as Mrs. Franklin would be able to function more independently and complete the termination phase of the nurse–patient relationship.

Approximately 9 months after hospitalization, Miss Maris discontinued the home visits and reassured Mrs. Franklin that she could keep in touch via the telephone. Mrs. Franklin is working as a secretary and is now dating a widower with two children.

SUGGESTED READINGS

American Nurses Association. *Standards: Psychiatric–Mental Health Nursing Practice*. Kansas City, Mo.: American Nurses Association, 1982.

Brink, P. J. Value Orientations as an Assessment Tool in Cultural Diversity. *Nursing Research*, Vol. 33, No. 4 (July/August, 1984), 198–203.

Carpenito, L. J. *Handbook of Nursing Diagnosis*. Philadelphia: Lippincott, 1984.

Ciminero, A. R., Calhoun, K. S., & Adams, H. E., (Eds.) *Handbook of Behavioral Assessment*. New York: Wiley, 1977.

Eggland, E. T. How To Take a Meaningful History. *Nursing '77*, Vol. 7, No. 7 (July, 1977), 22–30.

Eisenman, E., Backer, B. A., & Dubbert, P. M. The Mental Health Assessment Interview. In *Psychiatric/Mental Health Nursing: Contemporary Readings*. New York: D. Van Nostrand, 1978, 7–30.

Flaskerud, J. H. A Comparison of Perceptions of Problematic Behavior by Six Minority Groups and Mental Health Professionals. *Nursing Research*, Vol. 33, No. 4 (July/August, 1984), 190–197.

Hagey, R. S., & McDonough, P. The Problem of Professional Labeling. *Nursing Outlook*, Volume 32, Number 3 (May/June, 1984), 150–157.

King, J. M. The Initial Interview—Assessment of the Patient and His Difficulties. *Perspectives in Psychiatric Care*, Vol. 5, No. 8 (1967), 256–261.

Lamonica, E. L. *The Nursing Process: A Humanistic Approach*. Menlo Park, Calif.: Addison-Wesley, 1979.

Mahoney, E. A., Verdisco, L., & Shortridge, L. *How to Collect and Record a Health History*. New York: Lippincott, 1976.

Meissner, J. E. Uncovering Your Patient's Hidden Psychosocial Problems. *Nursing '80*, Vol. 10, No. 5 (May, 1980), 78–79.

Narrow, B. W. *Patient Teaching in Nursing Practice*. New York: Wiley, 1979.

Reimer, T. T., Brink, P. J., & Saunders, J. M. Cultural Assessment: Content and Process. *Nursing Outlook*, Vol. 32, No. 2 (March/April, 1984), 78–82.

Reynolds, J., & Logsdon, J. Assessing Your Patient's Mental Status. *Nursing '79*, Vol. 9, No. 8 (August, 1979), 26–33.

Sloboda, S. Understanding Patient Behavior. *Nursing '77*, Vol. 7, No. 9 (September, 1977), 74–77.

Snyder, C. J., & Wilson, M. F. Elements of a Psychological Assessment. *American Journal of Nursing*, Vol. 77, No. 2 (February, 1977), 235–239.

Stoll, R. S. Guidelines for Spiritual Assessment. *American Journal of Nursing*, Vol. 79, No. 9 (September, 1979), 1574–1577.

Stuart, M. The Nursing Care Plan: A Communication System That Really Works. *Nursing '78*, Vol. 8, No. 8 (August, 1978), 28–33.

Turnbull, Sister J. Shifting the Focus to Health. *American Journal of Nursing*, Vol. 76, No. 12 (December, 1976). 1985–1987.

Vasey, E. K. Writing Your Patient's Care Plan . . . Effectively. *Nursing '79*, Vol. 9, No. 4 (April, 1979), 67–71.

Watts, R. J. Dimensions of Sexual Health. *American Journal of Nursing*, Vol. 79, No. 9 (September, 1979), 1568–1572.

Wolberg, L. R. *Handbook of Short-Term Psychotherapy*. New York: Thieme-Stratton, 1980.

Yura, H., & Walsh, M. B. *The Nursing Process: Assessing, Planning, Implementing, Evaluating*. 4th ed. Norwalk, Conn.: Appleton-Century-Crofts, 1983.

GLOSSARY

Accountability. A professional quality mandating that the nurse be answerable for her practice to the patient, peers, other professionals, the public and, most importantly, to self.

Acting out. The behavioral expression of fantasies, feelings, or conflicts through unconventional actions.

Adaptation. The ability to vary responses to perceived needs and the demands exerted by the internal or external environment.

Addiction. Strong uncontrolled psychophysiological dependence on the effects of substances that when taken into the body provide temporary relief from emotional discomfort.

Advocacy. An attitude of support to protect the integrity and safeguard the rights of the patient.

Affect. A generalized, persistent, and pervasive feeling tone.

Aggression. Destructive goal-directed behavior closely associated with anger.

Agranulocytosis. A blood dyscrasia in which there is a marked reduction in the leukocyte count.

Akathisia. An extrapyramidal effect demonstrated as continuous, persistent, generalized body movement even while the client is in a position of rest.

Akinesia. Loss of movement for any reason.

Alcohol hallucinosis. A substance-induced organic mental disorder that occurs within 24 to 48 hours following the abrupt cessation of, or reduction in, alcohol ingestion. The chief characteristic is the presence of auditory hallucinations.

Alcohol withdrawal delirium. A substance-induced organic mental disorder that occurs after cessation of or reduction in alcohol ingestion. The defining characteristic is the presence of delirium as evidenced by delusions and vivid visual hallucinations. In addition there may be present bodily tremors, tachycardia, elevated blood pressure, and sweating.

Ambivalence. The simultaneous existence of contrary emotions, values, attitudes, or desires toward an object, person, or course of action.

Amnesia. An unconscious process of forgetting; may be manifested as a loss of personal identity or as a blocking out of periods or aspects of the past.

Anger. A disruptive emotion that usually evokes a negative response indicative of a state of displeasure, sense of frustration, or a position of conflict.

Anxiety. A feeling state in which the individual experiences pervasive, vague, intense sensations of apprehension or impending disaster.

Apathy. A state of indifference or absence of affective response.

Assertiveness. An expression of open, honest, direct, nondestructive, appropriate verbal and nonverbal behavior that communicates to others personal feelings, opinions, beliefs, wishes, wants, or needs.

Assessment. A process whereby the nurse gathers and examines all data pertinent to the patient and his illness.

Assurance. A sense of confidence in self. In psychiatric–mental health nursing, assurance is any nursing strategy designed to support the healthy aspects of the client's ego skills and level of confidence in self. The outcome is that the client experiences continued encouragement, trust, and hope.

Asylum. A protective, nurturing environment in which an individual has the opportunity for regrouping personal resources to better face and meet the demands of living.

Ataxia. Loss of power of muscular coordination.

Attitude. An affectively preconceived view of self, others, and the environment that gives direction to action as a person interacts and responds to life and living.

Autism. The complete exclusion of reality through preoccupation and absorption in fantasy within the self.

Autistic thought. Thought content derived from within the self, the meaning of which is known only to the self.

Behavior. A set of actions characteristic to an individual that can be observed and recorded.

Behavior modification. A treatment modality and process for changing behavior that has been identified as problematic.

Biofeedback. A strategy in which electronic monitoring equipment is used to heighten awareness so that the person learns to exercise control over automatic physiological responses to stressors.

Bipolar disorder. A major affective disorder characterized by the presence of both mania and depression.

Blocking. A sudden interruption in the stream of thought.

Blunting. A term used to describe affective behavior in which the individual displays a dulling of emotional response.

Body language. The expression of thoughts and feelings without verbalization.

Catatonic excitement. A state of hyperactivity characterized by severe agitation and explosive acting-out behavior. A clinical manifestation associated with schizophrenia, catatonic type.

Catatonic stupor. A state of psychomotor disturbance in which the individual appears to have lost control of motor and muscular functioning, resulting in marked rigidity or flexibility of the musculature.

Circumstantiality. A pattern of communication that is demonstrated by the speaker's inclusion of many irrelevant and nonessential details in his speech before he is able to come to the point.

Clang association. An associative thought disturbance observed in the speech of manic or agitated schizophrenic patients where the sound of words triggers a new train of unrelated thought, often exhibited in rhyming and punning.

Cognition. A process of logical thought leading to perceptual or intellectual knowing.

Cognitive dissonance. Incongruity of thought.

Cohesiveness. A group process term used to convey the extent or degree to which members of a group demonstrate affiliation and attachment between and among themselves.

Commitment. In nursing, a term used to describe a professional quality of the nurse. It is a pledge of self to the pursuit of ethical behavior and excellence in practice.

Communication. A social process involving an interchange of ideas between two or more people.

Compromise. A tactic in conflict resolution. It involves mutual concession that permits partial fulfillment of individual goals. Its use results in a lose-lose outcome.

Compulsion. The uncontrollable urge to perform repetitive acts despite one's better judgment.

Concreteness. A disturbance of association in which an individual focuses on the specific and is unable to engage in abstract ideation.

Confabulation. The unconscious invention and verbal recounting of plausible explanations to conceal memory gaps so as to preserve the integrity of the self-system.

Confidentiality. An ethical standard that speaks to the client's right to privacy and privileged communication.

Conflict. A feeling state, either conscious or unconscious, in which the individual experiences a clash between two or more equally strong, opposing forces. Can be experienced both intrapsychically and interpersonally.

Conflict resolution. A tension management strategy for dispelling discord and restoring harmony. It is a systematic process for promoting goal attainment.

Confrontation. A reality-based strategy for resolving an issue or problem that employs a direct, honest approach in a face-to-face encounter.

Confusion. A state of indecision relating to time, place, or person as well as an inability to distinguish clearly between thoughts.

Congruency. Consistency of expression as related to thoughts, feelings, and actions.

Conscious. That part of the mind or state of awareness that is necessary for adapting to and making use of one's environment.

Consensual validation. A communication technique that is used to arrive at mutual understanding and agreement regarding the meaning of a specific segment of communication.

Coping. The ability to adapt and adjust to changing life situations using various strategies, either consciously or unconsciously. Coping is a process by which an individual attempts to solve problems when confronted with an environmental demand.

Crisis. A situation or a problem with which the individual is not able to cope through usual or ordinary means.

Crisis intervention. Short-term treatment directed toward assisting the individual to solve his immediate problems.

Data base. A composite set of subjective and objective findings that serve as a foundation for analysis and interpretation, from which deductions can be made.

Deinstitutionalization. A trend in mental health care toward replacement of large institution and long-term institutional care with community mental health centers and community support systems.

Delirium. A condition characterized by a clouding of consciousness, confusion, and sensory impairment.

Delirium tremens. A common term used to describe alcohol withdrawal delirium.

Delusion. A fixed false belief that cannot be corrected through logical reasoning. Four common types include: (1) **delusion of grandeur**, a fixed false belief in which the patient portrays an exaggerated feeling of importance in terms of wealth, power, or influence; (2) **delusion of persecution**, a fixed false belief in which the patient claims that others are against him or are about to harm him; (3) **delusion of somatization**, a fixed false belief in which the patient maintains that his body is disturbed or disordered in one or all of its parts; and (4) **delusions of reference**, a fixed false belief in which the patient avows that the words or actions of others have special meaning and are specifically directed toward him.

Dementia. The impairment of memory or decrease in intellectual capacity due to structural brain damage or dysfunction.

Depersonalization. A denying of one's own personal identity; a feeling of being different, strange, or unreal.

Depression. An intense pervasive feeling of sadness or dejection.

Detoxification. A restoration of physiological homeostasis through removal of a toxic substance by physiological purification, substitution, or withdrawal.

Disorientation. An impaired recognition and understanding of temporal, spatial, or personal relationships.

Dissociation. Cutting off or compartmentalizing a segment of the personality from its entirety, which permits the existence of dual or multiple personalities.

Dissociative Disorders. A diagnostic category characterized by abrupt, time-limited changes in self-awareness, recollection of events, or customary behavior.

Dystonia. An extrapyramidal tract effect involving impairment in muscle tone resulting in an inability to coordinate voluntary muscle movement. Characteristically, the patient experiences rigidity and spasm of limb and neck muscles along with difficulty in speaking and swallowing.

Echograxia. Repetition of action.

Echolalia. Repetition of words or phrases.

Educational therapy. An adjunctive therapeutic modality in which the primary method of treatment is educational or vocational training. The individualized patient programs are designed to develop or increase self-esteem, strengthen group identification, or maximize school and occupational adjustments.

Ego. That part of the personality that maintains contact with and evaluates reality in order to establish or maintain a state of equilibrium with the self.

Ego boundaries. A psychoanalytic concept, used to explain the distinction betwene the self and nonself, which allows an individual to discriminate between reality and fantasy.

Ego-dystonic. Refers to any thought, feeling, or behavior that is identified as unacceptable and dissonant to the self.

Ego-syntonic. Refers to any thought, feeling, or behavior that is acceptable and compatible to and with the self.

Elation. An intense, unstable feeling of optimism, satisfaction, or joy.

Emotion. An intense, highly charged feeling.

Empathy. A sustained quality of objective feeling with and for another without loss of one's personal perspective.

Euphoria. An exaggerated sense of well-being.

Exercise therapy. An adjunctive therapeutic activity in which the primary method of treatment is that of corrective, physical activity. It is designed to promote physical fitness and alter psychopathologically induced physical appearance and body functioning. Activities include swimming in a therapeutic pool, calisthenics, exercycling, and group games.

Extrapyramidal effects. An autonomic nervous system response evidenced by skeletal muscle dysfunction.

Fear. An emotional response to an immediate, known and exaggerated, external, definite or perceived danger that produces within the individual a feeling of disequilibrium.

Feedback. A process of communication validation whereby the receiver indicates that the communicated message has been heard and understood.

Fixation. A psychoanalytic term developed by Freud to account for stagnation or arrest of the functional tasks associated with each stage of the developmental process. Fixation implies incomplete developmental progression.

Flight of ideas. A constant, rapid flow of disconnected verbalization, in which one idea is prompted by another or by environmental distractions.

Gain. Advantages derived from the presence of symptoms or illness.

Gain, primary. A reduction in the level of anxiety produced by the presence of symptoms.

Gain, secondary. The material, emotional, or social advantage acquired as a result of the presence of the symptom or illness; i.e., dependence, avoidance, comfort, or attention.

Grief. A subjective response to loss or severe deprivation.

Group. A unit of society composed of two or more people in interaction.

Group maintenance. Functions carried out as part of group process that are directed toward preservation of the group. These functions enable the group to grow, develop, and strengthen relationships among its members.

Group task. Functions carried out as a part of group process that are directed toward meeting the identified goals of the group. These functions enable the group to accomplish its designated task.

Hallucination. A false sensory perception for which there is no external stimuli. Five common types include: auditory (hearing); gustatory (tasting); olfactory (smelling); tactile (touching); and visual (seeing).

Hallucinogen. A chemical substance that produces defects in perception resulting in hallucinatory experiences.

Helplessness. A psychological feeling state of disequilibrium in which the individual experiences an overwhelming sense of powerlessness in obtaining need gratification.

Hopelessness. A feeling state based on a false cognitive process that leads one to believe that neither the self or others can aid in the resolution of disequilibrium.

Hostility. A feeling state in which the individual, consciously or unconsciously, experiences a sense of helplessness or hopelessness associated with persons or objects toward whom negative attitudes or actions are directed.

Hyperpyretic crisis. Elevation of systemic body temperature to 106°F or above; a drug reaction produced by concomitant administration of MAO inhibitors with tricyclic compounds.

Hypertensive crisis. A syndrome characterized by sudden elevation of the blood pressure associated with severe headache, nausea, vomiting, visual disturbances, transient neurological disturbances, disorientation, and drowsiness, which may progress to coma. The diastolic pressure is often as great as 150 mm Hg.

Id. The part of the mind that contains the primitive, instinctual impulses and urges and operates on the pleasure principle.

Illusion. A false perception leading to a misinterpretation of an external stimulus.

Immediacy of need. A nursing term used to indicate the manifestations and priority of need present within the client as extrapolated from the available data base through assessment and the exercise of professional judgmental conclusions.

Impulse. The translation of thoughts into actions without regard to consequences.

Industrial therapy. An adjunctive treatment program in which the primary method of treatment is the development of salable work skills. The selected activities are specifically designed to cultivate appropriate employee behavior such as attendance, promptness, consistent application of effort. An additional aspect of industrial programs includes assessment and evaluation of existing skills and readiness to learn new skills. Industrial therapy is of particular significance to those patients who are anticipating reentry into the work force.

Informed consent. The client's knowledgeable agreement based on understanding the risks and benefits of each and every alternative action available related to his care and treatment.

Insight. Self-understanding regarding motives, needs, wants, and actions.

Instinct. An innate, automatic reaction to a particular set of stimuli.

Interactive–interventive process. The nurse–patient relationship in operation.

Judgment. The ability to recognize the true, logical relationship between ideas so that a realistic, rational decision can be achieved.

Labile. Rapid, unprovoked, uncontrolled, and unexpected emotional changes. It is a symptom most often associated with organic mental disorders.

Limit setting. The establishment of boundaries.

Looseness of associations. A pattern of incongruent thought demonstrating a change of focus from one idea to another without any apparent connection between the two.

Mania. An elated or euphoric mood state characterized by instability, increased psychomotor activity, and rapidly shifting thoughts.

Manual arts therapy. An adjunctive therapeutic program in which the primary method of treatment is the development of selected manipulative skills. Particular activities such as lithography, photography, or woodworking are designed to develop hand-eye coordination as well as provide a potentially salable skill or leisure-time purposeful activity. It is often included under occupational or recreational therapy. It fosters within the patient a sense of satisfaction and accomplishment.

Memory. A complex mental function involving the ability to recall and reproduce mental images obtained or learned through sensory experiences.

Mental mechanisms. Intrapsychic coping devices of ego defense existing outside of and beyond conscious awareness.

Mind. A multisensory data bank that records, filters, processes, and integrates all input.

Mood. A perceived, sustained emotional state that influences functioning of the individual.

Need. An essential or requisite for the maintenance of life.

Negativism. A generalized opposition to requests, demands, or norms of others.

Neologism. New words coined by the psychotic individual that are meaningful to the patient but meaningless to the listener.

Noncompliance. A judgmental term used to describe a client's resistance to prescribed treatment.

Nonverbal communication. A form of communication without speech that includes gestures, facial expression, body posture, and nonsymbolic sounds.

Norm. A standard accepted for functioning.

Nursing care plan. A written outline containing a systematized assessment and identification of the patient's problems, objectives for care, and the methods or strategies for achieving the objectives.

Nursing diagnosis. A summary statement(s) or judgment(s) made by the nurse about the data gathered and prioritized during the assessment process. Each statement identifies an actual, potential, or possible patient problem that requires nursing intervention in order to be solved.

Nursing process. A system of planning the delivery of nursing care. It involves four major steps: assessment, planning, implementation, evaluation.

Observation. A deliberate, planned, and systematized process of obtaining objective and subjective data.

Obsession. Preoccupation with a persistent, repetitive thought.

Occupational therapy. An adjunctive therapeutic activity in which the primary method of treatment is that of purposeful occupation. The selected activities are specifically directed toward meeting the individual patient's need. It provides an opportunity for patients to work through unconscious conflicts through the mechanism of sublimation or by acting out. The product made or skill learned enhances self-concept and stimulates socialization.

Orthostatic hypotension. A sudden drop in blood pressure produced by abrupt changes in position, such as moving from a supine to erect position.

Panic. An acute, intense, and overwhelming feeling of anxiety which results in disorganization of various aspects of the personality.

Perception. The recognition and interpretation of sensations.

Phobia. An intense fear of some object or situation not ordinarily associated with danger.

Photosensitivity. Skin reactions that occur during therapy with antipsychotic drugs. Characterized by the development of a rash or exaggerated sunburn on exposure to ultraviolet rays (sunlight, fluorescent lighting). Reaction confined to uncovered areas of skin.

Prevention, primary. Actions taken to intervene with those populations identified as being at risk for breakdown, thereby reducing the potential for incidence of disease.

Prevention, secondary. The use of intervention strategies that facilitate the early detection and treatment of disease.

Prevention, tertiary. Interventions or actions designed to maintain optimal functioning and diminish the residual effects through rehabilitation.

Problem. An actual, potential, or possible difficulty or concern with which a patient is not coping satisfactorily. Identified problems are based on unmet needs.

Pseudoparkinsonism. An extrapyramidal tract effect with characteristic symptoms of muscular rigidity, tremor, and complete or partial loss of movement. Symptoms indicative of these characteristics are observed as drooling, swelling of the tongue, slurred speech, a masklike facial expression, pill-rolling movements of the fingers, or a shuffling gait.

Psychic energizer. A common term for chemotherapeutic agents that are used to stimulate or elevate mood; antidepressant agents.

Psychogenic. A term used to indicate that the pathological condition originates within the mind.

Psychomotor activity. Physical response to internal emotional stimuli.

Psychomotor retardation. A demonstrable lag between the perception of a stimulus and the corresponding behavioral or emotional response.

Rapport. A feeling state of mutual sharing, openness, and receptivity between individuals.

Reality. A culturally, perceptually, and environmentally defined term that identifies a person's objective world and his relationship within it.

Reality testing. The ability to evaluate and differentiate between one's internal and external environment.

Recreational therapy. An adjunctive therapeutic modality in which the primary method of treatment is that of free, voluntary and expressive motor, sensory, or mental activity. The selected activities are specifically directed toward encouraging the patient to develop pleasurable attitudes and engage in wholesome emotional release. It stimulates interest and broadens the scope of leisure-time activities.

Relationship. The existence of a connection or association between people.

Relaxation therapy. A cognitively and behaviorally based therapy designed to manage tension and reduce stress through the deliberate use of concentration, imagery, muscular relaxation, and deep breathing exercises.

Resistance. Instinctive or intentional opposition or withholding of information or involvement in the pursuit of problem resolution.

Resistance resource. A readily available means that a person possesses which can be used to facilitate that person's dealing with and overcoming a stressor. Resources can be material, artifactual, cognitive, emotional, physical, biochemical, valuative–attitudinal, interpersonal–relational, or macrosociocultural.

Respect. To hold in high regard.

Role playing. A simulation technique used to increase awareness and resolve human conflict.

Self-actualization. The epitome of maturation within each developmental phase.

Self-concept. The image that one holds about self.

Self-disclosure. The sharing of personal and private information about self that has the potential for increasing vulnerability.

Self-esteem. The degree to which one values self.

Separation anxiety. Anxiety that results from either anticipatory or real loss of a significant other or object.

Stress. A real or perceived pressure that produces physiological and psychological change within the organism.

Stressor. Any agent, condition, situation, goal, feeling, thought, or behavior that demands an increase in any vital activity within the autonomic or central nervous system of the individual.

Superego. That part of the personality that defines the value system under which the individual operates and acts as a censoring agent for all behavioral operations.

Sympathy. A momentary feeling engendered within the nurse that evokes an immediate interventive response to alleviate the distress.

Tardive dyskinesia. An irreversible extrapyramidal side effect of antipsychotic agents characterized by grimacing, choreiform or athetoid movements of fingers, arms, toes, and ankles along with tonic contractions of neck and back muscles.

Therapeutic use of self. The constructive use of the total personality of the nurse in a way that brings about a positive change for the patient.

Thought disorders. A disturbance of memory, judgment, and current perceptions resulting in interference with the individual's reasoning and problem-solving and decision-making ability.

Transactions. A term used in transactional analysis to connote communication patterns used by individuals when interacting with others. Observation and analysis of both verbal and nonverbal communication gives an indication regarding the particular ego state from which the individual is functioning at any given point in time.

Unconscious. That part of the mind that records and stores all knowledge, feelings, and experiences. Under ordinary circumstances this material is not readily accessible for recall to the conscious mind.

Value. The importance one places on a person, idea, or object.

Value clarification. A process used to identify what is meaningful or prized by an individual or society.

Withdrawal. A movement away from reality in which the individual attempts to avoid contact, involvement, and relatedness with others.

Word salad. A coded form of language whose mixture of words and phrases has no meaning.

APPENDIX I

DSM-III Classification: Axes I and II Categories and Codes

All official DSM-III codes and terms are included in ICD-9-CM. However, in order to differentiate those DSM-III categories that use the same ICD-9-CM codes, unofficial non-ICD-9-CM codes are provided in parentheses for use when greater specificity is necessary.

The long dashes indicate the need for a fifth-digit subtype or other qualifying term.

DISORDERS USUALLY FIRST EVIDENT IN INFANCY, CHILDHOOD OR ADOLESCENCE

Mental retardation

(Code in fifth digit: 1 = with other behavioral symptoms [requiring attention or treatment and that are not part of another disorder], 0 = without other behavioral symptoms.)

317.0(x) Mild mental retardation, ______

318.0(x) Moderate mental retardation, ______

318.1(x) Severe mental retardation, ______

318.2(x) Profound mental retardation, ______

319.0(x) Unspecified mental retardation, ______

Attention deficit disorder

314.01 with hyperactivity

314.00 without hyperactivity

314.80 residual type

Conduct disorder

312.00 undersocialized, aggressive

312.10 undersocialized, nonaggressive

312.23 socialized, aggressive

312.21 socialized, nonaggressive

312.90 atypical

Anxiety disorders of childhood or adolescence

309.21 Separation anxiety disorder

313.21 Avoidant disorder of childhood or adolescence

313.00 Overanxious disorder

Other disorders of infancy, childhood or adolescence

313.89 Reactive attachment disorder of infancy

313.22 Schizoid disorder of childhood or adolescence

Other disorders of infancy, childhood or adolescence (*cont.*)

313.23 Elective mutism
313.81 Oppositional disorder
313.82 Identity disorder

Eating disorders

307.10 Anorexia nervosa
307.51 Bulimia
307.52 Pica
307.53 Rumination disorder of infancy
307.50 Atypical eating disorder

Stereotyped movement disorders

307.21 Transient tic disorder
307.22 Chronic motor tic disorder
307.23 Tourette's disorder
307.20 Atypical tic disorder
307.30 Atypical stereotyped movement disorder

Other disorders with physical manifestations

307.00 Stuttering
307.60 Functional enuresis
307.70 Functional encopresis
307.46 Sleepwalking disorder
307.46 Sleep terror disorder (307.49)

Pervasive developmental disorders

Code in fifth digit: 0 = full syndrome present, 1 = residual state.

299.0x Infantile autism, ______
299.9x Childhood onset pervasive developmental disorder, ______
299.8x Atypical, ______

Specific developmental disorders
Note: These are coded on Axis II.

315.00 Developmental reading disorder
315.10 Developmental arithmetic disorder
315.31 Developmental language disorder
315.39 Developmental articulation disorder
315.50 Mixed specific developmental disorder
315.90 Atypical specific developmental disorder

ORGANIC MENTAL DISORDERS

Section 1. Organic mental disorders whose etiology or pathophysiological process is listed below (taken from the mental disorders section of ICD-9-CM).

Dementias arising in the senium and presenium

PRIMARY DEGENERATIVE DEMENTIA, SENILE ONSET,

290.30 with delirium
290.20 with delusions
290.21 with depression
290.00 uncomplicated

Code in fifth digit:
1 = with delirium, 2 = with delusions, 3 = with depression, 0 = uncomplicated.

290.1x Primary degenerative dementia, presenile onset, ______
290.4x Multi-infarct dementia, ______

Substance-induced

ALCOHOL

303.00 intoxication
291.40 idiosyncratic intoxication
291.80 withdrawal
291.00 withdrawal delirium
291.30 hallucinosis
291.10 amnestic disorder

Code severity of dementia in fifth digit:

1 = mild, 2 = moderate, 3 = severe, 0 = unspecified.

291.2x Dementia associated with alcoholism, ______

BARBITURATE OR SIMILARLY ACTING SEDATIVE OR HYPNOTIC

305.40 intoxication (327.00)
292.00 withdrawal (327.01)
292.00 withdrawal delirium (327.02)
292.83 amnestic disorder (327.04)

OPIOID

305.50 intoxication (327.10)
292.00 withdrawal (327.11)

COCAINE

305.60 intoxication (327.20)

AMPHETAMINE OR SIMILARLY ACTING SYMPATHOMIMETIC

305.70 intoxication (327.30)
292.81 delirium (327.32)
292.11 delusional disorder (327.35)
292.00 withdrawal (327.31)

PHENCYCLIDINE (PCP) OR SIMILARLY ACTING ARYLCYCLOHEXYLAMINE

305.90 intoxication (327.40)
292.81 delirium (327.42)
292.90 mixed organic mental disorder (327.49)

HALLUCINOGEN

305.30 hallucinosis (327.56)
292.11 delusional disorder (327.55)
292.84 affective disorder (327.57)

CANNABIS

305.20 intoxication (327.60)
292.11 delusional disorder (327.65)

TOBACCO

292.00 withdrawal (327.71)

CAFFEINE

305.90 intoxication (327.80)

OTHER OR UNSPECIFIED SUBSTANCE

305.90 intoxication (327.90)
292.00 withdrawal (327.91)
292.81 delirium (327.92)
292.82 dementia (327.93)
292.83 amnestic disorder (327.94)
292.11 delusional disorder (327.95)
292.12 hallucinosis (327.96)
292.84 affective disorder (327.97)
292.89 pesonality disorder (327.98)
292.90 atypical or mixed organic mental disorder (327.99)

Section 2. Organic syndromes whose etiology or pathophysiological process is either noted as an additional diagnosis from outside the mental disorders section of ICD-9-CM or is unknown.

293.00 Delirium
294.10 Dementia
294.00 Amnestic syndrome
293.81 Organic delusional syndrome
293.82 Organic hallucinosis
293.83 Organic affective syndrome
310.10 Organic personality syndrome
294.80 Atypical or mixed organic brain syndrome

SUBSTANCE USE DISORDERS

Code in fifth digit: 1 = continuous, 2 = episodic, 3 = in remission, 0 = unspecified.

305.0x Alcohol abuse, ______
303.9x Alcohol dependence (Alcoholism), ______
305.4x Barbiturate or similarly acting sedative or hypnotic abuse,
304.1x Barbiturate or similarly acting sedative or hypnotic dependence, ______
305.5x Opioid abuse, ______
304.0x Opioid dependence, ______

SUBSTANCE USE DISORDERS (*CONT.*)

305.6x Cocaine abuse, ______
305.7x Amphetamine or similarly acting sympathomimetic abuse, ______
304.4x Amphetamine or similarly acting sympathomimetic dependence, ______
305.9x Phencyclidine (PCP) or similarly acting arylcyclohexylamine abuse, ______ (328.4x)
305.3x Hallucinogen abuse, ______
305.2x Cannabis abuse, ______
304.3x Cannabis dependence, ______
305.1x Tobacco dependence, ______
305.9x Other, mixed or unspecified substance abuse, ______
304.6x Other specified substance dependence, ______
304.9x Unspecified substance dependence, ______
304.7x Dependence on combination of opioid and other non-alcoholic substance, ______
304.8x Dependence on combination of substances, excluding opioids and alcohol, ______

SCHIZOPHRENIC DISORDERS

Code in fifth digit: 1 = subchronic, 2 = chronic, 3 = subchronic with acute exacerbation, 4 = chronic with acute exacerbation, 5 = in remission, 0 = unspecified.

SCHIZOPHRENIA,
295.1x disorganized, ______
295.2x catatonic, ______
295.3x paranoid, ______
295.9x undifferentiated, ______
295.6x residual, ______

PARANOID DISORDERS

297.10 Paranoia
297.30 Shared paranoid disorder
298.30 Acute paranoid disorder
297.90 Atypical paranoid disorder

PSYCHOTIC DISORDERS NOT ELSEWHERE CLASSIFIED

295.40 Schizophreniform disorder
298.80 Brief reactive psychosis
295.70 Schizoaffective disorder
298.90 Atypical psychosis

NEUROTIC DISORDERS

These are included in Affective, Anxiety, Somatoform, Dissociative, and Psychosexual Disorders. In order to facilitate the identification of the categories that in DSM-II were grouped together in the class of Neuroses, the DSM-II terms are included separately in parentheses after the corresponding categories. These DSM-II terms are included in ICD-9-CM and therefore are acceptable as alternatives to the recommended DSM-III terms that precede them.

AFFECTIVE DISORDERS

Major affective disorders

Code major depressive episode in fifth digit: 6 = in remission, 4 = with psychotic features (the unofficial non-ICD-9-CM fifth digit 7 may be used instead to indicate that the psychotic features are mood-incongruent), 3 = with melancholia, 2 = without melancholia, 0 = unspecified.

Code manic episode in fifth digit: 6 = in remission, 4 = with psychotic features (the unofficial non-ICD-9-CM fifth digit 7 may be used instead to indicate that the psychotic features are mood-incongruent), 2 = without psychotic features, 0 = unspecified.

BIPOLAR DISORDER, (225)
296.6x mixed, ______
296.4x manic, ______
296.5x depressed, ______

MAJOR DEPRESSION, (228)
296.2x single episode, ______
296.3x recurrent, ______

Other specific affective disorders
301.13 Cyclothymic disorder
300.40 Dysthymic disorder (or Depressive neurosis)

Atypical affective disorders
296.70 Atypical bipolar disorder
296.82 Atypical depression

ANXIETY DISORDERS

PHOBIC DISORDERS (OR PHOBIC NEUROSES)
300.21 Agoraphobia with panic attacks
300.22 Agoraphobia without panic attacks
300.23 Social phobia
300.29 Simple phobia

ANXIETY STATES (OR ANXIETY NEUROSES)
300.01 Panic disorder
300.02 Generalized anxiety disorder
300.30 Obsessive compulsive disorder (or Obsessive compulsive neurosis)

POST-TRAUMATIC STRESS DISORDER
308.30 acute
309.81 chronic or delayed
300.00 Atypical anxiety disorder

SOMATOFORM DISORDERS

300.81 Somatization disorder
300.11 Conversion disorder (or Hysterical neurosis, conversion type)
307.80 Psychogenic pain disorder
300.70 Hypochondriasis (or Hypochondriacal neurosis)
300.70 Atypical somatoform disorder (300.71)

DISSOCIATIVE DISORDERS (OR HYSTERICAL NEUROSES, DISSOCIATIVE TYPE)

300.12 Psychogenic amnesia
300.13 Psychogenic fugue
300.14 Multiple personality
300.60 Depersonalization disorder (or Depersonalization neurosis)
300.15 Atypical dissociative disorder

PSYCHOSEXUAL DISORDERS GENDER IDENTITY DISORDERS

Indicate sexual history in the fifth digit of Transsexualism code: 1 = asexual, 2 = homosexual, 3 = heterosexual, 0 = unspecified.

302.5x Transsexualism, ______
302.60 Gender identity disorder of childhood
302.85 Atypical gender identity disorder

Paraphilias
302.81 Fetishism
302.30 Transvestism
302.10 Zoophilia
302.20 Pedophilia
302.40 Exhibitionism
302.82 Voyeurism
302.83 Sexual masochism
302.84 Sexual sadism
302.90 Atypical paraphilia

Psychosexual dysfunctions
302.71 Inhibited sexual desire
302.72 Inhibited sexual excitement
302.73 Inhibited female orgasm
302.74 Inhibited male orgasm
302.75 Premature ejaculation
302.76 Functional dyspareunia
306.51 Functional vaginismus

Psychosexual dysfunctions (*cont.*)

302.70 Atypical psychosexual dysfunction

Other psychosexual disorders

302.00 Ego-dystonic homosexuality
302.89 Psychosexual disorder not elsewhere classified

FACTITIOUS DISORDERS

300.16 Factitious disorder with psychological symptoms
301.51 Chronic factitious disorder with physical symptoms
300.19 Atypical factitious disorder with physical symptoms

DISORDERS OF IMPULSE CONTROL NOT ELSEWHERE CLASSIFIED

312.31 Pathological gambling
312.32 Kleptomania
312.33 Pyromania
312.34 Intermittent explosive disorder
312.35 Isolated explosive disorder
312.39 Atypical impulse control disorder

ADJUSTMENT DISORDER

309.00 with depressed mood
309.24 with anxious mood
309.28 with mixed emotional features
309.30 with disturbance of conduct
309.40 with mixed disturbance of emotions and conduct
309.23 with work (or academic) inhibition
309.83 with withdrawal
309.90 with atypical features

PSYCHOLOGICAL FACTORS AFFECTING PHYSICAL CONDITION

Specify physical condition on Axis III.

316.00 Psychological factors affecting physical condition

PERSONALITY DISORDERS

Note: These are coded on Axis II.

301.00 Paranoid
301.20 Schizoid
301.22 Schizotypal
301.50 Histrionic
301.81 Narcissistic
301.70 Antisocial
301.83 Borderline
301.82 Avoidant
301.60 Dependent
301.40 Compulsive
301.84 Passive-Aggressive
301.89 Atypical, mixed or other personality disorder

V CODES FOR CONDITIONS NOT ATTRIBUTABLE TO A MENTAL DISORDER THAT ARE A FOCUS OF ATTENTION OR TREATMENT

V65.20 Malingering
V62.89 Borderline intellectual functioning (V62.88)
V71.01 Adult antisocial behavior
V71.02 Childhood or adolescent antisocial behavior
V62.30 Academic problem
V62.20 Occupational problem
V62.82 Uncomplicated bereavement
V15.81 Noncompliance with medical treatment

V62.89 Phase of life problem or other life circumstance problem
V61.10 Marital problem
V61.20 Parent-child problem
V61.80 Other specified family circumstances
V62.81 Other interpersonal problem

ADDITIONAL CODES

300.90 Unspecified mental disorder (nonpsychotic)

V71.09 No diagnosis or condition on Axis I
799.90 Diagnosis or condition deferred on Axis I

V71.09	No diagnosis on Axis II
799.90	Diagnosis deferred on Axis II

(From American Psychiatric Association; Diagnostic and Statistical Manual of Mental Disorders. *3rd ed. Washington, D.C.: American Psychiatric Association, 1980. Reprinted with permission.)*

APPENDIX II

DSM-III-R Classification: Axes I and II Categories and Codes

*All official DSM-III-R codes and are included in ICD-9-CM. Codes followed by a * are used for more than one DSM-III-R diagnosis or subtype in order to maintain compatibility with ICD-9-CM.*

Numbers in parentheses are page numbers.

A long dash following a diagnostic term indicates the need for a fifth digit subtype or other qualifying term.

The term specify *following the name of some diagnostic categories indicates qualifying terms that clinicians may wish to add in parentheses after the name of the disorder.*

NOS = Not Otherwise Specified

The current severity of a disorder may be specified after the diagnosis as:

mild
moderate
severe — currently meets diagnostic criteria

in partial remission
(or residual state)
in complete remission

DISORDERS USUALLY FIRST EVIDENT IN INFANCY, CHILDHOOD, OR ADOLESCENCE

DEVELOPMENTAL DISORDERS

Note: These are coded on Axis II.

Mental Retardation (28)

317.00 Mild mental retardation
318.00 Moderate mental retardation
318.10 Severe mental retardation
319.00 Unspecified mental retardation

Pervasive Developmental Disorders (33)

299.00 Autistic disorder (38)
Specify if childhood onset

Pervasive Developmental Disorders (33) (*cont.*)

299.80 Pervasive developmental disorder NOS

Specific Developmental Disorders (39)

ACADEMIC SKILLS DISORDERS

315.10 Developmental arithmetic disorder (41)
315.80 Developmental expressive writing disorder (42)
315.00 Developmental reading disorder (43)

LANGUAGE AND SPEECH DISORDERS

315.39 Developmental articulation disorder (44)
315.31* Developmental expressive language disorder (45)
315.31* Developmental receptive language disorder (47)

MOTOR SKILLS DISORDER

315.40 Developmental coordiantion disorder (48)
315.90* Specific developmental disorder NOS

Other Developmental Disorders (49)

315.90* Developmental disorder NOS

Disruptive Behavior Disorders (49)

314.01 Attention-deficit hyperactivity disorder (50)

CONDUCT DISORDER, (53)

312.20 group type
312.00 solitary aggressive type
312.90 undifferentiated type
313.81 Oppositional defiant disorder (56)

Anxiety Disorders of Childhood or Adolescence (58)

309.21 Separation anxiety disorder (58)
313.21 Avoidant disorder of childhood or adolescence (61)
313.00 Overanxious disorder (63)

Eating Disorders (65)

307.10 Anorexia nervosa (65)
307.51 Bulimia nervosa (67)
307.52 Pica (69)
307.53 Rumination disorder of infancy (70)
307.50 Eating disorder NOS

Gender Identity Disorders (71)

302.60 Gender identity disorder of childhood (71)
302.50 Transsexualism (74)
Specify sexual history: asexual, homosexual, heterosexual, unspecified
302.85* Gender identity disorder of adolescence or adulthood, nontranssexual type (76)
Specify sexual history: asexual, homosexual, heterosexual, unspecified
302.85* Gender identity disorder NOS

Tic Disorders (78)

307.23 Tourette's disorder (79)
307.22 Chronic motor or vocal tic disorder (81)
307.21 Transient tic disorder (81)

Specify: single episode or recurrent
307.20 Tic disorder NOS

Elimination Disorders (82)
307.70 Functional encopresis (82)
Specify: primary or secondary type
307.60 functional enuresis (84)
Specify: primary or secondary type
Specify: nocturnal only, diurnal only, nocturnal and diurnal

Speech Disorders Not Elsewhere Classified (85)
307.00* Cluttering (85)
307.00* Stuttering (86)

Other Disorders of Infancy, Childhood, or Adolescence (88)
313.23 Elective mutism (88)
313.82 Identity disorder (89)
313.89 Reactive attachment disorder of infancy or early childhood (91)
307.30 Stereotypy/habit disorder (93)
314.00 Undifferentiated attention-deficit disorder (95)

ORGANIC MENTAL DISORDERS (97)

Dementias Arising in the Senium and Presenium (119)

PRIMARY DEGENERATIVE DEMENTIA OF THE ALZHEIMER TYPE, SENILE ONSET, (119)
290.30 with delirium
290.20 with delusions
290.21 with depression
290.00* uncomplicated
(Note: code 331.00 Alzheimer's disease on Axis III)

Code in fifth digit:
1 = with delirium, 2 = with delusions, 3 = with depression, 0* = uncomplicated

290.1x Primary degenerative dementia of the Alzheimer type, presenile onset, ______ (119)
(Note: code 331.00 Alzheimer's disease on Axis III)
290.4x Multi-infarctdementia, ______ (121)
290.00* Senile dementia NOS
Specify etiology on Axis III if known
290.10* Presenile dementia NOS
Specify etiology on Axis III if known (e.g., Pick's disease, Jakob-Creutzfeldt disease)

Psychoactive Substance-Induced Organic Mental Disorders (123)

ALCOHOL
303.00 intoxication (127)
291.40 idiosyncratic intoxication (128)
291.80 Uncomplicated alcohol withdrawal (129)
291.00 withdrawal delirium (131)
291.30 hallucinosis (131)
291.10 amnestic disorder (133)
291.20 Dementia associated with alcoholism (133)

AMPHETAMINE OF SIMILARLY ACTING SYMPATHOMIMETIC
305.70* intoxication (134)
292.00* withdrawal (136)
292.81* delirum (136)
292.11* delusional disorder (137)

CAFFEINE
305.90* intoxication (138)

CANNABIS
305.20* intoxication (139)
292.11* delusional disorder (140)

Psychoactive Substance-Induced Organic Mental Disorders (123) (*cont.*)

COCAINE
305.60* intoxication (141)
292.00* withdrawal (142)
292.81* delirium (143)
292.11* delusional disorder (143)

HALLUCINOGEN
305.30* hallucinosis (144)
292.11* delusional disorder (146)
292.84* mood disorder (146)
292.89* Posthallucinogen perception disorder (147)

INHALANT
305.90* intoxication (148)

NICOTINE
292.00* withdrawal (150)

OPIOID
305.50* intoxication (151)
292.00* withdrawal (152)

PHENCYCLIDINE (PCP) OR SIMILARLY ACTING ARYLCYCLOHEXYLAMINE
305.90* intoxication (154)
292.81* delirium (155)
292.11* delusional disorder (156)
292.84* mood disorder (156)
292.90* organic mental disorder NOS

SEDATIVE, HYPNOTIC, OR ANXIOLYTIC
305.40* intoxication (158)
292.00* Uncomplicated sedative, hypnotic, or anxiolytic withdrawal (159)
292.00* withdrawal delirium (160)
292.83* amnestic disorder (161)

OTHER OR UNSPECIFIED PSYCHOACTIVE SUBSTANCE (162)
305.90* intoxication
292.00* withdrawal
292.81* delirium
292.82* dementia
292.83* amnestic disorder
292.11* delusional disorder
292.12 hallucinosis
292.84* mood disorder
292.89* anxiety disorder
292.89* personality disorder
292.90* organic mental disorder NOS

Organic Mental Disorders associated with Axis III physical disorders or conditions, or whose etiology is unknown. (162)

293.00 Delirium (100)
294.10 Dementia (103)
294.00 Amnestic disorder (108)
293.81 Organic delusional disorder (109)
293.82 Organic hallucinosis (110)
293.83 Organic mood disorder (111)
Specify: manic, depressed, mixed
294.80* Organic anxiety disorder (113)
310.10 Organic personality disorder (114)
Specify if explosive type
294.80* Organic mental disorder NOS

PSYCHOACTIVE SUBSTANCE USE DISORDERS (165)

ALCOHOL (173)
303.90 dependence
305.00 abuse

AMPHETAMINE OR SIMILARLY ACTING SYMPATHOMIMETIC (175)
304.40 dependence
305.70* abuse

CANNABIS (176)
304.30 dependence
305.20* abuse

COCAINE (177)
304.20 dependence
305.60* abuse

HALLUCINOGEN (179)
304.50* dependence
305.30* abuse

INHALANT (180)
304.60 dependence
305.90* abuse

NICOTINE (181)
305.10 dependence

OPIOID (182)
304.00 dependence
305.50* abuse

PHENCYCLIDINE (PCP) OR SIMILARLY ACTING ARYLCYCLOHEXYLAMINE (183)
304.50* dependence
305.90* abuse

SEDATIVE, HYPNOTIC, OR ANXIOLYTIC (184)
304.10 dependence
305.40* abuse
304.90* Polysubstance dependence (185)
304.90* Psychoactive substance dependence NOS
305.90* Psychoactive substance abuse NOS

SCHIZOPHRENIA (187)

Code in fifth digit: 1 = subchronic, 2 = chronic, 3 = subchronic with acute exacerbation, 4 = chronic with acute exacerbation, 5 = in remission, 0 = unspecified.

SCHIZOPHRENIA,
295.2x catatonic, ______
295.1x disorganized, ______
295.3x paranoid, ______
Specify if stable type
295.9x undifferentiated, ______
295.6x residual, ______
Specify if late onset

DELUSIONAL (PARANOID) DISORDER (199)

297.10 Delusional (Paranoid) disorder
Specify type: erotomanic
grandiose
jealous
persecutory
somatic
unspecified

PSYCHOTIC DISORDERS NOT ELSEWHERE CLASSIFIED (205)

298.80 Brief rective psychosis (205)
295.40 Schizophreniform disorder (207)
Specify: without good prognostic features or with good prognostic features
295.70 Schizoaffective disorder (208)
Specify: bipolar type or depressive type
297.30 Induced psychotic disorder (210)
298.90 Psychotic disorder NOS (Atypical psychosis) (211)

MOOD DISORDERS (213)

Code current state of Major Depression and Bipolar Disorder with fifth digit:
1 = mild
2 = moderate
3 = severe, without psychotic features
4 = with psychotic features (*specify* mood-congruent or mood-incongruent)
5 = in partial remission
6 = in full remission
0 = unspecified

For major depressive episodes, *specify* if chronic and *specify* if melancholic type.

For Bipolar Disorder, Bipolar Disorder NOS, Recurrent Major Depression, and Depressive Disorder NOS, *specify* if seasonal pattern.

Bipolar Disorders

BIPOLAR DISORDER, (225)

Bipolar Disorders (*cont.*)

296.6x mixed, ______
296.4x manic, ______
296.5x depressed, ______
301.13 Cyclothymia (226)
296.70 Bipolar disorder NOS

Depressive Disorders

MAJOR DEPRESSION, (228)
296.2x single episode, ______
296.3x recurrent, ______
300.40 Dysthymia (or Depressive neurosis) (230)
Specify: primary or secondary type
Specify: early or late onset
311.00 Depressive disorder NOS

ANXIETY DISORDERS OR ANXIETY AND PHOBIC NEUROSES (235)

PANIC DISORDER (235)
300.21 with agoraphobia
Specify current severity of agoraphobic avoidance
Specify current severity of panic attacks
300.01 without agoraphobia
Specify current severity of panic attacks
300.22 Agoraphobia without history of panic disorder (240)
Specify with or without limited symptom attacks
300.23 Social phobia (241)
Specify if generalized type
300.29 Simple phobia (243)
300.30 Obsessive compulsive disorder (or Obsessive compulsive neurosis) (245)
309.89 Post-traumatic stress disorder (247)
Specify if delayed onset
300.02 Generalized anxiety disorder (251)
300.00 Anxiety disorder NOS

SOMATOFORM DISORDERS (255)

300.70* Body dysmorphic disorder (255)
300.11 Conversion disorder (or Hysterical neurosis, conversion type) (257)
Specify: single episode or recurrent
300.70* Hypochondriasis (or Hypochondriacal neurosis) (259)
300.81 Somatization disorder (261)
307.80 Somatoform pain disorder (264)
300.70* Undifferentiated somatoform disorder (266)
300.70* Somatoform disorder NOS (267)

DISSOCIATIVE DISORDERS OR HYSTERICAL NEUROSES, DISSOCIATIVE TYPE (269)

300.14 Multiple personality disorder (269)
300.13 Psychogenic fugue (272)
300.12 Psychogenic amnesia (273)
300.60 Depersonalization disorder (or Depersonalization neurosis) (275)
300.15 Dissociative disorder NOS

SEXUAL DISORDERS (279)

Paraphilias (279)
302.40 Exhibitionism (282)
302.81 Fetishism (282)
302.89 Frotteurism (283)
302.20 Pedophilia (284)
Specify: same sex, opposite sex, same and opposite sex
Specify if limited to incest
Specify: exclusive type or nonexclusive type
302.83 Sexual masochism (286)

302.84 Sexual sadism (287)
302.30 Transvestic fetishism (288)
302.82 Voyerusim (289)
302.90* Paraphilia NOS (290)

Sexual Dysfunctions (290)

Specify: psychogenic only, or psychogenic and biogenic (Note: if biogenic only, code on Axis III)
Specify: lifelong or acquired
Specify: generalized or situational

SEXUAL DESIRE DISORDERS (293)
302.71 Hypoactive sexual desire disorder
302.79 Sexual aversion disorder
Sexual arousal disorders (294)
302.72* Female sexual arousal disorder
302.72* Male erectile disorder
Orgasm disorders (294)
302.73 Inhibited female orgasm
302.74 Inhibited male orgasm
302.75 Premature ejaculation
Sexual pain disorders (295)
302.75 Dyspareunia
306.51 Vaginismus
302.70 Sexual dysfunction NOS

Other Sexual Disorders

302.90* Sexual disorder NOS

SLEEP DISORDERS (297)

Dyssomnias (298)

INSOMNIA DISORDER
307.42* related to another mental disorder (nonorganic) (330)
780.50* related to known organic factor (300)
307.42* Primary insomnia (301)
Hypersomnia disorder
307.44 related to another mental disorder (nonorganic) (303)
780.50* related to a known organic factor (303)
780.54 Primary hypersomnia (305)
307.45 Sleep-wake schedule disorder (305)
Specify: advanced or delayed phase type, disorganized type, frequently changing type

OTHER DYSSOMNIAS
307.40* Dyssomnia NOS

Parasomnias (308)

307.47 Dream anxiety disorder (Nightmare disorder) (308)
307.46* Sleep terror disorder (310)
307.46* Sleepwalking disorder (311)
307.40* Parasomnia NOS (313)

FACTITIOUS DISORDERS (315)

FACTITIOUS DISORDER
301.51 with physical symptoms (316)
300.16 with psychological symptoms (318)
300.19 Factitious disorder NOS (320)

IMPULSE CONTROL DISORDERS NOT ELSEWHERE CLASSIFIED (321)

312.34 Intermittent explosive disorder (321)
312.32 Kleptomania (322)
312.31 Pathological gambling (324)
312.33 Pyromania (325)
312.39* Trichotillomania (326)
312.39* Impulse control disorder NOS (328)

ADJUSTMENT DISORDER (329)

ADJUSTMENT DISORDER

ADJUSTMENT DISORDERS (329) (*cont.*)

309.24 with anxious mood
309.00 with depressed mood
309.30 with disturbance of conduct
309.40 with mixed disturbance of emotions and conduct
309.28 with mixed emotional features
309.82 with physical complaints
309.83 with withdrawal
309.23 with work (or academic) inhibition
309.90 Adjustment disorder NOS

PSYCHOLOGICAL FACTORS AFFECTING PHYSICAL CONDITION (333)

316.00 Psychological factors affecting physical condition
Specify physical condition on Axis III

PERSONALITY DISORDERS (335)

Note: These are coded on Axis II.

Cluster A
301.00 Paranoid (337)
301.20 Schizoid (339)
301.22 Schizotypal (340)

Cluster B
301.70 Antisocial (342)
301.83 Borderline (346)
301.50 Histrionic (348)
301.81 Narcissistic (349)

Cluster C
301.82 Avoidant (351)
301.60 Dependent (353)
301.40 Obsessive compulsive (354)
301.84 Passive aggressive (356)
301.90 Personality disorder NOS

V CODES FOR CONDITIONS NOT ATTRIBUTABLE TO A MENTAL DISORDER THAT ARE A FOCUS OF ATTENTION OR TREATMENT (359)

V62.30 Academic problem
V71.01 Adult Antisocial behavior

V40.00 Borderline intellectual functioning (Note: This is coded on Axis II.)

V71.02 Childhood or adolescent antisocial behavior
V65.20 Malingering
V61.10 Marital problem
V15.81 Noncompliance with medical treatment
V62.20 Occupational problem
V61.20 Parent-child problem
V62.81 Other interpersonal problem
V61.80 Other specified family circumstances
V62.89 Phase of life problem or other life circumstance problem
V62.82 Uncomplicated bereavement

ADDITIONAL CODES (363)

300.90 Unspecified mental disorder (nonpsychotic)
V71.09* No diagnosis or condition on Axis I
799.90* Diagnosis or condition deferred on Axis I

V71.09* No diagnosis or condition on Axis II
799.90* Diagnosis or condition deferred on Axis II

MULTIAXIAL SYSTEM

Axis I Clinic Syndromes V Codes

Axis II Developmental Disorders
Personality Disoders

Axis III Physical Disorders and Conditions

Axis IV Severity of Psychosocial Stressors

Axis V Global Assessment of Functioning

(*From American Psychiatric Association;* Diagnostic and Statistical Manual of Mental Disorders DSM-III-R. *3rd, rev. ed. Washington, D.C.: American Psychiatric Association Staff, 1987. Reprinted with permission.*)

INDEX